# WEIGHING

## THE OPTIONS

### Criteria for Evaluating Weight-Management Programs

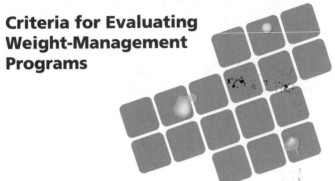

Committee to Develop Criteria for Evaluating the Outcomes
of Approaches to Prevent and Treat Obesity

Food and Nutrition Board

Paul R. Thomas, *Editor*

INSTITUTE OF MEDICINE

NATIONAL ACADEMY PRESS
Washington, D.C. 1995

NOTICE: The project that is the subject of this report was approved by the Governing Board of the National Research Council, whose members are drawn from the councils of the National Academy of Sciences, the National Academy of Engineering, and the Institute of Medicine. The members of the committee responsible for the report were chosen for their special competencies and with regard for appropriate balance.

This report has been reviewed by a group other than the authors according to procedures approved by a Report Review Committee consisting of members of the National Academy of Sciences, the National Academy of Engineering, and the Institute of Medicine.

The Institute of Medicine was chartered in 1970 by the National Academy of Sciences to enlist distinguished members of the appropriate professions in the examination of policy matters pertaining to the health of the public. In this, the Institute acts under both the Academy's 1863 congressional charter responsibility to be an adviser to the federal government and its own initiative in identifying issues of medical care, research, and education. Dr. Kenneth I. Shine is president of the Institute of Medicine.

This study was supported through internal funds of the National Academy of Sciences.

**Library of Congress Cataloging-in-Publication Data**

Weighing the options : criteria for evaluating weight-management
    programs / Committee to Develop Criteria for Evaluating the Outcomes
    of Approaches to Prevent and Treat Obesity, Food and Nutrition
    Board, Institute of Medicine ; Paul R. Thomas, editor.
       p.  cm.
    Includes bibliographical references and index.
    ISBN 0-309-05131-2
    1. Reducing diets—Evaluation. 2. Weight loss. I. Thomas, Paul
R., 1953- . II. Institute of Medicine (U.S.). Committee to
Develop Criteria for Evaluating the Outcomes of Approaches to
Prevent and Treat Obesity.
RM222.2.W2967   1995
613.2′5—dc20
                                         94-44625
                                            CIP

Printed in the United States of America

The serpent has been a symbol of long life, healing, and knowledge among almost all cultures and religions since the beginning of recorded history. The image adopted as a logotype by the Institute of Medicine is based on a relief carving from ancient Greece, now held by the Staatlichemuseen in Berlin.

**National Academy Press**
**2101 Constitution Avenue, NW**
**Washington, DC 20418**

## COMMITTEE TO DEVELOP CRITERIA FOR EVALUATING THE OUTCOMES OF APPROACHES TO PREVENT AND TREAT OBESITY

**JUDITH S. STERN** (*Chair*), Departments of Nutrition and Internal Medicine, University of California, Davis

**JULES HIRSCH** (*Vice Chair*),* Rockefeller University, New York, New York

**STEVEN N. BLAIR**, Cooper Institute for Aerobics Research, Dallas, Texas

**JOHN P. FOREYT**, Nutrition Research Clinic, Baylor College of Medicine, Houston, Texas

**ARTHUR FRANK**, Obesity Management Program, George Washington University, Washington, D.C.

**SHIRIKI K. KUMANYIKA**, College of Medicine, Pennsylvania State University, Hershey

**JENNIFER H. MADANS**, Division of Epidemiology, National Center for Health Statistics, Centers for Disease Control and Prevention, Hyattsville, Maryland

**G. ALAN MARLATT**, Addictive Behaviors Research Center, University of Washington, Seattle

**SACHIKO T. ST. JEOR**, Nutrition Education and Research Program, University of Nevada School of Medicine, Reno

**ALBERT J. STUNKARD**,* Department of Psychiatry, University of Pennsylvania, Philadelphia

### Food and Nutrition Board Liaison

**DENNIS M. BIER**, Children's Nutrition Research Center, Houston, Texas

### Staff

**PAUL R. THOMAS**, Project Director
**SHEILA A. MOATS**, Research Associate
**SUSAN M. KNASIAK**, Program Assistant

---

* Member, Institute of Medicine

iii

**ARTHUR H. RUBENSTEIN** (*Institute of Medicine Council Liaison*),* Department of Medicine, The University of Chicago, Chicago

### Staff

**ALLISON A. YATES**, Director (from July 1994)
**BERNADETTE M. MARRIOTT**, Acting Director (January–June 1994)
**CATHERINE E. WOTEKI**, Director (through December 1993)
**MARCIA S. LEWIS**, Administrative Assistant
**GAIL E. SPEARS**, Administrative Assistant
**SUSAN M. WYATT**, Financial Associate (through October 1994)
**JAMAINE L. TINKER**, Financial Associate (from October 1994)

The Food and Nutrition Board (FNB) was established in 1940 to study issues of critical national importance pertaining to the safety and adequacy of the nation's food supply, to establish principles and guidelines for adequate nutrition, and to render authoritative judgment on the relationships among food intake, nutrition, and health. The FNB responds to requests from federal agencies and others to initiate studies concerning food and nutrition, assigns them to standing or ad hoc committees, then oversees the work of these committees. The FNB is a unit of the Institute of Medicine, part of the National Academy of Sciences.

# Preface

For several years, the Food and Nutrition Board (FNB) of the Institute of Medicine (IOM), National Academy of Sciences (NAS) has wished to develop criteria that could be used by others to evaluate the effectiveness of various approaches to preventing and treating the problems of overweight and obesity. Nearly one-third of adults in the United States are obese. Individuals wanting to lose weight have a wide variety of programs, services, and advice from which to choose, ranging from over-the-counter diet aids and community-based classes to commercial weight-loss centers and treatment by individual health-care providers. To date, however, few carefully derived sets of criteria have been available for evaluating the plethora of programs and approaches for the treatment and prevention of obesity in a systematic, comprehensive, and consistent manner.

Given the need to develop such criteria, the NAS provided the FNB with funding to conduct a 1-year study with the following objectives:

- Identify direct measurements of outcomes of obesity treatment and prevention programs as well as their priorities and special uses.
- Identify program characteristics that should be specified and measured in program evaluation.
- Identify appropriate uses of indirect measurements of outcomes (especially risk of specific diseases) of large-scale weight-loss programs.
- Identify characteristics that contribute to clients' choices of programs and their outcomes with these programs.

- Identify the degree of weight loss needed to improve various health outcomes.
- Where information concerning these topics is limited, develop a specific agenda for research.

The Committee to Develop Criteria for Evaluating the Outcomes of Approaches to Prevent and Treat Obesity (hereafter termed the Obesity Committee), whose members wrote this report, consists of 10 scientists, most of whom are recognized leaders in obesity research and management. They work in a variety of settings, including public and private universities, medical schools, research centers, the federal government, and private practice. Brief biographies of the committee and project director can be found in Appendix E.

The committee met four times during the course of this study. Our draft report was formally reviewed under the auspices of the National Academy of Sciences' Report Review Committee by a panel of experts whose identities have not been revealed to the committee. In addition, members of the FNB reviewed the draft. The reviewers provided thoughtful, constructive critiques, and we have incorporated many of their suggestions in this report.

The focus of the report has been defined by the charges to the committee and our interpretation of them as well as the usual limits of time and resources. This report does not provide comprehensive descriptions and assessments of the various approaches to weight loss, nor does it discuss eating disorders such as anorexia or bulimia. In addition, we focused our work on obesity in adults and on obesity treatment rather than prevention. We have not neglected adolescent obesity and the prevention of obesity, but these are large topics that deserve special study by other committees.

This report has been prepared for a large audience, including biomedical researchers, clinicians, and public health specialists; individuals involved in the development, manufacture, or sale of weight-loss products and services; educators; federal, state, and local policymakers; and interested consumers. For the general public, a separate book on obesity and health, based on this report, is needed. That book would help readers evaluate the nature and causes of weight problems and help determine which, if any, type of weight-loss approach might be best for them and whether they need professional help.

## ACKNOWLEDGMENTS

This report would not have been possible without the help of the IOM staff. Special thanks go to our colleague Paul R. Thomas. Dr. Thomas served as Project Director and editor of this report, and we relied heavily on his in-depth knowledge of nutrition and his excellent writing and editing skills. We also appreciate the help provided by Project Assistant Susan M. Knasiak, whose substantial computer, technical, and organizational skills facilitated the preparation of this manuscript and arrangements for our meetings, travel, and conference calls, and Sheila A. Moats, Research Associate, for her skills at reference identification and verification and help with planning a workshop and drafting a section of the report. Catherine E. Woteki, former director of the FNB, was instrumental in developing the proposal that led to this study and in efforts to obtain funding. We are very grateful to the Executive Committee of the Governing Board of the National Research Council, NAS, for agreeing to provide the necessary financial support.

During the course of this study, several nutrition professionals, biomedical scientists, government representatives, and representatives of the weight-loss industry contributed to discussions about the content of this report. Some provided material or advice at our invitation, some participated in a workshop held at our second meeting, and others responded to specific questions we posed. We are very thankful for their help and carefully considered all comments. We wish to single out the following individuals by name:

*Representatives of government agencies*: Joan M. Conway, U.S. Department of Agriculture; Karen A. Donato, National Institutes of Health (NIH); Katherine M. Flegal, National Center for Health Statistics (NCHS); Van S. Hubbard, NIH; Richard Kelly, Federal Trade Commission; Barbara J. Moore, NIH; and the Division of Health Examination Statistics, NCHS.

*Representatives of the private sector*: L. Arthur Campfield, Hoffmann-La Roche; Linda Webb Carilli, Weight Watchers International, Inc.; David J. Goldstein, Eli Lilly & Company (also affiliated with the Indiana University School of Medicine); Karen Miller-Kovach, Weight Watchers International, Inc.; Bruce F. Trumm II, Abbott Laboratories; and Brenda L. Wolfe, Jenny Craig, Inc.

*Academics*: Kelly D. Brownell, Yale University; Sally M. Davis, University of New Mexico School of Medicine, Albuquerque; Robert W. Jeffery, University of Minnesota, Minneapolis; and Rena R. Wing, University of Pittsburgh School of Medicine.

*Others*: Gail L. Kaye and Francis J. Peterson.

Very special thanks are due the three nutrition scientists who prepared background papers for the committee's use. George L. Blackburn, Chief of the Nutrition/Metabolism Laboratory at New England Deaconess Hospital in Boston, prepared an algorithm of whom to treat for obesity and categories of treatment intensity. F. Xavier Pi-Sunyer, Chief of the Division of Endocrinology, Diabetes, and Nutrition at St. Luke's/Roosevelt Hospital Center in New York City, prepared a paper on the treatment of obesity with drugs; we used it to develop our statements and recommendations on the subject at various places in the report. Beatrice S. Kanders, an obesity specialist and now a private consultant in Atlanta, prepared a background paper on the prevention and treatment of obesity in childhood and adolescence. Because pediatric obesity is a very important subject that we were not able to address owing to time constraints, we have included an edited version of Dr. Kanders' paper in Appendix C.

We appreciate the assistance provided by the IOM's Reports and Information Office. Claudia Carl steered this report through formal review, and Mike Edington helped prepare the final manuscript for publication. Andrea Posner and Florence Poillon served ably as copy editors. Thanks are also due to the staff of the National Academy Press, particularly Sally Stanfield, Barbara Kline Pope, and Christine Chirichella, for their help in publishing and marketing the report and for their patience with us. Our acknowledgments would not be complete without thanking Kenneth I. Shine, IOM President; Enriqueta C. Bond, former IOM Executive Officer; Joseph S. Cassells, Interim IOM Executive Officer; Bernadette M. Marriott; Allison A. Yates; and the members of the FNB for their support, advice, and encouragement throughout the short life of this fast-track study.

Finally, as chair, I would like to thank my fellow committee members for their hard work and good cheer in meeting what often seemed to be impossible deadlines.

Judith S. Stern, *Chair*

# Contents

# APPENDIXES

# WEIGHING
## THE OPTIONS

**Criteria for Evaluating
Weight-Management
Programs**

# Summary

The United States is experiencing an epidemic of obesity among both adults and children. Approximately 35 percent of women and 31 percent of men age 20 and older are considered obese, as are about one-quarter of children and adolescents. While government health goals for the year 2000 call for no more than 20 percent of adults and 15 percent of adolescents to be obese, the prevalence of this often disabling disease is increasing rather than decreasing.

Obesity, of course, is not increasing because people are consciously trying to gain weight. In fact, tens of millions of people in this country are dieting at any one time; they and many others are struggling to manage their weight to improve their appearance, feel better, and be healthier. Many programs and services exist to help individuals achieve weight control. But the limited studies paint a grim picture: those who complete weight-loss programs lose approximately 10 percent of their body weight, only to regain two-thirds of it back within 1 year and almost all of it back within 5 years.

These figures point to the fact that obesity is one of the most pervasive public health problems in this country, a complex, multifactorial disease of appetite regulation and energy metabolism involving genetics, physiology, biochemistry, and the neurosciences, as well as environmental, psychosocial, and cultural factors. Unfortunately, the lay public and health-care providers, as well as insurance companies, often view it simply as a problem of willful misconduct—eating too much and exercising too little. Obesity is a remarkable disease in terms of the effort required

1

by an individual for its management and the extent of discrimination its victims suffer.

While people often wish to lose weight for the sake of their appearance, public health concerns about obesity relate to this disease's link to numerous chronic diseases that can lead to premature illness and death. The scientific evidence summarized in Chapter 2 suggests strongly that obese individuals who lose even relatively small amounts of weight are likely to decrease their blood pressure (and thereby the risk of hypertension), reduce abnormally high levels of blood glucose (associated with diabetes), bring blood concentrations of cholesterol and triglycerides (associated with cardiovascular disease) down to more desirable levels, reduce sleep apnea, decrease their risk of osteoarthritis of the weight-bearing joints and depression, and increase self-esteem. In many cases, the obese person who loses weight finds that an accompanying comorbidity is improved, its progression is slowed, or the symptoms disappear.

Healthy weights are generally associated with a body mass index (BMI; a measure of whether weight is appropriate for height, measured in kg/m$^2$) of 19–25 in those 19–34 years of age and 21–27 in those 35 years of age and older. Beyond these ranges, health risks increase as BMI increases. Health risks also increase with excess abdominal/visceral fat (as estimated by a waist-hip ratio [WHR] >1.0 for males and >0.8 for females), high blood pressure (>140/90), dyslipidemias (total cholesterol and triglyceride concentrations of >200 and >225 mg/dl, respectively), non-insulin-dependent diabetes mellitus, and a family history of premature death due to cardiovascular disease (e.g., parent, grandparent, sibling, uncle, or aunt dying before age 50). Weight loss usually improves the management of obesity-related comorbidities or decreases the risks of their development.

The high prevalence of obesity in the United States together with its link to numerous chronic diseases leads to the conclusion that this disease is responsible for a substantial proportion of total health-care costs. We estimate that today's health-care costs of obesity exceed $70 billion per year. To this figure can be added the more than $33 billion spent yearly on weight-reduction products (including diet foods and drinks) and services, for an estimated total of more than $100 billion per year as the economic costs of obesity. Such an estimate cannot include the psychosocial costs of obesity, which range from lowered self-esteem to the more serious binge-eating disorders and clinical depression.

Given the huge economic and personal costs of obesity, research must continue to identify the fundamental biological defects that underlie obesity and discover how to manage and ultimately treat them. At the same time, however, it is important to improve the success of obesity treatments available now. This report is directed to the latter purpose. Treatment cannot cure obesity, of course, but it can provide assistance, information, and reinforcement for the long-term management of this disease.

It is important to note that this report focuses on adult obesity. Given the relatively few data on evaluating and managing obesity in children and adolescents, as well as the time constraints under which we operated, little attention was paid to the subject. However, pediatric obesity is an important public health problem, and we have included a background paper on the subject in Appendix C of this report.

## TYPES OF PROGRAMS AND APPROACHES TO TREAT OBESITY

The wide variety of weight-loss programs can be placed along a continuum on the basis of many factors, including intensity of treatment, cost, the nature of the intervention(s), and degree of involvement of health-care providers. We chose to organize the plethora of programs into three major categories: do-it-yourself programs, nonclinical programs, and clinical programs:

- *Do-it-yourself programs* are individually formulated and therefore extraordinarily varied. This category includes any effort by an individual to lose weight by himself or herself or with a group of like-minded others through programs such as Overeaters Anonymous and TOPS (Take Off Pounds Sensibly) and community-based and work-site programs. Individual judgment, books, products, and group therapy may dispense good or bad advice. The common denominator of programs in this category is that outside resources are not used in a personalized or individualized manner.
- *Nonclinical programs* are popular and are often commercially franchised. They typically have a structure created by a parent company and often use instructional and guidance materials that are prepared in consultation with health-care providers. The qualifying characteristic of these programs is that they rely substantially on variably trained counselors (who are not health-care providers) to provide services to clients.
- *Clinical programs* are those in which services are provided by a licensed professional who may or may not have received special training to treat obese patients. The programs may or may not be part of a commercial franchise system. In some clinical programs, an individual professional provider works alone; in others, a multidisciplinary group of professional providers works together and systematically coordinates their efforts, records, and patient base. Clinical programs include such services as nutrition, medical care, behavior therapy, exercise, and psy-

chological counseling, and they may utilize very-low-calorie diets, medications, and surgery.

We have identified five broad approaches to treatment used by the do-it-yourself, nonclinical, and clinical programs: diet, physical activity, behavior modification, drug therapy, and gastric surgery. Not all approaches are used by, or available to, each category of programs. However, each program category uses one or more of these approaches.

Special attention is due drugs and surgery, because these options may offer help to individuals who have failed with other approaches. Data show that anti-obesity drugs help some people to lose weight and maintain weight loss. However, relatively few such drugs are available for this purpose, and their use is generally limited to several months. Standards for use of anti-obesity drugs should be liberalized so that these medications are treated similarly to those used for the treatment of other medical problems such as hypertension, where the presumption is that medication may be required for long periods of time and beneficial results are maintained only as long as the drug is taken. Such a change should stimulate research and development on new, more effective, medications. In regard to surgery, there is compelling evidence that comorbidities are reduced or delayed in severely obese patients who have lost weight as a result of gastric surgery. Therefore, it is puzzling that this treatment is not more widely used for severely obese individuals (BMI $\geq$35) at very high risk for obesity-related morbidity and mortality.

It is important to state that our recommendations are meant to apply to the weight-management programs that use data or testimonials in their advertising and promotional activities to suggest that weight loss is likely to be successful with them or that they are more effective than competing programs. Programs that engage in these activities should be held to some level of proof of their claims, so they must be encouraged to collect certain types of information in standardized ways and provide certain kinds of information to potential clients. Potential clients, in turn, should be encouraged to expect this information from programs, so that programs that do not comply may be put at a competitive disadvantage and thereby become motivated to rethink their position. This information is needed so that consumers can make informed choices and there can be reasonable oversight of programs by regulatory agencies such as the Federal Trade Commission, the Food and Drug Administration, and state agencies, as well as by interested biomedical scientists. Weight-management programs that do not make claims of success—such as classes provided by a community YMCA or YWCA, counseling by dietitians at a local hospital, or meetings of a local chapter of Overeaters Anonymous—

should not be required to assume the data-collection burdens and expense of meeting our recommendations, but should endeavor to do so if resources permit. Given that the loss of even a small amount of weight may benefit health, we want interested clients to have many options in their communities to receive help in achieving a healthful lifestyle.

## EVOLVING FROM WEIGHT LOSS TO WEIGHT MANAGEMENT

The facts summarized above provide compelling evidence of the need for a new perspective on obesity-treatment outcomes. This report has been developed in response to that need. **We recommend that the definition of success that is applied in evaluating weight-loss programs be broadened and made more realistic based on the research findings that small weight losses can reduce the risks of developing chronic diseases. Specifically, the goal of obesity treatment should be refocused from weight loss alone, which is often aimed at appearance, to *weight management*, achieving the best weight possible in the context of overall health.** In contrast to weight loss, the primary purpose of weight management is to achieve and maintain good health. This concept includes weight loss but is not limited to it. **We recommend that weight-loss programs evolve into weight-management programs and be judged more by their effects on the overall health of participants than by their effects on weight alone.** The recommendations set forth in this report are framed around weight management.

This report is organized around a simple conceptual overview of decisionmaking—an individual making a decision about an option and then experiencing an outcome and evaluating it—that we adapted and expanded and from which we developed criteria and a model for evaluating obesity-treatment programs. Our *Weighing the Options* model (see Figure 1) provides a framework for the conduct of programs and behavior of individuals that should help consumers choose more wisely from among available programs. Its health-based approach to weight management should also help them to be more successful at weight loss.

Figure 1 illustrates the model in such a way that each of its major components is associated with a criterion, and each criterion is discussed as it pertains to both weight-management programs and consumers seeking such programs. Our discussion of this model and recommendations derived from it is organized by the three criteria: (1) match between program and consumer, (2) soundness and safety of the program, and (3) outcome of the program.

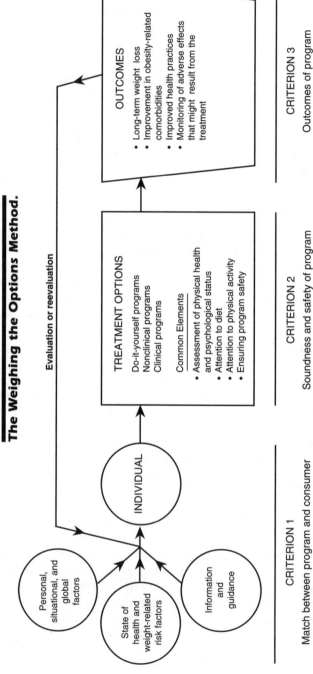

**The Weighing the Options Method.**

Evaluation or reevaluation

OUTCOMES

- Long-term weight loss
- Improvement in obesity-related comorbidities
- Improved health practices
- Monitoring of adverse effects that might result from the treatment

TREATMENT OPTIONS

Do-it-yourself programs
Nonclinical programs
Clinical programs

Common Elements

- Assessment of physical health and psychological status
- Attention to diet
- Attention to physical activity
- Ensuring program safety

INDIVIDUAL

Personal, situational, and global factors

State of health and weight-related risk factors

Information and guidance

CRITERION 1

Match between program and consumer

PROGRAM: Who is appropriate for this program?
CONSUMER: Should I be in this program, given my goals and characteristics?

CRITERION 2

Soundness and safety of program

PROGRAM: Is my program based on sound biological and behavioral principles, and is it safe for its intended participants?
CONSUMER: Is the program safe and sound for me?

CRITERION 3

Outcomes of program

PROGRAM: What is the evidence for success of my program?
CONSUMER: Are the benefits I am likely to achieve from the program worth the effort and cost?

FIGURE 1

### Weighing the Options Criterion 1: The Match Between Program and Consumer

Matching, which pertains to the first part of our model, has long been a key aspect of medical treatment. Chapter 5 reviews several schemes for matching in the obesity field, all of which we found useful although limited for our purposes. We approached the matching of individuals to treatments by identifying four sets of factors that may influence decision-making:

- *Personal, situational, and global factors:* Personal factors include demographic ones, such as age and gender, that cannot be changed as well as psychosocial ones, such as motivation and readiness to change, that one can alter. Situational factors can be changed by the individual's actions; an example is using the stairs whenever appropriate rather than the elevator. Global factors are those that influence the environment in which an individual lives, such as culture and views about weight; they typically change slowly over time from the efforts of large numbers of people. The availability and cost of a weight-loss program are two global factors that often influence a person's decision about whether or not to undertake a particular weight-loss program.
- *Health status and weight-related risk factors* are factors that, as they worsen, may become an individual's primary motivation for losing weight. These factors are described in the section on Criterion 2.
- *Information and guidance* come from a variety of sources, including the media (information and advertising); family, friends, and acquaintances (who relay their opinions and experiences with the various options); and health-care providers. The information and guidance may be sound or unsound, well intentioned or intended to deceive, and empowering or provoking inaction. They may also be incomplete or biased toward a particular program or approach that may not be suitable.
- *Experiencing a successful, partially successful, or unsuccessful outcome from an obesity-treatment program:* This factor applies to those who have already gone through a program and are deciding whether to continue with the same program or try another one.

In some cases, it is possible to identify mismatches of individuals with weight-loss programs, at least in the sense of excluding people from particular options. For example, a healthy young woman with a BMI of 28 is no candidate for gastric surgery, whereas a very obese male with a BMI of 40 and hypertension—who has not lost weight despite many attempts—is not likely to be helped by a do-it-yourself diet book or exercise video. However, for most people who wish to lose weight, there is general agreement that it is not yet possible to match people with programs to significantly improve their chances of success. The complex interactions that occur between an individual and the many factors that influence program choice are beyond the current ability of biomedical science to explain, much less predict. Nevertheless, it is possible to make some prudent qualitative recommendations to increase the likelihood of a successful match. They are described below and summarized in Table 1.

### Program's Perspective on Criterion 1: Who Is Appropriate for This Program?

Each program decides what types of clients are appropriate and inappropriate given its specific philosophies, protocols, and treatment approaches. Pregnant women and individuals who are underweight or anorectic are inappropriate candidates for any weight-loss program. Nonclinical programs should require (and do-it-yourself programs should advise) that lactating women, children, and adolescents, as well as those with bulimia; significant cardiovascular, renal, or psychiatric disease; diabetes; or other significant medical problems undertake weight loss only under medical supervision or in consultation or partnership with their health-care provider. Nonclinical programs should encourage clients with obesity-related comorbidities or other health problems to maintain contact with their health-care provider for the duration of the program. Both nonclinical and clinical programs should obtain some information on the state of health and weight-loss goals of potential clients to determine if they are appropriate for a specific program and what types of individualized attention they may require.

Do-it-yourself programs such as those provided in diet books, diet plans in magazines, or over-the-counter weight-loss devices or products should provide information in the text or other instructional materials on who should and who should not use the program. Since there is usually no legal obligation that this information be provided or that it be true and complete, the publisher or manufacturer of the program should be responsible for providing it voluntarily.

### Consumer's Perspective on Criterion 1: Should I Be in This Program, Given My Goals and Characteristics?

Because consumers decide on their own or with the help of others whether to enter a weight-loss program and which one to choose, they must consider carefully their weight-loss goals and whether they are ap-

**TABLE 1**  Summary of Recommendations Pertaining to Criterion 1

| | Program Perspective | | |
| --- | --- | --- | --- |
| | Do-It-Yourself Program | Nonclinical Program | Clinical Program |
| Decide what clients are appropriate for program | Yes | Yes | Yes |
| Provide information in text or other instructional materials on who can and who should not use program | Publisher or manufacturer of program should provide information voluntarily | Yes | Yes |
| Obtain information on state of health and weight-loss goals of potential clients | Generally cannot do | Yes | Yes |
| Weight loss for individuals with obesity-related comorbidities or other health problems | Encourage contact with health-care provider for duration of program | | Yes |
| Weight loss for lactating women, children, and adolescents; and those with bulimia, significant cardiovascular, renal, or psychiatric disease; diabetes; or other significant medical problems | Advise against without medical supervision | Require medical supervision as condition of entry | May be appropriate |
| Weight loss for pregnant women and individuals who are underweight or anorectic | Discourage | Discourage entry | |

Consumer Perspective

Consider carefully your weight-loss goals and whether you are an appropriate candidate for weight loss.

Decide whether the time is right to be able to devote the considerable attention and effort required to succeed at weight loss.

Be evaluated by a health-care provider (or have been in recent past) before undertaking a do-it-yourself or nonclinical program. Discuss program or product with health-care provider.

Expect that programs will provide sufficient information so you can assess whether you are appropriate or inappropriate as a potential candidate.

propriate candidates for weight loss, and decide whether the time is right for them to devote the considerable attention and effort required to succeed. Individuals should expect a program to provide them with sufficient information to help assess whether they are appropriate or inappropriate potential candidates. We recommend that those contemplating a do-it-yourself or nonclinical program be evaluated first by a health-care provider (or have been assessed in the recent past) before proceeding. They should discuss the program or product with a knowledgeable health-care provider to determine whether it is sound and appropriate.

### Weighing the Options Criterion 2:
### The Soundness and Safety of the Program

The programs themselves and their characteristics constitute the center section of the *Weighing the Options* model. Earlier, we described the three types of programs into which all options were placed: do-it-yourself, nonclinical, and clinical programs. Insofar as the vast majority of dieters choose to join weight-loss services or select do-it-yourself options, there is an almost total absence of controls for the efficacy and safety of weight-loss methods as actually practiced throughout the population. Because health risks may attend obesity and the process of losing weight, we believe that all programs should meet some minimum expectations. Specifically, we recommend that four critical areas be addressed by all weight-loss and weight-management programs: (1) assessment of physical health and psychological status, (2) attention to diet, (3) attention to physical activity, and (4) ensuring program safety. These critical areas are discussed in detail in Chapter 6 and summarized below.

• *Assessment of physical health and psychological status:* Individuals considering a do-it-yourself or nonclinical program to lose weight should have some basic knowledge about their overall state of health before they begin. This is important not only because we believe that all adults should assume some responsibility for their health care, but because this self-assessment should help them determine which programs might be best for them. Many nonclinical programs screen potential clients by measuring height and weight and asking questions about health status. Ideally, however, obese individuals should have a physician review their health history and provide a physical examination, with particular attention to obesity comorbidities, prior to beginning a program. Individuals are almost always assessed by physicians as part of a clinical program.

• *Diet:* How much one eats (and, to some extent, what one eats) is a major determinant of body weight. Therefore, food intake should play a central role in all weight-management efforts. The overall goal in obesity treatment is to obtain a negative energy balance by reducing energy intake (i.e., eating less), increasing energy expenditure (i.e., performing more physical activity), or preferably both. Programs that promise results without dieting and physical activity will surely be ineffective over the long term. Generally, weight loss requires decreasing total energy intake and utilizing, as much as possible, a variety of available foods. The federal government's dietary guidance plan, the Food Guide Pyramid, is a useful tool to help individuals meet dietary recommendations. Decreasing alcohol intake, foods of minimal nutritional value, and fats and simple sugars is a good strategy for reducing energy intake without eliminating essential nutrients. A weight-reduction diet should contain adequate protein to maintain nitrogen balance and limit the loss of lean body mass. Energy intakes of less than 1,200 kcal/day may not meet nutrient requirements, and a dietary supplement may be needed. Individuals consuming such low-calorie diets should seek the advice of a health-care provider (e.g., a physician or dietitian). Diets of less than 800 kcal/day should not be used except under a physician's supervision. A health-care provider knowledgeable about obesity and its treatment and about the physiology of weight loss can help an individual develop a nutritionally adequate diet plan tailored to his or her weight-loss goals and appropriate to factors such as gender, age, dietary preferences, and level of physical activity.

• *Physical activity:* As with diet, activity level should play a central role in all weight-management efforts. Physical activity can lead to weight loss, may help prevent weight regain after a weight-loss program, and helps reduce some of the comorbidities associated with obesity (e.g., dyslipidemias and hyperglycemia). Because most obese persons are inactive, physical activity interventions in this group should be approached with low starting levels and slow progression to higher levels of activity. We recommend that a gradual reshaping of a participant's physical activity pattern over time be the focus of intervention, rather than providing a strict, regimented, and specific dose of activity in an exercise prescription. The most feasible mode of activity for most adults is walking. Each person should develop a realistic goal for increasing activity, perhaps with professional guidance, which can be modified over time as activity levels increase. It is reasonable to suggest a gradual progression up to 1 hour of moderate-intensity activity (e.g., brisk walking) each day, accumulated over the course of a day. As participants become more physically fit, they will be capable of more activity; they may ultimately engage in more vigorous activities such as cycling, jogging, or other vigorous sports and recreational activities and thereby achieve their caloric-expenditure goals in a shorter period of time. Selection of activity goals and the type of activities to be used are highly individualized matters. Persons should be encouraged to find what works for them and should evaluate different approaches until a sustainable activity plan is developed.

•   *Ensuring program safety:* Generally, the more restrictive the diet, the greater are the risks of adverse effects associated with weight loss. Do-it-yourself and nonclinical programs must be relatively safe (i.e., carry minimal risk) for their clients. Clinical programs must also be as safe as reasonably possible, given that they are likely to be designed for the very obese with comorbidities and health problems. Programs must insist that clients with one or more obesity-related comorbidities be monitored. A client should expect a program to provide detailed information about any potential risks that could occur. Special attention must be paid to the safety of programs for children, pregnant women, and the elderly. There are a variety of minor and major risks associated with dieting. For example, there is an increase in the risk of gall bladder disease among people who lose weight rapidly on very-low-fat diets. Risks to health from weight loss vary with the individual and the type of program.

Our recommendations related to Criterion 2 are described below and summarized in Table 2.

### Program's Perspective on Criterion 2: Is My Program Based on Sound Biological and Behavioral Principles, and Is It Safe for Its Intended Participants?

All providers should take steps to ensure that their programs are safe and sound. Nonclinical and clinical programs can provide information about the qualifications and training of staff, appropriate corporate managers, and, if desired, consultants involved in developing the program. Authors and other originators of do-it-yourself programs should cite their credentials, qualifications, and experiences in managing obesity.

Clinical programs should be able to assess the physical and psychological health of their patients. Nonclinical and do-it-yourself programs, in contrast, can only encourage clients to have such an assessment conducted by their health-care providers. All programs should encourage individuals to know their blood pressure and blood lipid concentrations; whether or not they have diabetes, osteoarthritis in weight-bearing joints, or sleep apnea; and whether a family member has died prematurely from coronary heart disease. Do-it-yourself and nonclinical programs should strongly encourage individuals who have one or more of these risk factors to be under the care of a health-care provider. These programs should develop simple checklists for clients to highlight the importance of rou-

**TABLE 2**   Summary of Recommendations Pertaining to Criterion 2

| | Program Perspective | | |
| --- | --- | --- | --- |
| | Do-It-Yourself Program | Nonclinical Program | Clinical Program |
| Take steps to ensure that program is safe and sound | Yes | Yes | Yes |
| Encourage individuals to know their blood pressure and blood lipid concentrations; whether or not they have diabetes, osteoarthritis in weight-bearing joints, or sleep apnea; and whether a family member has died prematurely (before age 50) from coronary heart disease | Yes | Yes | Yes |
| Encourage individuals who have one or more risk factors (see above) to be under care of health-care provider • | Yes | Yes | NA (not applicable) |
| Assess clients for risk factors (see above) | NA | NA | Yes |
| Develop simple checklists for clients to highlight importance of routinely monitoring health status | Yes | Yes | NA |
| Inform about the known and hypothetical risks of program | Yes | Yes | Have special responsibilities to assess and manage potential risks, especially when special diets, drugs, or surgery are used |
| Qualifications and training | Cite credentials, qualifications, and experiences in managing obesity | Provide this information about staff, appropriate corporate managers, and if desired, consultants involved in developing the program | |

*continued on next page*

**TABLE 2** Continued

| | Program Perspective | | |
|---|---|---|---|
| | Do-It-Yourself Program | Nonclinical Program | Clinical Program |
| Height and weight of clients and calculation of body mass index and waist-to-hip ratio | Encourage clients to take these measurements and make calculations. Instruct how to do so and explain results. | Make measurements and calculations; provide and interpret results | |
| Assessment of physical and psychological health of clients | Encourage clients to have assessment performed by their health-care provider | | Perform assessment |
| Psychological assessment | Provide test such as Dieting Readiness Test; give explicit guidance how to use and score it | Administer test such as Dieting Readiness Test | Administer test such as Dieting Readiness Test along with the General Well-Being Schedule |
| Diet and physical activity assessment | Inform clients of importance of attention to these factors; give explicit guidance how to do so | Clients should have these evaluated at the beginning and end of treatment phase of program and at least every 6 months during any maintenance phase | |

Consumer Perspective

Have a good understanding of program and what to expect from it through treatment and any maintenance phase.

Monitor weight weekly and continue to assess (or have assessed) diet and physical activity patterns at 6-month intervals or more frequently after the weight-loss phase of program.

Expect that program will be a safe and sound one.

Expect that do-it-yourself programs will provide the credentials and qualifications of the author/originator. Nonclinical and clinical programs will make available information about the qualifications and training of staff.

tinely monitoring health status. Clinical programs should assess all clients for these risk factors.

Nonclinical and clinical programs should measure the height and weight of clients and calculate their BMI and WHR, providing both the results and the information to interpret those results. Do-it-yourself programs should encourage their clients to take these measurements and make these calculations, instruct them how to do so, and explain the results.

Clients in nonclinical and clinical programs should have their diets and physical activity patterns evaluated at least at the beginning and end of the treatment phase of the program and every 6 months during any maintenance phase (various assessment tools are described in Appendix A). Nonclinical programs should assess the psychological status of clients with a questionnaire such as the Dieting Readiness Test; clinical programs should use this type of questionnaire along with a second questionnaire such as the General Well-Being Schedule (both questionnaires are provided in Appendix B). Do-it-yourself programs should inform clients about the importance of attention to diet, physical activity, and psychological assessment (by providing the Dieting Readiness Test or a similar questionnaire), and give explicit guidance in how to do so.

Since no weight-loss attempt is risk free, it is incumbent on each program to inform potential clients about the known and hypothetical risks of that program. Clinical programs have special responsibilities to assess and manage potential risks, especially when special diets (e.g., very-low-calorie diets), drugs, or surgery are used as part of the treatment.

## Consumer's Perspective on Criterion 2: Is the Program Safe and Sound for Me?

Given the limitations of do-it-yourself and nonclinical programs to assess health compared to clinical programs, consumers choosing the former have a greater responsibility for self-monitoring their health. Consumers should have a good understanding of the program of interest and what they can expect from it throughout the treatment and any maintenance phase. They should have access to information about the qualifications and training of staff in nonclinical and clinical programs and the credentials and qualifications of the author/originator of a do-it-yourself program.

Clients should expect that the program of interest will be a safe and sound one (by meeting our recommendations for them as detailed above). We recommend that they monitor their weight weekly and continue to assess (or have assessed) their diet and physical-activity patterns at 6-

month intervals or more frequently after the weight-loss phase of a program. This will act as a useful periodic check on these two major influences of weight and will help to maintain weight loss.

### Weighing the Options Criterion 3: Outcomes of the Program

The third portion of the model focuses on the outcomes of the program. We have identified four components of successful weight management: (1) long-term weight loss, (2) improvement in obesity-related comorbidities, (3) improved health practices, and (4) monitoring of adverse effects that might result from the program. We believe that weight-loss programs should be judged by how well individuals do in these four areas, and potential clients should expect that a high-quality program will attend to, or urge attention be paid to (since most of these components are not under the direct control of the program), each of these areas. We recommend that the following be used as guidelines to determine if these goals are met:

• *Long-term weight loss:* Long-term means 1 year or more, and weight loss of any significance is the loss of ≥5 percent of body weight or a reduction in BMI by 1 or more units.
• *Improvement in obesity-related comorbidities:* One or more associated risk factors (e.g., high blood pressure; elevated blood concentrations of cholesterol, triglycerides, or glucose; and non-insulin-dependent diabetes mellitus), if present, should be improved to a degree considered clinically significant.
• *Improved health practices:* Obtaining health-related knowledge may be assessed indirectly by evaluating whether basic information about obesity is presented by the program and whether the individual reads or hears it. Engaging in good eating habits may be assessed by using a dietary assessment tool such as those cited in Appendix A or evidence that the individual meets the recommendations of the Food Guide Pyramid on at least 4 of 7 days. Engaging in regular physical activity involves one-half hour or more of moderate-intensity activity (e.g., brisk walking) four or more times a week and preferably daily. Obtaining regular medical attention includes seeing a physician at yearly intervals, particularly if the individual has not achieved a healthy weight. Regular screening of these individuals by a health-care provider will help to identify as early as possible the presence of comorbid conditions and lead to the initiation or continuation of appropriate treatment. Improved well-being can be assessed through questionnaires described in Appendix A. For all programs, we recommend a test such as the Dieting Readiness Test prior to

initiation and, in addition, for clinical programs only, a test such as the General Well-Being Schedule to screen for eating disorders and psychiatric pathologies (see Appendix B).

• *Monitoring adverse effects that might result from program:* Clinical and nonclinical programs should question their clients periodically about any changes in health while on the program and should encourage them to volunteer such information if changes do occur. A do-it-yourself program should inform consumers that because the program may potentially have adverse health effects, they should be attentive to any changes in their health while on it.

As stated earlier, most people fail at weight management over the course of a year or more. Research shows that for the small numbers of people who do maintain their losses, the most important factors associated with long-term success include a regular habit of exercise, continued contact with the treatment program, normalization of eating patterns, continued self-monitoring of diet and exercise, and a positive, problem-solving attitude toward life's stressors. Family dysfunction and negative life events are associated strongly with weight rebound.

Our recommendations for Criterion 3 are described below and summarized in Table 3.

### Program's Perspective on Criterion 3: What Is the Evidence for Success of My Program?

It is not cost effective or practical for most do-it-yourself programs to evaluate their outcomes. Nevertheless, they can make sure that they cover the importance of long-term weight loss and the reduction of obesity-related comorbidities, provide information and guidance on improving health behaviors, and discuss in detail the potential health risks from weight loss in general and their program in particular.

Because clients come physically to nonclinical and clinical programs, the programs can monitor and document their weight loss over time. Such programs should have quality control procedures in place to ensure that protocols are adhered to by staff and to modify those protocols as warranted given the experiences and feedback of clients. They should also have mechanisms to evaluate the success of their programs. If the company is organized as a franchise, mechanisms should be available to evaluate the program as a whole and at individual sites.

All programs should also provide information and guidance on improving health behaviors and should discuss the potential risks of dieting, including those from their programs. Do-it-yourself and nonclinical programs should encourage clients (and strongly encourage those with

**TABLE 3** Summary of Recommendations Pertaining to Criterion 3

| | Program Perspective | | |
| --- | --- | --- | --- |
| | Do-It-Yourself Program | Nonclinical Program | Clinical Program |
| Be judged primarily on success in achieving long-term weight loss, including small losses that are maintained | Yes | Yes | Yes |
| Be judged on ability to empower clients to eat a healthful diet and become more active, reduce obesity-related comorbidities, improve objective and subjective measures of quality of life, and make desired changes in health-related knowledge and attitudes | Yes | Yes | Yes |
| Provide information and guidance on improving health behaviors and discuss potential risks of dieting, including those from their programs | Yes | Yes | Yes |
| Contact with health-care provider for monitoring and disposition of any obesity-related comorbidities | Encourage clients, especially those with obesity-related comorbidities | | Provide medical assessment and monitoring |
| Evaluate outcomes | Probably not cost effective or practical. Make sure to cover the importance of long-term weight loss and the reduction of obesity-related comorbidities, provide information and guidance on improving health behaviors, and discuss potential health risks from weight loss in general and their program in particular. | Monitor and document weight loss of clients over time. Have quality control procedures in place to ensure that protocols are adhered to by staff, and modify protocols given the feedback and experiences of clients. Have mechanisms to evaluate success of program. | |

**TABLE 3**   Continued

Consumer Perspective

You and the program have joint responsibilities for your final outcome.

Have realistic expectations of program and be willing to devote the time and effort required.

Choose a program in light of your own short- and long-term goals for weight management. Reevaluate your goals every 3 to 6 months.

Choose programs that focus on long-term weight management; provide instruction in healthful eating, increasing activity, and improving self-esteem; and explain thoroughly the potential health risks from weight loss.

Look for programs that devote considerable effort to helping people change their behaviors through information, guidance, and skills training.

For do-it-yourself programs, look through program literature for information (beyond testimonials or other anecdotal evidence) that program is successful.

If you are in a do-it-yourself or nonclinical program, be in touch with a health-care provider who can monitor any changes in your health.

Expect that at 3- to 6-month intervals, a program will evaluate whether you are meeting your goals and whether the goals or treatment should be modified.

---

obesity-related comorbidities) to have regular contact with a health-care provider throughout the treatment and maintenance phases of their weight loss so that their overall health can be monitored as well as the disposition of any comorbidities. Clinical programs should be expected to provide this medical assessment and monitoring.

It is appropriate that weight-management programs continue to be judged primarily on their success in achieving long-term weight loss (including small weight losses that are maintained). However, in addition, programs should be judged on their ability to empower their clients to eat a healthful diet and become more active, reduce obesity-related comorbidities, improve objective and subjective measures of quality of life, and make desired changes in health-related knowledge and attitudes.

### Consumer's Perspective on Criterion 3: Are the Benefits I Am Likely to Achieve from the Program Worth the Effort and Cost?

When they begin a weight-management program, consumers must recognize that they and the program have responsibilities for the final outcome. To improve their chances for success, consumers should choose programs that focus on long-term weight management; provide instruction in healthful eating, increasing activity, and improving self-esteem; and explain thoroughly the potential health risks from weight loss. Individuals interested in a specific do-it-yourself program should search in the program literature for evidence that the program is successful; if information on success is absent or consists primarily of testimonials or other anecdotal evidence (including, in the case of programs by health-care providers, only their own clients or patients), the program should be viewed with suspicion.

Consumers should look for programs that devote considerable effort to helping people change their behaviors through information, guidance, and skills training. To make the most of the weight-management effort, however, consumers should have realistic expectations of a program and be willing to devote the time and effort required. Those in do-it-yourself and nonclinical programs should be in touch with a health-care provider who can monitor the status of any obesity-related comorbidities and changes in health.

When individuals choose a program, it should be in light of their short- and long-term goals for weight management. Our *Weighing the Options* model (see Figure 1) is a dynamic one that incorporates periodic reevaluation by the client and program to assess whether an individual and a program are meeting these goals and whether the goals or the treatment should be modified. We recommend these evaluations every 3 to 6 months.

## Truth and Full Disclosure

It is important to determine the nature and amount of information to be disclosed to individuals considering a weight-management program. Information on program disclosure should be sufficient to enable the client to make informed choices among the program options and, we hope, decrease unrealistic expectations. Our recommendations, if put into practice, should also lead to decreases in unsubstantiated claims and thus highlight any unethical behavior by the programs themselves. The background for these recommendations is the extensive literature on informed voluntary consent that has become a key element in research on human subjects and several sets of guidelines described in Chapter 1: the truth-in-dieting regulation in New York City, the weight-loss guidelines for Michigan, actions by the Federal Trade Commission to regulate deceptive claims by weight-loss programs, and National Institutes of Health guidelines for evaluating weight-loss programs and choosing a weight-loss program.

Any weight-management program has a responsibility to prospective clients to provide truthful and unambiguous information that is not misleading or subject to misinterpretation. This includes a written (and, for nonclinical and clinical programs, oral) description of the risks and benefits of treatment and an opportunity to ask questions. To assist individuals in making informed choices from the many nonclinical and clinical programs, information made available should include the nature of a given program, its structure and management, and a description of its staff, including training; all costs, including effort and time; the type of client typically served by the program; and the short- and long-term treatment outcomes. Key elements of these recommendations are provided in Table 4. Obviously there can be no such standardization for do-it-yourself programs, given the nature of the individual's interaction with these programs, the wide variety of approaches that they encompass (e.g., books, devices, products, and dietary supplements), and their almost unlimited freedom to make statements and claims.

To facilitate comparisons between programs, we recommend that weight-management programs collect the data summarized in Table 5. At the current time, it is difficult to compare different programs, in part

**TABLE 4**   Program Disclosure of Information

All potential clients of weight-management programs should receive information such as the following:

• A truthful, unambiguous, and nonmisleading statement of the approach and goals of the program. Part of such a statement might read, for example, "We are a program that emphasizes changes in lifestyle, with group instruction in diet and physical activity."

• A brief description of the credentials of staff, with more detailed information available on request. For example, "Our staff is composed of one physician (M.D.), two registered nurses (R.N.s), three registered dietitians (R.D.s), one master's-level exercise physiologist, and one Ph.D.-level psychologist. At your first visit, you will be seen by the physician. At each visit you will be seen by a dietitian and exercise physiologist and after every five visits by the psychologist. Résumés of our staff are available on request."

• A statement of the client population and experiences over a period of 9 months or more. For example, "To date, we have seen 823 clients for at least three visits each. Although only 26 clients have participated in this program for more than 1 year, they have maintained an average weight loss of 12 pounds."

• A full disclosure of costs. For example, "If you avail yourself of all our facilities with one weekly visit for a period of 1 year, the total cost to you will be between $2,000 and $2,500." Costs should include the initial cost; ongoing costs and additional cost of extra products, services, supplements, and laboratory tests; and costs paid by the average client. Programs may also wish to provide information on the experiences clients have had in recovering their costs from third-party payers.

• A statement of procedures recommended for clients. For example, "We urge that each of our clients see a physician before joining our program. If you have high blood pressure or diabetes, you should see your physician at intervals of his or her choosing while with our program."

**TABLE 5** Collection of Data by Weight-Management Programs

---

1. The number of people attending the first treatment session. (This is the group of potential clients and those who will become actual clients.)

2. Number of clients attending their first two treatment sessions (a gauge of those who have really begun a program) and percentage continuing to participate in the program at 1, 3, 6, and 12 months. (These timepoints seem reasonable but are selected somewhat arbitrarily, for while there is no set of ideal timepoints, it is important to have a set for standardization and comparison among programs. Programs may, of course, use additional timepoints.)

3. Average weight, height, body mass index (BMI), and waist-to-hip ratio (WHR) of clients attending the first two sessions and average change in these variables at 1, 3, 6, and 12 months in the program. (These data should be assembled by gender and, if possible, by race, age, and starting weight or BMI.)

4. The percentage of actual clients who complete each of the stages of the treatment program. This means either the number of clients that complete the program's prescribed number of sessions (e.g., 8 weeks for an 8-week program) or the number of clients in treatment at 3 months.

5. The percentage of actual clients who re-enroll in the same program for further treatment. (This figure should not necessarily be interpreted as a measure of client failure in a program; it may indicate satisfaction with the program.)

---

because of differences in the clients selected and in the data collected and reported.

If programs make claims for long-term maintenance of weight loss, the percentage of clients who have lost weight and maintained it for 1 and 2 years should be provided (along with the percentage of clients for whom the information is available) as well as the average weight loss. Many companies use testimonials, often from prominent people, to show a program's success at achieving weight loss. In these cases, they should also cite the experience of their clients in general (as noted above) or cite the general experience of similar dieters taken from reports in the scientific literature.

## Implications of Our Recommendations

We are well aware that our recommendations will elicit a variety of reactions. Some will consider them to be overly general and not providing sufficiently detailed guidance to consumers for selecting a program and to programs for improving the quality of their services. Others will see the recommendations as being too prescriptive—too much like implicit standards of care that regulatory agencies or consumer-protection bodies at the national, state, or local levels might turn into regulations resulting in potentially onerous and expensive limitations on the conduct of major commercial weight-loss programs. We developed our recommendations without engaging in this debate and based them on the scientific research available and the deliberative judgment of the committee. As one expert committee, we think it likely that implementing our recommendations will help more people to lose weight successfully and keep it off over the long term. How they are implemented, however, should be decided not by us but by broad constituencies through an interactive process of public discussion. Consumers, weight-management programs, researchers, and regulatory agencies should all find these recommendations of use in somewhat different ways.

Given the billions of dollars consumers currently spend on weight-loss programs, we believe strongly that these programs require special attention and evaluation. Unfortunately, our health-care system has not treated obesity as a chronic disease requiring long-term management, even as the prevalence of this disease continues to increase. We believe that a new concept of obesity treatment is needed, and this report represents a first effort by a group of biomedical experts convened by the Food and Nutrition Board of the Institute of Medicine to stimulate this process. This report provides clients, obesity-management programs, researchers, and policymakers with recommendations by which to evaluate programs and outcomes. Although there will undoubtedly be discussion about the specific details of our recommendations, we believe that consensus exists about the need for them.

## THE FUTURE OF WEIGHT MANAGEMENT

Successful weight management ultimately includes preventing obesity from developing in the first place or delaying its onset and keeping somewhat overweight individuals from becoming obese, subjects addressed in Chapter 9. At this time, the tools are not available to prevent obesity, and most prevention programs to date have ended in failure. Programs to prevent obesity and encourage the adoption of healthier lifestyles among adults at work sites and in community programs produce modest results at best. Very few studies have investigated preventing obesity in children, for example, through school-based programs or by modeling healthy eating behaviors in the family. We recommend that money not be spent on large obesity prevention programs; smaller-scale research programs on prevention should be focused, perhaps according to stages of life at which obesity is more likely to occur, such as adolescence, or among high-risk groups, such as black females. Given the disappointing results of obesity prevention programs, more studies are needed on how to conduct large-scale intervention studies more effectively and to produce more desirable results.

Chapter 10 describes our research and policy recommendations. Continued research to understand the fundamental causes of obesity, particularly at the molecular and genetic levels, is enormously important. In addition, the behavioral and environmental influences on the expression of obesity need to be much better understood. The genetic and environmental determinants of obesity and its associated comorbidities vary among population groups, and the variation and reasons for this variation are important areas of research. In addition, research is needed on cognitive-behavioral approaches to increase success at long-term weight loss and maintenance and to further understand the contributions of diet and physical activity in achieving successful weight management. Furthermore, it would be useful to determine the mechanisms by which anti-obesity drugs and gastric surgery promote weight loss.

While research should eventually uncover the causes of obesity and lead to this disease being better managed, prevented, and treated, the application of scientific findings alone is rarely enough to resolve public health problems. Public policies are needed to translate the research findings to the lay public and to apply what is already known about successful weight management. We have three major public-policy recommendations:

- Obesity should be acknowledged as one of this country's most important nutrition-related diseases, which has important consequences for the funding of research by government, foundations, and private agencies; for health-care reform; and for oversight of the weight-loss industry by regulatory agencies.
- There must be increased recognition and support for obesity research at the genetic, molecular, and cellular levels that will aid our understanding of the causes of obesity and its associated comorbidities.
- A more aggressive policy is required to inform the public and health-care providers about the nature of obesity, the difficulties inherent in treating this disease, and the need for susceptible individuals to take steps to prevent its occurrence or minimize its development. Health-care providers in particular should learn more about obesity and its treatment.

Because successful weight management has proven an elusive goal for most obese individuals in the United States, the marketplace has provided many legitimate as well as unfounded products and services. Improving the rate of success at weight management requires would-be dieters to understand that gimmicks, from weight-loss pills to esoteric diets, either are totally ineffectual or are no more than small countermeasures to an incompletely understood disorder of energy balance. Furthermore, dieters should stay away from programs that claim more than they can substantiate or state that their unique methods ensure permanent weight loss. For its part, the scientific community must continue research to provide a fundamental understanding of the causes of obesity, leading to the design of maximally successful treatments and means to more effectively prevent this disease.

# 1

## Introduction and Background

In spite of our ever-increasing knowledge of the health risks of obesity, people in the United States are getting fatter. This country is in the midst of an epidemic of obesity, as described in Chapter 2, with 35 percent of women and 31 percent of men aged 20 and older considered obese. The prevalence is even higher among those with lower levels of education, black women, and Mexican-Americans of both sexes.

Many individuals want to lose weight for a variety of reasons that include improving appearance, feeling better, and being healthier. Often a person's primary motivation for weight loss is to increase his or her perceived attractiveness and self-esteem. Health-care providers are most likely to recommend weight loss to help obese people decrease their risks of developing, and improve the management of, a variety of medical problems and chronic diseases that includes diabetes, hypertension, other cardiovascular diseases, sleep apnea, and osteoarthritis of weight-bearing joints.

It is paradoxical that obesity is increasing in the United States while more people are dieting than ever before, spending, by one estimate, more than $33 billion per year on weight-reduction products (including diet foods and soft drinks, artificial sweeteners, and diet books) and services (e.g., fitness clubs and weight-loss programs) (U.S. Congress, 1990). The majority of dieters have designed their own weight-loss programs (95 percent of men and 87 percent of women, according to one survey [Levy and Heaton, 1993]), which may be based on popular books, include over-the-counter diet aids, and consist of self-directed modifications of diet and exercise. Despite efforts to improve the efficacy of treatments for obesity, no methods have emerged that offer a substantial chance of long-term weight loss except for surgery among the extremely obese. The fact is that despite the billions of dollars spent, few people reduce their body weight to a desirable or healthy level and even fewer maintain the weight lost beyond 2 or 3 years.

Chapter 3 describes the abundance of weight-control services, programs, and products currently available, which range from popular books and over-the-counter diet aids to medically supervised weight-management programs, drugs, and surgery. For practical purposes, we have grouped the options into three major categories of programs: do-it-yourself, nonclinical, and clinical programs. We also identify and describe five broad approaches to treatment used by these programs: diet, physical activity, behavior modification, drug therapy, and gastric surgery. The related Appendixes A and B provide examples of assessment instruments that might be used in obesity treatment in clinical and research settings.

Chapter 4 presents a simple conceptual overview of the factors relevant to decisionmaking, in this case, by a person making decisions about weight loss. It consists of the individual's choosing one or more weight-loss programs, undertaking the program, and experiencing the outcome of the undertaking. Three criteria were developed to be used by individuals in evaluating weight-loss programs: (1) the match between the program and consumer, (2) the soundness and safety of the program, and (3) outcomes of the program. Together, these criteria provide guidance for consumers to increase their chances of success at weight loss and for weight-loss programs to increase their ability to help individuals lose weight.

Criterion 1, the subject of Chapter 5, pertains to the match between the individual and the program (i.e., trying to predict, with some degree of precision, which individuals will succeed in a given program). We describe many factors that influence the program choices of individuals and review a number of matching schemes proposed by others. Chapter 6 addresses Criterion 2, the soundness and safety of the program. A sound weight-loss program should give attention to diet and physical activity, be as safe as reasonably possible, and encourage clients to have some knowledge of their weight-related physical health and psychological status. Chapter 7 presents Criterion 3, the outcomes of the program. Here we identify the psychological and physiological factors associated with long-term success at weight loss. This chapter also presents a new concept of obesity treatment focused on the achievement or maintenance of health rather than on simple weight reduction. The concept is based on the scientific literature documenting that obese individuals do not need to lose all or even most of their excess weight in order to improve risk factors (e.g., blood pressure and blood cholesterol and glucose concentrations) and, presumably, their health. Therefore, a primary goal of weight-loss programs in the future should be to help people lose enough weight to reduce the health risks associated with obesity rather than achieve a culturally defined ideal or desirable body weight. In effect, we are recommending that weight-loss programs evolve into weight-management programs.

Chapter 8 synthesizes the criteria presented in Chapters 4–7 in the form of a model. Our *Weighing the Options* model can be used by an individual wishing to lose weight, ideally with the help of a health-care provider, to learn the legitimate options available, identify weight-management goals, and reevaluate goals and options on the basis of results obtained from specific programs. We hope our criteria and model will serve several purposes: (1) enable outside parties to evaluate programs in a consistent and comprehensive fashion, (2) stimulate programs to disclose important information to consumers as a matter of policy and to improve the quality of the programs, and (3) help consumers make informed choices in program selection with a focus on long-term weight management rather than simple weight loss. The chapter presents a framework for the conduct of weight-management programs so that they can be evaluated more uniformly and consumers can make informed choices.

Current understanding in the treatment of obesity has led to questioning traditional beliefs about long-term weight management (i.e., the maintenance of weight loss)—particularly the view that successful weight loss requires a period of intense management that can be followed by much less attention during the maintenance phase. To the extent that powerful biological and environmental forces are at work to regain lost weight, weight can be kept down only by dealing with obesity as one would manage any chronic disease—by continuous treatment, lifelong efforts, and vigilance. We use the term *weight management* in this report to refer to weight loss over both the short term (the period of actual weight loss) and the long term (the long, indefinite period of effort aimed at minimizing the amount and rate of regain of lost weight).

Successful weight management ultimately includes preventing obesity from developing in the first place. Chapter 9 focuses on the prevention of new cases of this disease at three levels by targeting (1) the general population, (2) high-risk subgroups, and (3) individuals who are overweight but not yet obese or who are otherwise known to be predisposed to obesity. Unfortunately, work-site- and community-based prevention programs have produced results no better than those of obesity treatment programs. Hopes had been high that these low-cost programs, which have attracted large numbers of individuals, would be effective.

The most optimistic feature of this report is surely found in the research agenda in Chapter 10. Learning more about how health-related behaviors develop and can be modified, together with the rapid growth of knowledge and better tools in areas such as molecular genetics and metabolic regulation, gives promise that at some point we will understand the underlying causes of obesity. This should ultimately lead to the development of programs that treat the underlying causes of obesity and not just the symptoms.

## INFLUENCING THE PRACTICES OF WEIGHT-LOSS COMPANIES

Our charge was to develop criteria for evaluating weight-loss programs, and this is the focus of the middle and main section of our report. We began our efforts by reviewing earlier and ongoing efforts to influence and regulate the practices and advertising claims of the weight-loss industry. Specifically, we reviewed criteria for weight-loss programs established by the New York City Department of Consumer Affairs (Winner, 1991) and the Michigan Task Force to Establish Weight Loss Guidelines (Drewnowski, 1990); actions by the Federal Trade Commission to regulate deceptive claims by weight-loss programs (see, for example, Clark, 1993a, b); and guidelines from the National Institutes of Health (NIH) for evaluating weight-loss methods and programs (NIH Technology Assessment Conference Panel, 1993) and for choosing a weight-loss program (NIDDK, 1993a). We also considered an accreditation system for weight-management programs (see Appendix D).

These important examples of efforts to influence or regulate the activities of the weight-loss industry do not imply any endorsement on our part, though they helped us in various ways in developing our recommendations throughout this report. Within the scientific community, there are varying opinions about the correctness and appropriateness of some of the statements and recommendations contained in these examples.

### New York City Department of Consumer Affairs (DCA)

The DCA first documented some of the deceptive practices used by rapid-weight-loss centers by having DCA staff, posing as potential clients, visit 14 weight-loss centers. Staff members reported that (1) the vast majority of centers did not discuss potential risks even when asked, (2) some centers counseled underweight individuals to lose weight, and (3) some centers made false and misleading statements going beyond scientific evidence and engaged in quackery (Winner, 1991).

As a result of this 1991 investigation, the DCA put into effect the nation's first "Truth-in-Dieting" regulation on May 17, 1992. The ruling applies to more than 130 weight-loss centers in New York City that promote rapid weight loss. Rapid weight loss, using the DCA criteria, referred to "weight loss of more than $1\frac{1}{2}$ pounds to 2 pounds per week or weight loss of more than 1 percent of body weight per week after the second week of participation in a weight-loss program." The requirements of the four-step ruling included (1) posting of a "Weight-Loss Consumer Bill of Rights" sign; (2) handing the potential client a "palm-size" copy of the sign; (3) disclosing all the costs of the program, including those associated with purchase of products or laboratory tests; and (4) disclosing the duration of the recommended program (Winner, 1991). The required "Bill of Rights" sign was to state:

> 1. WARNING: Rapid weight loss may cause serious health problems. (Rapid weight loss is weight loss of more than $1\frac{1}{2}$ to 2 pounds per week or weight loss of more than 1 percent of body weight per week after the second week of participation in a weight-loss program.)
> 2. Only permanent lifestyle changes—such as making healthful food choices and increasing physical activity—promote long-term weight loss.
> 3. Consult your personal physician before starting any weight-loss program.
> 4. Qualifications of this provider's staff are available on request.
> 5. You have a right to
> * ask questions about the potential health risks of this program, its nutritional content, and its psychological-support and educational components;
> * know the price of treatment, including the price of extra products, services, supplements, and laboratory tests; and
> * know the program duration that is being recommended for you.

Although it is not required, at least one commercial program has been distributing the Bill of Rights sign to clients outside the New York City area (personal communication with Linda Webb Carilli, M.S., R.D., General Manager, Corporate Affairs, Weight Watchers International, Inc.).

## Michigan Department of Public Health

In 1990, a task force appointed by the Michigan Department of Public Health developed a set of guidelines for adult weight-loss programs in that state (Drewnowski, 1990; Petersmarck, 1992). The guidelines, listed in Table 1-1, apply to nonclinical and clinical programs and are quite

**TABLE 1-1**   Weight-Loss Guidelines for Michigan, 1990

*Screening*
The client should be screened to verify that there are no medical or psychological conditions which could make weight loss inappropriate.
The client's level of health risk should be identified: low-risk, moderate-risk, or high-risk.

*Level of Care*
The weight-loss program should provide the level of care appropriate to the client's level of health risk: Levels of Care 1, 2, or 3.

*Individualized Treatment Plan*
Factors contributing to the client's weight status should be identified. These factors should serve as the bases for each client's individualized weight-loss plan, which may include the weight goal, and plans for nutrition, exercise, behavioral change, medical monitoring or supervision, and health supervision.

*Staffing*
Weight-loss service providers should be trained and supervised adequately for the level of health risk of clients receiving care.

*Full Disclosure*
The client should give informed consent, having been informed of potential physical and psychological risks from weight loss and regain, likely long-term success of the program, full cost of the program, and credentials of the weight-loss care providers.

*Reasonable Weight Goal*
The weight goal for the client should be based on personal and family weight history, *not* exclusively on height and weight charts.

*Rate of Weight Loss*
The advertised and actual rate of weight loss, after the first two weeks, should not exceed an average of two pounds per week.

*Calories per Day*
The daily caloric level should be adjusted so that each client can achieve but not exceed the recommended rate of weight loss. The daily caloric intake should not be lower than 1,000 calories at Level 1; 800 calories at Level 2; and 600 calories at Level 3. If the daily caloric level is below 800 calories, additional safeguards should be in place.

**TABLE 1-1** Continued

---

*Diet Composition*
 • Protein: between 0.8 and 1.5 grams of protein per kilogram of goal body weight, but no more than 100 grams of protein per day.
   • Fat: 10–30 percent of calories as fat.
   • Carbohydrate: at least 100 grams per day for Level 1; at least 50 grams per day for Level 2.
   • Fluid: at least one quart of water daily.

*Nutritional Adequacy*
 The food plan should allow the client to obtain 100 percent of the client's Recommended Dietary Allowances (RDA). If nutrition supplements are used, nutrient levels should not greatly exceed 100 percent of the RDA.

*Nutrition Education*
 Nutrition education encouraging permanent healthful eating patterns should be incorporated into the weight-loss program.

*Formula Products*
 The food plan should consist of a variety of foods available from the conventional food supply. Formula products are not recommended for the treatment of moderate obesity, and should not be used at low-calorie formulations without specialized medical supervision.

*Exercise Component*
 The weight-loss program should include an exercise component that is safe and appropriate for the individual client:

 • The client should be screened for conditions which would make medical clearance before exercise appropriate.
 • The client should be instructed to recognize and deal with potentially dangerous physical responses to exercise.
 • The client should work toward 30–60 minutes of continuous exercise 5–7 times per week, with gradual increases in intensity and duration.

*Psychological Component*
 Behavior modification techniques appropriate for the specific client should be taught.

*Appetite Suppressants*
 Appetite suppressant drugs are not recommended, and should not take the place of changes in diet, exercise, and behavior.

*Weight Maintenance*
 A maintenance phase should be included in the treatment program.

---

SOURCE: Drewnowski, 1990. Reprinted with permission.

detailed. They have the advantage of screening prospective clients to assess their level of health risk and, on that basis, recommending individualized, multidisciplinary approaches that include nutrition, exercise, and behavior modification. The Michigan guidelines attempt to forge a match between program and client that is dictated by the client's health needs. It was the hope of the task force that its guidelines would be adopted as standards of health care in weight-loss programs throughout Michigan. Adoption of the guidelines would mandate that potential clients be screened for health risks prior to beginning a calorie-restricted diet and that weight-loss programs and clinics be staffed by qualified professionals capable of delivering appropriate levels of health care.

### Federal Trade Commission

In contrast to guidelines aimed at defining essential components of programs, the Federal Trade Commission's (FTC) efforts address and challenge specific, allegedly deceptive advertising claims that companies have made to promote their weight-reduction programs and diet aids. The FTC actions seek to place the companies under an order designed to remedy those allegedly deceptive claims. By the end of December 1993, the FTC had either begun litigation or settled complaints it had issued against 11 commercial weight-loss companies (personal communication with Richard F. Kelly, Esq., Assistant Director for the Division of Service Industry Practices, Federal Trade Commission).

In each of the cases that have been settled through a consent agreement, the FTC's order requires that any statements made about "success of participants of any weight loss program in achieving or maintaining weight loss or weight control" be based on data representative of either all participants or a clearly-defined subset of participants (personal communication with Richard F. Kelly, Esq.). When a claim is made that participants in a program successfully maintain lost weight, the order requires in most instances that the claim be accompanied by a disclosure of data that reflects the actual experience of program participants and a general statement about the temporary nature of most weight loss. An example given by FTC of "acceptable disclosure" is: "participants maintain an average of 60% of weight loss 22 months after active weight loss (includes 18 months on maintenance program). For many dieters weight loss is temporary" (FTC, 1993).

### NIH Guidelines for Evaluating Weight-Loss Programs

The NIH Technology Assessment Conference on methods for voluntary weight loss and control provided guidelines for evaluating weight-loss methods and programs (NIH Technology Assessment Conference Panel, 1993). According to the guidelines, information about program success that should be obtained includes the following:

- the percentage of all beginning participants who complete the program;
- the percentage of those completing the program who achieve various degrees of weight loss;
- the proportion of weight loss that is maintained at 1, 3, and even 5 years; and
- the percentage of participants who experienced adverse medical or psychological effects and the kind and severity.

Valid and reliable statistics of this kind are important, but they are not routinely provided by commercial diet plans or programs. Such data, preferably in the form of peer-reviewed published studies, should be available for all supervised programs, including those based in hospitals, clinics, or private practice.

According to the guidelines, additional information on program characteristics that should be obtained includes

- the relative mix of diet, exercise, and behavior modifications;
- the amount and kind of counseling: both individual counseling and closed groups (membership does not change except by attrition) are more successful than open groups (in which members may come and go);
- the nature of available multidisciplinary expertise (including medical, nutritional, psychological, physiologic, and exercise);
- the training provided for relapse prevention to deal with high-risk emotional and social situations;
- the nature and duration of the maintenance phase; and
- the flexibility of food choices and suitability of food types, and whether weight goals are set unilaterally or cooperatively with the program director.

## NIH Guidelines for Choosing a Weight-Loss Program

The Obesity Task Force at the National Institutes of Health developed consumer guidelines for choosing a safe and successful weight-loss program (NIDDK, 1993a). The five program features include the following:

- The diet should be safe and include all of the Recommended Dietary Allowances for vitamins, minerals, and protein.
- The program should be directed towards a slow, steady weight loss unless a more rapid weight loss is medically indicated.
- A doctor should evaluate health status if the client's weight-loss goal is greater than 15–20 pounds, if the client has any health problems, or if the client takes medication on a regular basis.
- The program should include plans for weight maintenance.
- The program should give the prospective client a detailed list of fees and costs of additional items.

## CONCLUDING REMARKS

In this country, where successful weight management has proven an elusive goal for most obese individuals, the marketplace has provided many legitimate, as well as unfounded, products and services. The latter play legal tag with governmental regulatory agencies while taking financial advantage of a public desperate for answers. Improving the rate of success of weight management requires that would-be dieters understand that methods from thigh creams to esoteric diets must be substantiated by validated evidence of efficacy. They may represent no more than small countermeasures to an incompletely understood disorder of energy balance. In addition, obese individuals must learn to stay away from programs that give false hopes by suggesting that, compared to the programs of legitimate competitors, they are more effective at weight loss and that their unique methods ensure permanent loss. For its part, the scientific community must continue research that will provide us with a fundamental understanding of the basic causes of obesity; this understanding is essential if we are to design maximally effective obesity treatments and develop the means for preventing the disease.

# 2

## The Nature and Problem of Obesity

The pressing need for criteria for evaluating weight-loss programs stems from the scope of the problem of obesity in this country and the evidence that it is worsening, in spite of extensive individual and programmatic efforts to achieve weight control. In its *Healthy People 2000* report published in 1991, the federal government proposed that no more than 20 percent of adults in this country aged 20 and older and no more than 15 percent of adolescents aged 12 through 19 should be overweight by the turn of the twenty-first century (DHHS, 1991; see Figure 2-1). Studies over the past two decades, however, show that our country is moving farther from, rather than closer to, this goal. As shown later in this chapter, the prevalence of overweight and obesity is rising, not falling, among most population groups as characterized by gender, age, and race.

Paradoxically, at the same time as the prevalence of obesity is increasing, tens of millions of people in this country are dieting at any given time. An obese individual faces a continuous, lifelong struggle with no expectation that the struggle required will diminish with time. For most people, even a brief abatement in effort will be met with a significant setback in control. Studies in controlled settings show that individuals who complete weight-loss programs lose approximately 10 percent of their body weight, but gain two-thirds of it back within 1 year and almost all of it back within 5 years (NIH Technology Assessment Conference Panel, 1993).

Obesity is one of the most prevalent diet-related health problems in

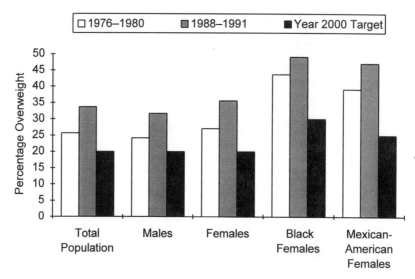

**Prevalence of overweight
among U.S. adults
aged 20–74.**

FIGURE 2-1    Data are from the National Health and Nutrition Examination
Surveys (NHANES) II (1976–1980) and III (Phase 1, 1988–1991), conducted by the
National Center for Health Statistics, and target goals are from *Healthy People
2000* (DHHS, 1991).

the United States, increasing the population's risk for chronic diseases
such as hypertension, other cardiovascular and cerebrovascular diseases,
some forms of cancer, and non-insulin-dependent diabetes mellitus. Obesity is a heterogeneous disease in which genetic, environmental, psychological, and other factors are involved. It occurs when energy intake exceeds the amount of energy expended over time. Only in a small minority
of cases is obesity caused by illnesses such as hypothyroidism or the
result of taking medications, such as steroids, that can cause weight gain.

One remarkable feature of obesity is that its management requires a
great deal of effort from the individual. Health-care providers or counselors can offer only advice and technical support at this time. In virtually
every other field that involves a chronic disease, there is the expectation
that drugs are required and may be effective in treating and possibly
curing these diseases. While researchers expect that the development and
long-term use of new drugs and combinations of drugs will help in the
chronic management of obesity, few drugs are available at present. For

the relatively small number of very obese individuals, there are favorable long-term outcomes with gastric surgery (NIH, 1992). However, for the majority of obese individuals, there is currently no hope of a cure or spontaneous resolution, no expectation that the disease will stabilize, and no hope that the symptoms can be diminished. There are few diseases in which health-care providers can offer so little for those who struggle so much.

Another remarkable feature of obesity is that its victims suffer discrimination. Perhaps most laypersons, health-care providers, and even obese individuals themselves do not perceive the metabolic nature of the disease and thus view obesity as a problem of willful misconduct—eating too much and exercising too little (Stunkard and Sørensen, 1993). For example, a survey by Price et al. (1987) found that two-thirds of 318 responding family practice physicians believed their obese patients to lack self-control; 39 percent described them as "lazy," and 34 percent characterized them as "sad." Another study found third-year medical students to perceive very obese individuals as "unpleasant, worthless, and bad," even after direct contact with them in a psychiatry rotation over 8 weeks (Blumberg and Mellis, 1985). We believe strongly that it is important for the lay public and health-care providers alike to change the common misperception that the obese are largely responsible for their disorder and deserve to be discriminated against if they do not reduce to a more socially desirable weight.

In this chapter, we provide an overview of the problem of overweight and obesity in the United States, its incidence and prevalence, and the weight-loss practices of individuals. We then review current findings about the specific benefits of weight loss and summarize the tremendous personal and societal costs of obesity.

## OBESITY IN THE UNITED STATES

There is a surprising amount of variation in the terminology used to describe excess weight and in the definition of these terms (see box titled "Obesity and Its Measurement"). This variation leads to difficulties in estimating precisely the extent of these disorders and in trying to compare the results of different studies. Not only are the terms *overweight* and *obesity* often used interchangeably, there is considerable disagreement concerning how to identify those at increased risk from excess weight (Kuczmarski, 1992).

The problems involved in defining obesity are similar to those encountered in defining physical activity, hypertension, and hypercholesterolemia, in which continuous variables such as weight, blood pressure, energy expenditure, and blood cholesterol concentration are categorized into distinct risk groups. While there is a general increase in risk as the measure increases, categorizing these variables assumes that, at one or more points on the distribution, risk increases substantially.

There are two ways to identify the points of increased risk. First, empirical examination of the relationship between the risk factor and the health outcome can identify the appropriate cutoff points. Alternatively, it is possible to base the cutoff on the distribution of the risk factor itself and to identify those at the upper end of the distribution as being in the high-risk category.

---

### OBESITY AND ITS MEASUREMENT

Overweight and obesity are terms that have distinct though related meanings and are often used interchangeably. Overweight refers to an excess amount of total body weight that includes all tissues (e.g., fat, bone, and muscle) and water. Obesity refers specifically to an excess of body fat. It is possible to be overweight without being obese, as might be the case with a body builder who gains a substantial amount of muscle mass. It is also possible, though not as common, to be obese without being overweight, a situation that might affect sedentary "couch potatoes" and some elderly persons. For practical purposes, however, most overweight people are also obese.

Obesity can be measured by several methods, such as weighing a person underwater, measuring skinfold thickness in several parts of the body, scanning by dual-energy X-ray absorptiometry (DEXA), and using bioelectric impedance analysis (which involves sending a very small amount of electric current through the body) and total body electrical conductivity (TOBEC) analysis (based on an interaction between the body and a varying magnetic field). Because some of these tests require sophisticated equipment and experienced, trained personnel, they are not practical in most settings. When total body fat is used as an index, men with more than 25 percent and women with more than 30 percent body fat are considered to be obese (NIDDK, 1993b). The most common and easily determined indirect techniques for assessing obesity are the body mass index (BMI) and weight-for-height tables. In this report, we will use the term obesity consistently in referring to the condition of excess body weight.

The body mass index (BMI) is a mathematical formula correlated highly with body fat. It is the measurement of choice used by health-care providers and investigators studying obesity. BMI is expressed as weight in kilograms divided by height in meters squared (BMI = $kg/m^2$). Table 2-1 presents BMI values on the basis of the more familiar height in inches and weight in pounds.

NOTE TO TABLE 2-1: Body mass index, originally referred to as the Quetelet Index (QI), is weight in kilograms divided by height in meters squared. Each entry gives the body weight in pounds for a person of a given height and body mass index. Pounds have been rounded off. To use the table, find the appropriate height in the left-hand column. Move across the row to a given weight. The number at the top of the column is the body mass index for that weight and height.

**TABLE 2-1** Body Weight (in pounds) According to Height (in inches) and Body Mass Index

Body Mass Index

| Height | 19 | 20 | 21 | 22 | 23 | 24 | 25 | 26 | 27 | 28 | 29 | 30 | 31 | 32 | 33 | 34 |
|---|---|---|---|---|---|---|---|---|---|---|---|---|---|---|---|---|
| | | | | | | | Body Weight | | | | | | | | | |
| 58 | 91 | 95 | 100 | 105 | 110 | 114 | 119 | 124 | 129 | 133 | 138 | 143 | 148 | 152 | 157 | 162 |
| 59 | 94 | 99 | 104 | 109 | 114 | 119 | 124 | 129 | 134 | 139 | 144 | 149 | 154 | 159 | 164 | 169 |
| 60 | 97 | 102 | 107 | 112 | 117 | 122 | 127 | 132 | 138 | 143 | 148 | 153 | 158 | 163 | 168 | 173 |
| 61 | 101 | 106 | 111 | 117 | 122 | 127 | 132 | 138 | 143 | 148 | 154 | 159 | 164 | 169 | 175 | 180 |
| 62 | 103 | 109 | 114 | 120 | 125 | 130 | 136 | 141 | 147 | 152 | 158 | 163 | 168 | 174 | 179 | 185 |
| 63 | 107 | 113 | 119 | 124 | 130 | 135 | 141 | 147 | 152 | 158 | 164 | 169 | 175 | 181 | 186 | 192 |
| 64 | 111 | 117 | 123 | 129 | 135 | 141 | 146 | 152 | 158 | 164 | 170 | 176 | 182 | 187 | 193 | 199 |
| 65 | 114 | 120 | 126 | 132 | 138 | 144 | 150 | 156 | 162 | 168 | 174 | 180 | 186 | 192 | 198 | 204 |
| 66 | 118 | 124 | 131 | 137 | 143 | 149 | 156 | 162 | 168 | 174 | 180 | 187 | 193 | 199 | 205 | 212 |
| 67 | 121 | 127 | 134 | 140 | 147 | 153 | 159 | 166 | 172 | 178 | 185 | 191 | 198 | 204 | 210 | 217 |
| 68 | 125 | 132 | 139 | 145 | 152 | 158 | 165 | 172 | 178 | 185 | 191 | 198 | 205 | 211 | 218 | 224 |
| 69 | 128 | 135 | 142 | 149 | 155 | 162 | 169 | 176 | 182 | 189 | 196 | 203 | 209 | 216 | 223 | 230 |
| 70 | 133 | 140 | 147 | 154 | 161 | 168 | 175 | 182 | 189 | 196 | 203 | 210 | 217 | 224 | 231 | 237 |
| 71 | 136 | 143 | 150 | 157 | 164 | 171 | 179 | 186 | 193 | 200 | 207 | 214 | 221 | 229 | 236 | 243 |
| 72 | 140 | 148 | 155 | 162 | 170 | 177 | 185 | 192 | 199 | 207 | 214 | 221 | 229 | 236 | 244 | 251 |
| 73 | 143 | 151 | 158 | 166 | 174 | 181 | 189 | 196 | 204 | 211 | 219 | 226 | 234 | 241 | 249 | 257 |
| 74 | 148 | 156 | 164 | 171 | 179 | 187 | 195 | 203 | 210 | 218 | 226 | 234 | 242 | 249 | 257 | 265 |
| 75 | 151 | 159 | 167 | 175 | 183 | 191 | 199 | 207 | 215 | 223 | 231 | 239 | 247 | 255 | 263 | 271 |
| 76 | 156 | 164 | 172 | 181 | 189 | 197 | 205 | 214 | 222 | 230 | 238 | 246 | 255 | 263 | 271 | 279 |

continued on next page

**TABLE 2-1** Continued

| | | | | | | | | Body Mass Index | | | | | | | | |
|---|---|---|---|---|---|---|---|---|---|---|---|---|---|---|---|---|
| Height | 35 | 36 | 37 | 38 | 39 | 40 | 41 | 42 | 43 | 44 | 45 | 46 | 47 | 48 | 49 | 50 |
| | | | | | | | | Body Weight | | | | | | | | |
| 58 | 167 | 172 | 176 | 181 | 186 | 191 | 195 | 200 | 205 | 210 | 214 | 219 | 224 | 229 | 233 | 238 |
| 59 | 174 | 179 | 184 | 188 | 193 | 198 | 203 | 208 | 213 | 218 | 223 | 228 | 233 | 238 | 243 | 248 |
| 60 | 178 | 183 | 188 | 194 | 199 | 204 | 209 | 214 | 219 | 224 | 229 | 234 | 239 | 244 | 250 | 255 |
| 61 | 185 | 191 | 196 | 201 | 207 | 212 | 217 | 222 | 228 | 233 | 238 | 244 | 249 | 254 | 260 | 265 |
| 62 | 190 | 196 | 201 | 206 | 212 | 217 | 223 | 228 | 234 | 239 | 245 | 250 | 255 | 261 | 266 | 272 |
| 63 | 198 | 203 | 209 | 214 | 220 | 226 | 231 | 237 | 243 | 248 | 254 | 260 | 265 | 271 | 277 | 282 |
| 64 | 205 | 211 | 217 | 223 | 228 | 234 | 240 | 246 | 252 | 258 | 264 | 269 | 275 | 281 | 287 | 293 |
| 65 | 210 | 216 | 222 | 228 | 234 | 240 | 246 | 252 | 258 | 264 | 270 | 276 | 282 | 288 | 294 | 300 |
| 66 | 218 | 224 | 230 | 236 | 243 | 249 | 255 | 261 | 268 | 274 | 280 | 286 | 292 | 299 | 305 | 311 |
| 67 | 223 | 229 | 236 | 242 | 248 | 255 | 261 | 268 | 274 | 280 | 287 | 293 | 299 | 306 | 312 | 319 |
| 68 | 231 | 238 | 244 | 251 | 257 | 264 | 271 | 277 | 284 | 290 | 297 | 304 | 310 | 317 | 323 | 330 |
| 69 | 236 | 243 | 250 | 257 | 263 | 270 | 277 | 284 | 290 | 297 | 304 | 311 | 317 | 324 | 331 | 338 |
| 70 | 244 | 251 | 258 | 265 | 272 | 279 | 286 | 293 | 300 | 307 | 314 | 321 | 328 | 335 | 342 | 349 |
| 71 | 250 | 257 | 264 | 271 | 279 | 286 | 293 | 300 | 307 | 314 | 321 | 329 | 336 | 343 | 350 | 357 |
| 72 | 258 | 266 | 273 | 281 | 288 | 295 | 303 | 313 | 317 | 325 | 332 | 340 | 347 | 354 | 362 | 369 |
| 73 | 264 | 272 | 279 | 287 | 294 | 302 | 309 | 317 | 324 | 332 | 340 | 347 | 355 | 362 | 370 | 377 |
| 74 | 273 | 281 | 288 | 296 | 304 | 312 | 319 | 327 | 335 | 343 | 351 | 358 | 366 | 374 | 382 | 390 |
| 75 | 279 | 287 | 294 | 302 | 310 | 318 | 326 | 334 | 342 | 350 | 358 | 366 | 374 | 382 | 390 | 398 |
| 76 | 287 | 296 | 304 | 312 | 320 | 328 | 337 | 345 | 353 | 361 | 370 | 378 | 386 | 394 | 402 | 411 |

SOURCE: Adapted and expanded from NIDDK, 1993b.

Both methods have been used to assess obesity. Weight-for-height tables are examples of the empirical approach. Based on these tables, the suggested weight for an adult 35 years or older at a height of 5 feet, 7 inches is 134 to 172 pounds. Such a person weighing more than the cutoff point of 172 pounds would be considered to have exceeded a desirable or healthy weight. While cutpoints are useful because they are conceptually easy to understand, they present some methodological problems. Inconsistencies in the results obtained from different empirical studies make it difficult to identify a single cutpoint representing excess risk. These inconsistencies can result from differences across studies in the definition of endpoints, the duration of follow-up, and the inclusion of other covariates (e.g., how fat is distributed on the body or whether obesity is associated with other chronic diseases). Cutpoints derived from empirical studies will also tend to change over time as the science on which they are based advances.

An alternative approach to establishing points of increased risk is used by the National Center for Health Statistics (NCHS), which identifies two categories of excess weight: overweight and severe overweight. The term *obesity* is not used. Given that weight generally increases with age and that this weight gain represents a potential health risk, NCHS uses the extremes of the distribution of BMI for young adults (aged 20–29 years) to identify those at most risk of being overweight. Data from the Second National Health and Nutrition Examination Survey (NHANES II) conducted during 1976–1980 are used to identify the cutpoints. The cutpoints for overweight and severe overweight correspond to the sex-specific 85th and 95th percentiles of BMI, respectively (27.8 and 31.1 for males; 27.3 and 32.3 for females), in the 1976–1980 survey. Of course, BMI distributions in other populations or in other years could result in different cutpoints if populations differ in how BMI is distributed, as is usually the case, or if there is a change over time in the weight of a population. NCHS uses these cutpoints from NHANES II as the reference against which to compare results from its other surveys. Although the NCHS cutpoints are based on the observed distribution of BMI, these cutpoints are closely related to those derived from studies of the relationship between BMI and health outcomes. They are comparable to a body weight 20 and 40 percent, respectively, above the so-called ideal body weight derived from the popular weight-for-height tables issued by Metropolitan Life Insurance Company in 1983.

The meaning of the term *healthy weight* as well as how best to measure it remains the subject of scientific debate. Research on identifying optimal weights continues (see, for example, AIN, 1994; Hammond and Garfinkel, 1969; Lew and Garfinkel, 1979; Lindsted et al., 1991; Society of Actuaries, 1980; Sorkin et al., in press; Waaler, 1984) and should be encouraged. However, given the complexity of the relationships between weight and health outcomes, it may only be possible to develop general guidelines as to what constitute healthy weights. Care must be taken in applying weight standards to individuals, and it may not be possible to set weight goals for particular individuals by using a single table or set of cutpoints.

## THE CLASSIFICATION OF OBESITY

What is a "healthy" or "unhealthy" weight? There is no sure answer to this question. The National Institutes of Health (NIH) National Task Force on Prevention and Treatment of Obesity stated that, in general, individuals are obese if their BMI is 25 or more through age 34 and 27 or more beyond age 34 (NIDDK, 1993b). Obesity is also assessed by using weight-for-height tables. Some of the most widely used tables come from the life insurance industry, which has height, weight, and mortality data on some 5 million individuals who have chosen to obtain life insurance policies. The 1959 and 1983 Metropolitan Life Insurance Company tables of desirable weight are still among the most popular in use. In 1990, the federal government issued a table of suggested weights for adults based on height and age. Table 2-2 provides a generous range of "healthy" weights for a given height. For individuals 19–34 years of age, the BMI range given is 19 to 25; for those age 35 and older, the BMI range is 21 to 27. These figures suggest that it is acceptable for weight to increase with age (see also Andres et al., 1993), though there is disagreement about this point (see, for example, Willett et al., 1991, and Bray, 1993a). One criticism of the NIH and federal government guidelines is that they imply that it is acceptable to gain some 10–20 pounds after age 34; critics argue that individuals who gain small amounts of weight over time should learn better lifestyle habits that might eliminate or minimize weight gain. As the scientific discourse about this matter continues, we have adopted the recommendations of the NIH National Task Force.

We will often use the term comorbidity in this report to refer to the concomitant pathologic processes and diseases associated with obesity. Comorbidities linked to obesity include coronary heart disease, stroke, hypertension, obstructive sleep apnea, diabetes mellitus, gout, dyslipidemia, osteoarthritis of weight-bearing joints (such as the knees and hips), gallstones and cholecystitis, reduced fertility, reduced physical agility and increased risk of accidents, and impaired obstetrical performance (IFT, 1994; Pi-Sunyer, 1993a).

Some of these health risks of obesity are more likely to occur when fat is concentrated in the abdominal or visceral area rather than the gluteal area. A measurement called the waist-to-hip ratio (WHR) is used clinically to assess whether weight is collected primarily in the hips and buttocks (producing what is known as a "pear" shape, common in females) or in the abdomen (an "apple" shape, common in males). The WHR is determined by measuring the waist with a non-stretchable tape measure at its smallest point (between the rib cage and navel) and the hips at their widest point (around the buttocks). (See Figure 2-2 to calculate WHR.) A WHR of more than 1.0 in males and 0.8 in females suggests a weight distribution that poses increased risks to health compared to the excess weight alone. Abdominal diameter in the saggital plane is a marginally better measure than WHR, and scanning techniques (such as dual-energy x-ray absorptiometry) are even more accurate in evaluating abdominal obesity.

**TABLE 2-2**   Suggested Weights for Adults

| Height[a] | Weight (pounds)[b] | |
| | 19–34 Years Old | 35 Years Old and Over |
| --- | --- | --- |
| 5'0" | 97–128 | 108–138 |
| 5'1" | 101–132 | 111–143 |
| 5'2" | 104–137 | 115–148 |
| 5'3" | 107–141 | 119–152 |
| 5'4" | 111–146 | 122–157 |
| 5'5" | 114–150 | 126–162 |
| 5'6" | 118–155 | 130–167 |
| 5'7" | 121–160 | 134–172 |
| 5'8" | 125–164 | 138–178 |
| 5'9" | 129–169 | 142–183 |
| 5'10" | 132–174 | 146–188 |
| 5'11" | 136–179 | 151–194 |
| 6'0" | 140–184 | 155–199 |
| 6'1" | 144–189 | 159–205 |
| 6'2" | 148–195 | 164–210 |
| 6'3" | 152–200 | 168–216 |
| 6'4" | 156–205 | 173–222 |
| 6'5" | 160–211 | 177–228 |
| 6'6" | 164–216 | 182–234 |

NOTE: The higher weights in the ranges generally apply to men, who tend to have more muscle and bone; the lower weights more often apply to women, who have less muscle and bone.

[a]Without shoes.
[b]Without clothes.

SOURCE: USDA and DHHS, 1990.

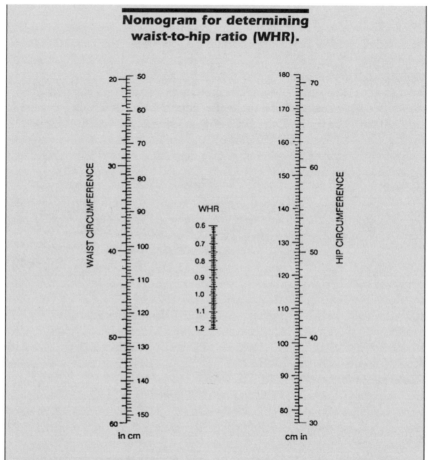

**Nomogram for determining waist-to-hip ratio (WHR).**

FIGURE 2-2  Place a ruler between the column for waist circumference and the column for hip circumference and read the ratio from the point where the ruler crosses the WHR line. SOURCE: Reprinted by permission of the Western Journal of Medicine. Bray, G.A., and D.S. Gray; Obesity: Part 1—Pathogenesis; 1988, volume 149, pages 429–441.

## INCIDENCE AND PREVALENCE

The most recent data on the prevalence of obesity in the United States come from the Third National Health and Nutrition Examination Survey (NHANES III) conducted by NCHS. Although the survey will not be completed until the end of 1994, information on BMI from the first 3 years of data collection (Phase 1, 1988–1991) has been reported (Kuczmarski et al., 1994). If NCHS's BMI cutpoints are used, 33 percent of the U.S. population aged 20 and over is overweight, and 14 percent is severely overweight. We believe that this large prevalence of obesity qualifies as an epidemic, using the common definition of this term—affecting many individuals in a population.

The prevalence of overweight varies considerably by age, gender, race, and socioeconomic status (SES). Data from 1988 to 1991 show that among those 20 years of age and over, the percent overweight increases with age, with the highest rates occurring in the 60–69-year-old group among males (42.2 percent overweight) and the 50–59-year-old group among females (52.0 percent). Based on age-adjusted data from this time period, 31.6 percent of white, non-Hispanic males and 32.1 percent of white, non-Hispanic females were overweight, as were 31.2 percent of black, non-Hispanic males; 48.5 percent of black, non-Hispanic females; 39.1 percent of Mexican-American males; and 47.2 percent of Mexican-American females (Kuczmarski et al., 1994). There is also great variability in percent overweight by SES. When educational attainment is used as an indicator of SES, 39 percent of those with less than a high-school education were overweight, compared to 36 percent of those with a high-school degree and 29 percent of those with some college education. These SES differentials hold for both genders (unpublished data from NHANES III, Phase 1, 1988–1991, provided by NCHS).

There also has been a dramatic increase in the prevalence of overweight over time, as shown from surveys conducted by NCHS. Because of differences in population coverage across the surveys, comparisons here are limited to those 20–74 years of age. Compared to the 33.3 percent of the population considered overweight in 1988–1991, only 24.4 percent was so defined in 1960–1962. This increase occurred among males and females and among blacks and whites (NCHS, 1994). Figures 2-3 and 2-4 show the increase in the prevalence of overweight over time among females and males, respectively, at various ages. The proportion overweight is highest in the 1988–1991 period in all age groups for both males and females; proportions overweight were relatively similar for the two earlier periods (1971–1974 and 1976–1980). For males, the greatest differential over time occurs in the older age groups, whereas for females the differential is smallest among those aged 65–74. It is clear that the U.S. population is rapidly moving further away from the government's public health goal that no more than 20 percent of adults be overweight by the turn of the century (see Figure 2-1).

Changes in prevalence of obesity over time can occur in many ways. For example, there could be a general shift to the right in the distribution of BMI, indicating that the total population is getting heavier, or there could be a more limited movement from the categories just below overweight into the overweight group. An examination of the total BMI dis-

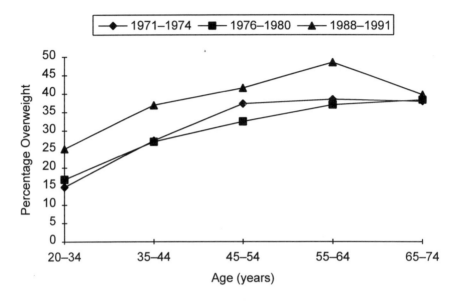

**Percentage of overweight females
20–74 years of age.**

**FIGURE 2-3**    Data are from NHANES I (1971–1974), II (1976–1980), and III (during 1988–1991), conducted by NCHS. Overweight individuals are those at or above the 85th percentile for persons 20–29 years, age and gender specific, in NHANES II.

tribution reveals that the former has taken place. There has been a decrease in the proportion of the population at healthier weights (e.g., BMI <25 was 57.2 percent in 1960–1962, 54.2 percent in 1971–1974, 54.4 percent in 1976–1980, and 48.1 percent in 1988–1991) and a general increase in the group at risk for weight-related problems (see Figure 2-5). The change in the BMI distribution can also reflect changes in the distribution of other behaviors. For example, smoking is highly related to weight and weight gain, and there has been a general decline in the proportion of the U.S. population that smokes (NCHS, 1994). However, adjusting for the effects of changes in smoking prevalence does not account for the increase in the proportion overweight from 1976–1980 to 1988–1991 (unpublished data from NHANES III, Phase 1, 1988–1991, provided by NCHS).

Cross-sectional data give valuable information on the status of the U.S. population at a given point in time, but longitudinal data are needed

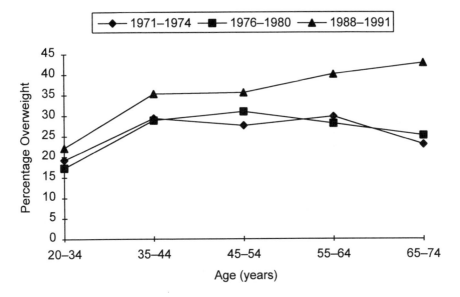

**Percentage of overweight males 20–74 years of age.**

FIGURE 2-4   Data are from NHANES I (1971–1974), II (1976–1980), and III (during 1988–1991), conducted by NCHS. Overweight individuals are those at or above the 85th percentile for persons 20–29 years, age and gender specific, in NHANES II.

to describe weight change patterns adequately. Williamson et al. (1990) analyzed data from a national sample in which subjects were weighed at two points 10 years apart. Among those 25–74 years old at the initiation of the study, the incidence of major weight gain (defined as an increase in BMI by 5 or more points) was highest in those 25–34 years old and then decreased with age. This pattern holds for both men and women, but the incidence of major weight gain was approximately twice as high among women within all age groups. The magnitude of gain decreased with increasing age until age 55, after which both men and women lost weight over the 10-year period. Among the nonoverweight group, men and women 35–44 years old were most likely to become overweight, with the incidence of overweight decreasing with increasing age. Compared to white females, black women 35–44 years old gained more weight on average, were more likely to have experienced a major weight gain, and were more likely to become overweight (Williamson et al., 1990).

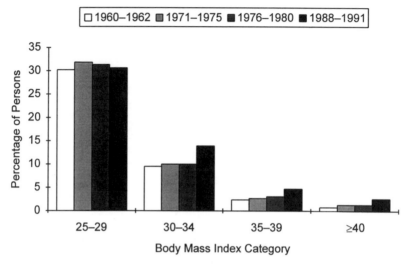

**Percentage distribution
of overweight persons
aged 20–74 years.**

FIGURE 2-5    The change in distribution of individuals with a BMI <25 was 57.2 percent in 1960–1962, 54.2 percent in 1971–1974, 54.4 percent in 1976–1980, and 48.1 percent in 1988–1991. Data are from NHES (National Health Examination Survey, Cycle 1, 1960–1962) and NHANES I (1971–1974), II (1976–1980), and III (Phase 1, 1988–1991), conducted by NCHS.

Figure 2-6 provides a schematic illustration of the problem of obesity in this country. While the prevalence of obesity is of epidemic proportions, the gradation indicates that most individuals are not obese, most obese persons are not severely so, and even some severely obese individuals may not have obesity-related comorbidities. An individual at any given BMI is at increased risk when one or more comorbidities are present or family history is positive for these comorbidities (see Figure 2-7). Prevention of obesity, of weight regain after loss, and of further weight gain is discussed in detail in Chapters 7 and 9.

While obesity has been increasing in the U.S. population as a whole and among major demographic subgroups, relevant comorbidities have not shown the same trend. Data from Phase I of NHANES III indicate that the prevalence of hypertension has declined over the past two decades. For example, 38.3 percent of the U.S. population aged 20–74 years (age adjusted) either had elevated blood pressure or were taking antihypertensive medication in 1971–1974. In 1988–1991, the hypertension

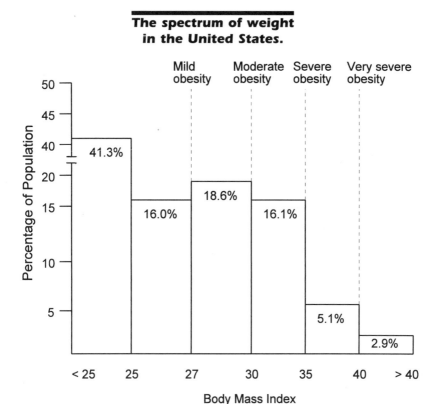

**The spectrum of weight in the United States.**

FIGURE 2-6 The various descriptors of the degree of obesity apply to individuals aged 35 and older and are associated with particular BMIs (mild obesity at a BMI of approximately 27, moderate obesity at 30, severe obesity at 35, and very severe obesity at approximately 40 or more). Approximately 41.3 percent of the population has a BMI of <25. Obesity may or may not be associated with one or more comorbidities except at the stage of severe obesity and beyond, when at least one comorbidity is almost always present. Younger adults are more likely to have no comorbidities (except for psychosocial ones) associated with their obesity. However, obese persons are at increased risk for developing comorbidities, especially over time as they get older.

prevalence declined to 23.4 percent. This decline was evident among both men and women, in all age groups, among non-Hispanic whites and African-Americans, but not among Mexican-Americans (NCHS, 1994). A similar trend has been found for blood cholesterol concentrations. In 1971–1974, 27.2 percent of the U.S. population 20–74 years of age (age adjusted) had cholesterol concentrations ≥240 mg/dl, decreasing to 19.7

**Health risks of obesity.**

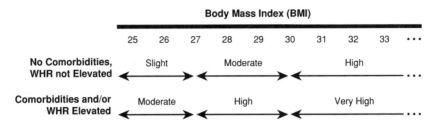

FIGURE 2-7   The risks are increased when adipose tissue is concentrated in the abdominal or visceral region (which is clinically assessed by calculating the waist-to-hip ratio [>1.0 for males and >0.8 for females]) and the presence of comorbidities such as high blood pressure (>140/90), lipid concentrations (cholesterol >200 mg/dl; triglycerides >225 mg/dl), non-insulin-dependent diabetes mellitus, osteoarthritis, sleep apnea, and premature death in the family from coronary heart disease. This figure presents general guidelines; each obese person requires individual evaluation.

percent in 1988–1991. As with hypertension, only Mexican-Americans did not share in this decline (NCHS, 1994).

The question naturally arises as to why the prevalence of obesity has increased substantially over the last several decades. Unfortunately there is no satisfactory answer at the present time since the underlying causes of this imbalance between energy intake and expenditure are still largely unknown. It is undoubtedly true that obesity is a complex, multifactorial disease of appetite regulation and energy metabolism involving the disciplines of genetics, physiology, biochemistry, and neuroscience as well as environmental, psychosocial, and cultural factors.

One explanation often advanced for the increased prevalence of obesity is that obesity is a disease of affluence. Dr. Bernadine Healy, a former director of the National Institutes of Health, made the point as follows: "One might say that overweight has been the deadly undertow of our nation's rising tide of prosperity in the 20th century" (Healy, 1993). The paradox is that it is the poor and disadvantaged in affluent, westernized countries who suffer disproportionately from obesity; the affluent themselves are usually much less affected.

For most people in the United States and in other westernized countries, the food supply is plentiful and savory, many people eat more than they need, and one can generally live well without being physically active. Our diet is relatively high in fat and calories and low in fiber-rich plant products. National surveys show that total energy and fat intakes in this country are increasing (Lenfant and Ernst, 1994) and that no more than one in five adults can be considered to be vigorously physically active (DHHS, 1991). What is also clear, however, is that obesity involves defects in fundamental biological processes that are genetic in nature (Bouchard and Pérusse, 1993b). This is shown by many animal studies, by the well-known observation that obesity runs in families, and from both twin and adoption studies (Meyer and Stunkard, 1993).

It is sometimes suggested that the generally poor results of efforts to prevent obesity may be the result of the powerful influence of genetic factors (Bouchard, 1994). It is true that estimates of genetic influences on human obesity, based on twin studies, yielded very high estimates of heritability (Meyer and Stunkard, 1993). More recent adoption and segregation analyses, however, have agreed on a more modest estimate of heritability, on the order of 33 percent (Vogler et al., in press). Although it is clear that genetics has a modest influence on obesity on a population basis, by far the largest amount of the variance in body weight is due to environmental influences. Fortunately, the environment can be changed, but the results of efforts at preventing obesity to date suggest that we have not been very successful in changing it (see Chapter 9).

Genetic influences largely determine whether a person can become obese, with environmental influences determining whether and to what extent he or she does become obese (Meyer and Stunkard, 1993). While research continues to identify the fundamental biological defects that underlie obesity and how to manage and ultimately repair them, we must at the same time endeavor to improve the success of obesity treatments available now. This report is directed to the latter purpose. It may well turn out, however, that the best way to substantially decrease the prevalence of obesity in affluent countries in the long run will be through a better understanding of biomedicine in the future.

## WEIGHT-LOSS PRACTICES

Many people in the United States desire to lose weight; their reasons include improving their appearance, increasing self-esteem, feeling better, reducing the risks of disease, and reducing the severity of medical problems and diseases that already exist. Of course, depending on the choice of the weight-loss approach and the number of pounds one wants to lose, the effort can be appropriate or inappropriate and improve health or make it worse. The National Health Interview Survey conducted by NCHS in 1990 concluded that approximately 44 million persons 25 years and older (23.3 percent of men and 40.1 percent of women) were trying to lose weight by eating less, increasing their physical activity, or both (Horm and Anderson, 1993). In fact, the actual figure is higher, since these estimates excluded persons who were told to lose weight by their physicians.

Since 1985, the proportion trying to lose weight by increasing physical activity has increased, while those trying to lose weight by eating less has remained constant (Horm and Anderson, 1993). Commercial weight-loss centers report that, over the course of a year, people are most likely to join their programs in January (just after the festive season) and May (shortly before the summer bathing-suit season) (personal communication with Barbara J. Moore, Ph.D., Special Expert, Division of Nutrition Research Coordination, National Institutes of Health).

In the NCHS survey, approximately 45 percent of the population considered themselves to be overweight; of this group, 58.6 percent were trying to lose weight. However, 4.0 percent of those who considered themselves to be underweight and 11.4 percent of those who thought their weight was about right were also trying to lose weight. Of particular concern, the proportion of those considering themselves to be underweight yet trying to lose weight increased from 0.7 to 4.0 percent between 1985 and 1990 (Horm and Anderson, 1993). There is a segment of normal-weight or slightly overweight women in this country who are obsessed with dieting and weight loss (Horm and Anderson, 1993). Sociocultural factors, which change over time, are driving the current emphasis on thinness in this and many other affluent countries, particularly among females, and affect the weight-related attitudes of all (Rodin, 1993). This is not to say, however, that slightly overweight individuals who wish to reduce to improve their appearance and enhance self-esteem should be dissuaded from doing so. Some of them may be at the first stages of disease, and treatment might prevent further problems. Some may be individuals who were formerly obese and now are only somewhat overweight, struggling to sustain their weight loss. In addition, some of them may in fact be at medical risk for comorbidities, depending, for example, where on the body their excess fat tends to aggregate.

The 1992 Weight Loss Practices Survey sponsored by the U.S. Food and Drug Administration and the National Heart, Lung, and Blood Institute found that 13 percent of adult males and 15 percent of adult females trying to lose weight were using commercial meal replacements (Levy and Heaton, 1993). Of these, 7 and 14 percent, respectively, were using over-the-counter and prescription weight-loss pills, and 5 and 13 percent, respectively, were in organized weight-loss programs. Approximately 40 percent of the sample said they had checked with their doctor before trying to lose weight; the likelihood of checking increased with increasing BMI. Other popular weight-loss approaches include cutting down on high-calorie and high-fat foods, using low-fat and low-calorie foods and drinks, and skipping meals (CCC, 1993).

## BENEFITS OF WEIGHT LOSS

Obese individuals who lose even small amounts of weight are likely to improve their health in the short run by reducing their risk of co-morbidities associated with obesity. The long-term benefits of weight loss are not yet well studied, although important new data are becoming available from randomized, controlled clinical trials.

### Small Weight Losses Linked to Health Benefits

Small weight losses, of as little as 10 to 15 percent of initial body weight, can generally help reduce obesity-related comorbidities (e.g., hypertension, abnormal glucose tolerance, and abnormal lipid concentrations), decrease the risk of depression, and increase self-esteem. In many cases, the obese person finds that weight loss helps to resolve the symptoms of a comorbidity or slow its progression.

#### Diabetes

Non-insulin-dependent diabetes mellitus (NIDDM) affects approximately 10 million people in this country. Approximately 80–90 percent of them are obese (NIH, 1987). The direct costs of NIDDM in 1990 were $15.5 billion, of which $8.8 billion can be attributed to diabetes resulting from obesity (Wolf and Colditz, 1994). Individuals with NIDDM show improvements in their blood glucose levels within days of starting a weight-loss program—be it from conventional diets of 1,200–1,500 kcal/day (Doar et al., 1975; Hadden et al., 1975) or very-low-calorie diets of 300–800 kcal/day (Amatruda et al., 1988; Anderson et al., 1992; Genuth et al., 1974; Henry et al., 1986). The short-term effect of dieting in reducing blood glucose concentrations is probably a direct result of lowered energy intake. However, as weight loss is maintained, insulin sensitivity improves, as shown by lowered blood glucose concentrations and decreased concentrations of glycosylated hemoglobin (Wing et al., 1991a). Fitz et al. (1983) reported that many diabetic patients who lost an average of 9.3 kg were able to discontinue taking insulin or oral antidiabetic agents. Similarly, Kirschner et al. (1988) reported that, after a 23-kg weight loss (22 percent of initial body weight), all patients taking oral glucose-lowering agents and 87 percent of those requiring daily insulin injections were able to discontinue the medication. In addition, a 10-year follow-up of 479 very obese patients who had gastric bypass surgery revealed that, of the 101 patients with NIDDM and 62 who had impaired glucose tolerance prior to surgery, 141 reverted to normal and only 22 continued to have problems in controlling their carbohydrate metabolism (Pories et al., 1992). Preliminary results from the Swedish Obesity Study reveal that among severely obese but healthy patients followed for 2 years, only 0.5 percent of those who underwent gastric surgery for their obesity and lost an average of 30 percent of initial weight developed NIDDM. This was in comparison to 7.8 percent in the control group who developed NIDDM (Sjöström et al., 1994a).

Recent studies in nonhuman primates with a propensity to develop obesity and NIDDM have shown that preventing obesity can delay indefinitely or prevent the development of overt NIDDM. These data are promising for the likely impact of the prevention of obesity on a large portion of NIDDM in humans (Hansen and Bodkin, 1993).

### Hypertension

Hypertension is usually defined as a systolic blood pressure (SBP) ≥140 mm Hg, a diastolic blood pressure (DBP) ≥90 mm Hg, or both. High normal blood pressure is classified as an SBP of 130–139 mm Hg and a DBP of 85–89 mm Hg (JNCDETHBP, 1993). Epidemiological studies validate the association between increased body weight and hypertension (Dustan, 1983), and the experimental evidence is conclusive that hypertension improves in overweight persons who lose weight. Hypertension accounts for more physician office visits in this country than any other disorder, and antihypertensive medications are the most frequently prescribed drugs (Kanders and Blackburn, 1992). In the largest study on hypertension and weight loss, Schotte and Stunkard (1990) found that a weight loss of 10.4 kg among obese hypertensive patients not receiving antihypertensive medication reduced their blood pressure by 15.8 mm Hg systolic and 13.6 mm Hg diastolic. Furthermore, blood pressure rose more slowly than did body weight in those patients who subsequently regained weight. Results from the Framingham study showed a 15 percent decrease in weight to be associated with a 10 percent reduction in systolic blood pressure (Kannel et al., 1967). In the Evans County longitudinal study, obese individuals who lost an average of 8 kg with the help of a weight-loss program had an average decrease of 18 and 13 mm Hg in their systolic and diastolic blood pressures, respectively (Tyroler et al., 1975). Reisin and colleagues (1978) reported that patients who averaged a weight loss of 10.5 kg on a diet of 800–1,200 kcal/day (without salt restriction) showed decreases in both systolic and diastolic blood pressures of approximately 20 mg Hg. Even though these patients did not reach their normal weight, about three-quarters had their blood pressure return to normal. MacMahon and colleagues (1985) reported a 1 mm Hg decrease in both systolic and diastolic blood pressure per kilogram of weight loss in a group of young, obese women. Eliahou et al. (1981) found that two-thirds of obese, hypertensive patients who followed their program became normotensive, even though as a group they only lost about half their excess weight. Foley et al. (1992) studied the impact of gastric restrictive surgery on hypertension and found hypertension resolved in 66 percent of the patients, even though their follow-up weights averaged 133 to 170 percent of their ideal body weights. So clear are the benefits of weight loss to lowering blood pressure that the Fifth Joint National Committee on Detection, Evaluation, and Treatment of High Blood Pressure continues to advise weight reduction as an important goal for obese, hypertensive individuals (NHBPEP, 1993). A companion report also recommends weight reduction for the primary prevention of hypertension (NHBPEPWG, 1993).

## Cardiovascular Disease

Many obese individuals have elevated blood triglycerides, reduced high-density lipoprotein cholesterol (HDL-C), and an elevated ratio of low-density lipoprotein cholesterol (LDL-C) to HDL-C, putting them at increased risk of cardiovascular disease (CVD). The direct costs of obesity-related CVD in 1990 were estimated to be $29.4 billion (Wolf and Colditz, 1994). CVD risk-factor profiles are often improved with weight loss. In particular, small weight losses of 5 to 10 percent of initial weight will increase blood HDL concentrations (Schwartz, 1987; Wood et al., 1988). In a study of cholesterol levels in obese patients, Osterman et al. (1992) found that the percentage decrease in total serum cholesterol positively correlated with the amount of weight loss in those with hypercholesterolemia. Weight loss associated with a lower total fat and calorie intake can favorably affect serum lipoprotein levels (Grundy et al., 1979; Kesaniemi and Grundy, 1983). In a study of 41 people on a 6-week, low-calorie (1,200 kcal for women, 1,500 kcal for men), low-fat diet, Seim and Holtmeier (1992) found that weight loss averaged 4.7 kg (5.8 percent of their average original weight), BMI decreased 6.0 percent for women and 5.3 percent for men, total cholesterol decreased 16 percent, LDL-C decreased 12 percent, and HDL-C decreased 18 percent.

## Sleep Apnea

One of the most serious complications of obesity is sleep apnea, defined as very brief periods of time during sleep when breathing ceases, occurring as often as 100 or more times a night. Not only does sleep apnea contribute to somnolence and impaired alertness during the day, it is also a risk factor for premature death (Young et al., 1993). Obesity is the single most important cause of sleep apnea, and weight reduction is remarkably effective in its control (Young et al., 1993). Unfortunately, a major problem with sleep apnea is that it is often not recognized by those suffering from it. Such recognition entails first becoming aware of the possibility of its occurrence and then enlisting the help of someone who sleeps with the individual. Alerted to the phenomenon, helpers have little difficulty in making a provisional diagnosis that can be readily confirmed by study in a sleep laboratory. The possibility of using obesity treatment programs as a means of identifying cases of sleep apnea has great potential as a public health measure. We recommend that these programs conduct such a brief (and effective) case-finding measure.

### Osteoarthritis

Joint symptoms, in particular osteoarthritis of the knee, hip, and back, are strongly associated with obesity (Anderson and Felson, 1988; de Gennes, 1993). Weight loss significantly reduced the risk of developing symptomatic knee osteoarthritis among women participating in the Framingham Knee Osteoarthritis Study (Felson et al., 1992). Weight loss decreases the symptoms and improves the management of osteoarthritis in other weight-bearing joints.

## Long-Term Benefits of Weight Loss Are Uncertain

While excess weight has been shown to be related to adverse health outcomes, the literature on the long-term health effects of weight loss is less consistent (Andres et al., 1993; Pamuk et al., 1992, 1993; Williamson et al., 1993). Most of the current information is derived from observational cohort studies that use mortality as an endpoint, although some data exist on other health outcomes.

Many of the epidemiologic studies of mortality suggest that weight loss is associated with increased risk (Andres et al., 1993; Pamuk et al., 1992; Williamson et al., 1993). Data from the NHANES I Epidemiologic Follow-up Study, a longitudinal study of persons examined as part of NHANES I (1971–1975), show that for men and women whose maximum BMI was between 26 and 29, the risk of death as of 1987 increased with increasing weight loss. Those who lost 15 percent or more of their maximum weight had more than twice the mortality risk of those who lost less than 5 percent, after adjustment for age, race, smoking, parity, preexisting illness, and maximum BMI. For those with BMIs of 29 or greater, weight losses of 5 to 14 percent were protective for men but not for women, for whom mortality risk increased with amount of weight lost (Pamuk et al., 1992). A relationship between weight loss and incident disability was also found in this cohort among those 60–74 years of age at baseline. While increasing BMI was associated with increasing incidence of disability, weight loss was associated with a twofold risk of disability among those 60–74 at baseline. Weight change was not associated with incident disability among those 45–59 years of age at baseline (Launer, 1994).

Several methodological problems of observational studies limit their generalizability. It is often difficult to determine the reason for the weight loss in observational studies, and it is possible that weight loss itself is an indicator of subclinical disease. Changes in smoking status could also affect the relationship between weight loss and mortality because those who stop smoking would be less likely to lose weight and would have a survival advantage. Many of the studies showing increased mortality with weight loss have attempted to eliminate these methodological problems by eliminating deaths in the early years of follow-up and controlling for smoking status. These controls generally do not eliminate the risk associated with weight loss (Pamuk et al., 1993). It is also possible that unhealthy dieting practices are putting those losing weight at additional risk, although the data on the effects of weight cycling are inconclusive (see box titled "Weight Cycling").

Preliminary results of a clinical study just being reported provide possible evidence of the long-term health benefits of weight loss. The ongoing two-part Swedish Obesity Study (SOS) consists of a registry study to examine the health of 10,000 severely obese subjects and an intervention study examining the long-term effects on morbidity and mortality of weight loss by surgical means (e.g., gastric banding, vertical-banded gastroplasty, and gastric bypass) among 2,000 subjects compared to weight loss by conventional means (n = 2,000) (Nabro et al., 1994). Between 1987 and 1992, a nationwide sample of obese subjects (n = 3,700) from 37 to 59 years of age was recruited, from which 856 candidates for surgical weight reduction and 856 matched controls were selected (Lissner et al., 1994). Initial BMI among these candidates and controls averaged 37.5 in men and 40.6 in women. Among 442 surgical cases followed for 2 years, body weight decreased from 121 ± 16 to 93 ± 17 kg compared to only a 0.6 ± 8.9 kg decrease among controls (Sjöström et al., 1994b). Although the SOS is not yet complete, preliminary results in initially healthy obese subjects showed that the highest BMI was associated with the highest relative risk of all-cause mortality (Lissner et al., 1994). Fat distribution, fasting blood insulin concentrations, and smoking were

## WEIGHT CYCLING

Some concerns have been raised that the repeated loss and regain of weight, a process known as weight cycling, may pose additional risks to health or have detrimental effects on body composition and energy metabolism. (Weight cycling is popularly called "yo-yo dieting" when the cause is due to repeated failed attempts at long-term weight loss.) Several prospective epidemiological studies show increased risk for all-cause and cardiovascular-disease mortality in individuals with large variations in body weight when compared to those whose weights are stable (Blair et al., 1993; Hamm et al., 1989; Lee and Paffenbarger, 1992; Lissner et al., 1991). These results are paradoxical given the established direct association between body composition and clinical status (e.g., blood pressure, lipid profile, and glucose tolerance) and risk of chronic diseases such as NIDDM, hypertension, and coronary heart disease. At least two other studies show no association between weight cycling and mortality (Lissner et al., 1990; Stevens and Lissner, 1990). Therefore, the application of the weight-variation and weight-loss study findings is unclear with respect to implications for clinical practice or public health policy.

Although the weight-variation and weight-loss study results are intriguing, the evidence is not sufficient to warrant ignoring overweight as a health risk or to recommend against appropriate weight-loss efforts in overweight persons. Furthermore, in studies with experimental animals, food restriction in both genetically lean and obese animals is associated with decreased mortality and increased median life span (Lane and Dickie, 1958; Masoro et al., 1982). In ongoing studies with nonhuman primates, food restriction is associated with decreased morbidity, specifically NIDDM (Hansen and Bodkin, 1993). Further study of these provocative issues is needed, with particular emphasis on elucidating possible biological mechanisms and with improved designs and methods in epidemiological studies of humans. Three recent reviews of the subject are NTF, 1994b; Reed and Hill, 1993 (which focuses on weight cycling in animals); and Wing, 1992 (weight cycling in humans).

also independent predictors of mortality. Obesity-related risk factors improved only in the surgical group. Marked improvements in current health, mood patterns, and obesity-specific problems were also found in 346 of the surgical cases compared to 346 controls (Sullivan et al., 1994). These results suggest that in a severely obese population, significant weight reduction decreases morbidity and ultimately should decrease mortality. They are consistent with the results of studies in experimental animals where restricting the food intake of genetically obese mice results in decreased mortality compared to obese controls fed ad libitum (Lane and Dickie, 1958). Further research is needed to confirm that sustained weight loss in the obese reduces the overall risks of morbidity and premature death over time.

Despite the fact that additional research on the relationship between weight loss and mortality is needed, we believe that it is prudent for obese individuals to lose weight to improve their health and to maintain the weight loss over time, particularly if they have one or more comorbidities associated with their obesity. Although supporting data are unavailable, it seems reasonable that weight loss is most likely to be safe and successful if done by following reputable programs and approaches and with the help of, or at least under the supervision of, a health-care provider with training in weight management. Even without weight loss, obese individuals are likely to derive health benefits from improving their health-care practices and dietary patterns and incorporating more physical activity into their lives.

## THE COSTS OF OBESITY

The high prevalence of obesity in this country together with its link to numerous chronic diseases leads to the conclusion that this disease is responsible for a substantial proportion of total health-care costs. Herman et al. (1987), for example, estimated that half of all NIDDM could be prevented by controlling obesity. Colditz (1992) calculated the economic costs of obesity in relation to NIDDM, cardiovascular disease, gall bladder disease, hypertension, and breast and colon cancer. Costs were measured as both direct costs (resources that could be allocated to other uses in the absence of disease, such as professional services and hospital care) and indirect ones (the value of lost output because of cessation or limitation of productivity, such as wages lost or the present value of future earnings lost by people who die prematurely). Colditz estimated conservatively that obesity was responsible for $39.3 billion, or 5.5 percent, of the costs of illness in 1986. If musculoskeletal disorders such as osteoarthritis were included, the economic costs of obesity increased to 7.8 percent of the costs of illness in 1986.

Further work by Colditz and a colleague led them to an estimate of $68.8 billion as the economic cost of obesity in 1990 (Wolf and Colditz, 1994). To this figure can be added the more than $33 billion spent yearly on weight-reduction products and services, for an estimated total of more than $100 billion per year as the economic cost of obesity.

This estimate does not include the psychosocial costs of obesity, which can range from lowered self-esteem to the more serious binge-eating disorders and clinical depression. A recent prospective study examined the social and economic consequences of obesity among a national random sample of obese adolescents and young adults (6 to 24 years of age) in 1981 who were reinterviewed in 1988 (Gortmaker et al., 1993). Compared to subjects of normal weight who were healthy and to those who suffered from other chronic health conditions, the obese female subjects over the 7-year period were significantly less likely to be married, had lower household incomes, and had a higher rate of household poverty, independent of their baseline socioeconomic status and aptitude-test scores. The overweight men fared somewhat better since they were only less likely to be married.

People, including physicians, have an unfortunate tendency to ascribe personal failings to the obese on the basis of discredited notions as to how this disorder comes about (Stunkard, 1993). The idea that self-indulgence or hedonism is a cause of obesity assaults obese people every day and, we believe, leads to discrimination. "Fat is the last preserve for unexamined bigotry," notes one obese professional woman (Coleman, 1993). Given the fact that treatment of obesity under the most optimal conditions is often unsuccessful in the long run, health-care providers must be especially sensitive to the weight-related intentions of obese individuals.

At this time, it is too early to know when and what kind of health-care reform bill will be passed by Congress and become law, so one cannot know whether and to what extent obesity treatment provided by or monitored by physicians, dietitians, psychologists, or other allied health professionals will be part of a benefits package. It is notable, however, that many managed-care programs and health insurance plans specifically exclude obesity treatment from their benefits package (personal communication with F. Xavier Pi-Sunyer, M.D., M.P.H., Director of the Obesity Research Center at St. Luke's-Roosevelt Hospital Center in New York City). At least one managed-care program has begun to offer special health-promotion packages that include incentives for weight loss by discounting the costs of a nonclinical weight-loss program and offering reimbursements for the costs of a program for achieving and maintaining weight loss (personal communication with Linda Webb Carilli, M.S., R.D., General Manager, Corporate Affairs, Weight Watchers International, Inc.). Some insurance companies will reimburse for the surgical treatment of morbid obesity, but Oregon's uniform health coverage no longer includes gastric bypass surgery (Chase, 1994). This is in the face of scientific evidence that such surgery can produce significant weight loss that can be maintained by many morbidly obese patients for long periods of time (NIH, 1992). Weight loss in the very obese improves functional status, reduces work absenteeism, decreases the prevalence and severity of sleep apnea, decreases blood pressure, reduces hyperglycemia, and improves social interaction (NIH Technology Assessment Conference Panel, 1993). As this country debates how to reform its health-care system, it is important that obese individuals not be discriminated against in receiving appropriate treatment and care for their disease that is covered by insurance.

The intractability of obesity has spawned an antidieting movement that advocates greater acceptance of individuals regardless of their weight and defends the rights of the obese to be protected from job discrimination and social biases (Brownell and Rodin, 1994). The movement questions whether effective obesity treatments exist and points out the potential negative consequences of dieting on psychological and physical well-being. An International No-Diet Day has been organized each year since 1992 to encourage people to appreciate the varied sizes and shapes of human bodies (Tufts, 1994). We agree, of course, that there should be more appreciation and acceptance of diversity in the physical attributes of people, more discouragement of dieting in vain attempts to attain unrealistic physical ideals, and no obsession with weight loss by individuals who are at or near desirable or healthy weights. However, it is inappropriate to argue that obese individuals should simply accept their body weight and not try to reduce, particularly if the obesity is increasing their risk for developing other medical problems or diseases.

## CONCLUDING REMARKS

This chapter has laid the foundation for what is to come in the remainder of this report. While the bad news is that the prevalence of obesity in this country is increasing, the good news is that obese individuals do not need to return to some ideal, non-obese weight to improve the risk factors, including hypertension and hypercholesterolemia, that predispose them to developing a variety of chronic diseases. Several studies demonstrate that small losses in general (approximately 10 to 15 percent of initial body weight) help reduce obesity-related comorbidities and that improvements in these risk factors persist with maintenance of these modest weight losses. They are an important component of the foundation for a new perspective on obesity-treatment outcomes that we present later in this report. The following chapter provides some additional background on the types of obesity treatment programs currently available and discusses the broad approaches to treatment used by them.

# 3

## Programs for and Approaches to Treating Obesity

The wide variety of weight-loss interventions can be placed along a continuum on the basis of many factors, including intensity of treatment, cost, nature of the intervention(s), and degree of involvement of health-care providers. So numerous are the options from which a person wishing to lose weight can choose that we consider them here only in summary form, illustrating three major categories of programs:

- Do-it-yourself programs
- Nonclinical programs
- Clinical programs

This grouping is not meant to imply that one should progress from one category to the next (i.e., one with a higher level of treatment intensity) if weight loss was not successful or only somewhat so. The next treatment option to try depends on the individual's state of health, the amount of weight to lose, his or her evaluation of the need for outside help, and other considerations.

The first part of this chapter consists of brief descriptions of do-it-yourself, nonclinical, and clinical programs. Following this, we discuss the broad approaches to treating obesity used within each of these categories of programs. These approaches include diet, physical activity, behavior modification, drug therapy, and gastric surgery.

## TYPES OF WEIGHT-LOSS PROGRAMS

### Do-It-Yourself Programs

Do-it-yourself programs are individually formulated and therefore extraordinarily varied. This category includes any effort by an individual to lose weight by himself or herself or with a group of like-minded others, through programs such as Overeaters Anonymous and TOPS (Take Off Pounds Sensibly) or community-based and work-site programs. Individual judgment, books, products, and group therapy may dispense good or bad advice. The common denominator of programs in this category is that outside resources are not used in a personalized or individualized manner. We have identified five general subcategories of self-help programs:

One subcategory includes the individual who is losing weight with a personally formulated low-calorie program with or without exercise, regardless of the safety or other characteristics of this effort. A second subcategory involves those who derive guidance from popular published materials such as books or magazines with diet instructions. A third subcategory includes those who use any of a number of popularly promoted products such as diet aids, low-calorie foods, and meal replacements. A fourth subcategory includes those who participate in a group as a source of counseling, advice, structure, or reinforcement. The fifth subcategory includes those participating in community-based and work-site programs.

### Nonclinical Programs

Nonclinical programs are popular and are often commercially franchised. They typically have a structure created by a parent company and often use instructional and guidance materials that are prepared in consultation with health-care providers. The qualifying characteristic of these programs is that they rely substantially on variably trained counselors (who are not health-care providers by our definition) to provide services to the individual client. However, these programs are often managed or advised by qualified and licensed health-care providers. They may or may not sell prepared food products, meal replacements, or other products to their clients. Many popular weight-loss centers offer advice on nutrition, physical activity, and behavior modification, which is provided at weekly classes or meetings. Specific outcomes of any of these programs are unknown, since little or no published data are available (Stunkard, 1992).

## Clinical Programs

In clinical programs, services are provided by a licensed professional who may or may not have received special training to treat obese patients. The programs may or may not be a part of a commercial franchise system. There are two subgroups within this category. One is the program in which an individual professional provider is working alone. It is assumed that, although the provider has the ability to refer the patient for special consultation, the services are in fact provided by the individual professional (psychologist, dietitian, physician, etc.) who is the focus of the therapeutic effort. The service provider may be providing such services as a very-low-calorie (formula) diet or medications. The other subcategory is a program that includes a multidisciplinary group of professional providers working together and systematically coordinating their efforts, records, and patient base. Their efforts may include such services as nutrition, medical care, behavior therapy, exercise, and psychological counseling, and they may utilize very-low-calorie diets, medications, and surgery. For the most part, specific outcomes of these individual programs are unknown.

We have provided characteristics of specific, well-known weight-loss programs in Table 3-1. We adapted and expanded this table, originally presented in Ward (1994), using materials and comments supplied by most of the programs described. The reader should not misconstrue this information as an endorsement or rejection by us of any of these programs. It was not the intent of this report to evaluate specific programs.

**TABLE 3-1**　A Comparison of Popular Weight-Loss Programs

---

**DO-IT-YOURSELF PROGRAMS**

**Overeaters Anonymous (OA)**

Approach/Method

Nonprofit international organization that provides volunteer support groups worldwide patterned after the 12-step Alcoholics Anonymous program. Addresses physical, emotional, and spiritual recovery aspects of compulsive overeating. Members encouraged to seek professional help for individualized diet/nutrition plan and for any emotional or physical problems.

Clients

Individuals who define themselves as compulsive eaters.

*continued on pp 67–80*

**TABLE 3-1** Continued

Staff

Nonprofessional volunteer group members who meet specific criteria lead meetings, sit on the board, and conduct activities.

Expected Weight Loss/Length of Program

Makes no claims for weight loss. Unlimited length.

Cost

Self-supporting with member contributions and sales of publications (includes workbooks, tapes, newsletters, and sponsor outreach programs. Its international monthly journal, *Lifeline*, costs $12.99/year.

Healthy Lifestyle Components

Recommends emotional, spiritual, and physical recovery changes. Makes no exercise or food recommendations.

Comments

Inexpensive. Provides group support. No need to follow a specific diet plan to participate. Minimal organization at the group level, so groups vary in approach. No health-care providers on staff.

Availability

10,500 groups in 47 countries. Headquarters: Rio Rancho, NM (505) 891-2664.

### TOPS (Take Off Pounds Sensibly)

Approach/Method

Nonprofit support organization of 310,000 members who meet weekly in groups. Does not prescribe or endorse particular eating or exercise regimen. Mandatory weigh-in at weekly meetings. Provides peer support. Uses award programs for healthy lifestyle changes; special recognition given to best weight losers. Members who maintain their goal weight loss for 3 months become members of KOPS (Keep Off Pounds Sensibly).

Clients

Members must submit weight goals and diets obtained from a health professional in writing.

Staff

Each group elects a volunteer (non-health professional) to direct and organize activities

**TABLE 3-1**   Continued

---

for one year. Health professionals, including R.D.s and psychologists, may be invited to speak at weekly meetings. Organization consults with a medical advisor.

### Expected Weight Loss/Length of Program

No claims made for weight loss. Unlimited length.

### Cost

First visit free. $16 annual fee ($20 in Canada) for the first 2 years; $14 annually thereafter ($18 in Canada). Includes 40-page quarterly magazine from company headquarters. Weekly meetings cost 50 cents to $1.

### Healthy Lifestyle Components

No official lifestyle or exercise recommendations, but endorses slow, permanent lifestyle changes. Members encouraged to consult health-care provider for an exercise regimen to meet their needs.

### Comments

Inexpensive form of continuing group support. Used as adjunct to professional care. Nonprofit and noncommercial, so no purchases required. Encourages long-term participation. Lacks professional guidance at chapter level since meetings run by volunteers. Groups vary widely in approach.

### Availability

11,700 chapters in 20 countries, mostly U.S. and Canada. Headquarters: Milwaukee, WI (800) 932-8677.

### NONCLINICAL PROGRAMS

### Diet Center

### Approach/Method

Focuses on achieving healthy body composition through diet and personalized exercise recommendations under the name *Exclusively You Weight Management Program*. Diet based on regular supermarket food; Diet Center prepackaged cuisine is optional. Body-fat analysis via electrical impedance taken at start of program and every 4 to 6 weeks thereafter. Clients encouraged to visit center daily for weigh-in. Calorie levels individualized to meet client needs and goals. Minimum level: 1,200 kcal/day. Four phases: 2-day conditioning phase prepares dieter for reducing. Reducing phase used until goal achieved. Stabilization, the third phase, has clients adjusting calories and physical activity to maintain weight. Maintenance, the fourth phase, lasts for 1 year. One-to-one counseling. Some group meetings available.

**TABLE 3-1**   Continued

### Clients

Not allowed to join: pregnant, lactating, anorectic, bulimic, and underweight individuals, and those under 18 years of age. Require physician's written approval: those with more than 50 pounds to lose, kidney or heart disease, diabetes, cancer, or emphysema.

### Staff

Clients consult with nonprofessional counselors who typically are program graduates trained by Diet Center. Two staff R.D.s and scientific advisors made up of a variety of health professionals design program at corporate level.

### Expected Weight Loss/Length of Program

Not more than 1.5 to 2 pounds weekly. Length will vary with individualized client goals, but 1-year maintenance program strongly encouraged.

### Cost

Varies. Ranges from about $35 to $50/week. The 1-year maintenance is a one-time flat fee ranging from $50 to $200. Some centers charge additional one-time fee for all body composition analyses and adjustments in diet and exercise goals.

### Healthy Lifestyle Components

*Exclusively Me* behavior management, as an ongoing part of the program, includes an activity book, audio tapes, and counseling. Used in conjunction with regular one-to-one sessions; counselor helps client design personal solutions to weight-control problems.

### Comments

Emphasizes body composition, not pounds, as a measure of health. Does not require the purchase of Diet Center food for participation. Professional guidance lacking at the client level. Little group support available. Vitamin supplement required.

### Availability

700 centers in U.S., Canada, Bermuda, Guam, and South America. Headquarters: Pittsburgh, PA (800) 333-2581.

### Jenny Craig

### Approach/Method

*Personal Weight Management* menu plans based on Jenny Craig's cuisine with additional store-bought foods. Diet ranges from 1,000 to 2,600 kcal, depending on client needs. Mandatory weekly one-to-one counseling; group workshops. After clients lose half their goal, they begin planning their own meals using their own foods.

## TABLE 3-1  Continued

### Clients

Not allowed to join: individuals who are underweight, pregnant, or those below age 13; those with celiac disease, diabetes (who inject more than twice daily or who are under 18 years of age), or allergies to ubiquitous ingredients in company's food products. Require physician's written permission: individuals with 18 additional conditions. Regardless of condition, clients encouraged to communicate with personal physician throughout program.

### Staff

Program developed by corporate R.D.s and psychologists. Company consults with advisory board of M.D.s, R.D.s, and Ph.D.s on program design. Consultants trained by Jenny Craig to implement program and offer support and motivational strategies. Corporate dietitians available for client questions or concerns at no extra charge.

### Expected Weight Loss/Length of Program

Clients encouraged to set reasonable weight goals based on personal history and healthy weight standards. Program designed to produce weight loss of 1 to 2 pounds/week. A separate, 12-month maintenance program is also offered.

### Cost

To join: $99 to $299, depending on option. Prices vary per inclusion of home audio- and videocassettes. Most expensive price includes *Lifestyle Maintenance* program. Jenny Craig cuisine costs average $70 weekly.

### Healthy Lifestyle Components

Clients use program guides to learn cognitive behavioral techniques for relapse prevention and problem management for lifestyle changes. Based on individual priorities, clients address major factors involved with weight management (e.g., exercise, which is addressed through a physical activity module and a walking program). Individual consultations; group workshops provide motivation and peer exchange. The *Lifestyle Maintenance* program addresses issues such as body image and maintaining motivation to exercise.

### Comments

Little food preparation. Vegetarian and kosher meal plans available; also plans for diabetic, hypoglycemic, and breastfeeding clients. Recipes provided. Must rely on Jenny Craig cuisine for participation. Lack of professional guidance at client level.

### Availability

800 centers in five countries; 650 centers in U.S. Headquarters: Del Mar, CA (800) 94-JENNY.

**TABLE 3-1** Continued

### Nutri/System

#### Approach/Method

Menu plans based on Nutri/System's prepared meals with additional grocery foods. Clients receive individual calorie levels ranging from 1,000 to 2,200 kcal/day. Multivitamin-mineral supplement available for clients. Personal counseling and group sessions available.

#### Clients

Not allowed to join: individuals who are pregnant, under 14 years of age, underweight, or anorectic. Require physician's written permission: lactating women and those with a variety of conditions including diabetes (if require insulin shots), heart disease (that limits normal activity), and kidney disease.

#### Staff

Staff dietitians, health educators, and Ph.D.s develop program at corporate level. Scientific Advisory Board consisting of M.D.s and Ph.D.s employed for program design. Counselors with education and experience in psychology, nutrition, counseling, and health-related fields provide weekly guidance to clients. Certified Personal Trainers administer the Personal Trainer Program developed in conjunction with Johnson & Johnson Advanced Behavioral Technologies, Inc. R.D.s available through a toll-free number to address client questions.

#### Expected Weight Loss/Length of Program

Averages 1.5 to 2 pounds/week. Clients select weight goal based on a recommended weight range using standard tables. Program length varies with weight-loss goals.

#### Cost

Varies. Clients can lose all desired weight for $99. Unlimited service program costs $249. Food costs average $49/week. Vitamin-mineral supplements, at-home cholesterol test, motivational audiotapes, and exercise audio/videocassettes available at additional cost.

#### Healthy Lifestyle Components

Wellness and Personal Trainer services developed in conjunction with Johnson & Johnson Health Management have been added to the program.

#### Comments

Few decisions about what to eat; relatively rigid diet with company foods. Portion-controlled Nutri/System foods allow dieters to focus more on making lifestyle changes than on the reducing diet. Program provides both Wellness and Personal Trainer services. Little contact with health professionals.

**TABLE 3-1** Continued

### Availability

650 centers in U.S. and Canada. Headquarters: Horsham, PA (215) 442-5411.

### Weight Watchers

#### Approach/Method

Emphasis on portion control and healthy lifestyle habits. Dieters choose from regular supermarket food, *Weight Watchers Personal Cuisine* (available in select markets to members only), or both. Reducing phase: Women average 1,250 kcal daily; men, 1,600 daily. Levels for weight maintenance determined individually. Weekly group meetings with mandatory weigh-in. Must need to lose at least 5 pounds to join.

#### Clients

Not allowed to join: those not weighing at least 5 pounds above the lowest end of their healthy weight range and those with a medically diagnosed eating disorder. Require physician's written approval: pregnant and lactating women and children under 10 years of age.

#### Staff

Group leaders are non-health professional graduates of program (Lifetime Members) trained by Weight Watchers. Program developed by corporate R.D.s. Company consults with medical advisor and advisory board consisting of M.D.s and Ph.D.s on program design. Health professionals at corporate level, including R.D.s, direct program.

#### Expected Weight Loss/Length of Program

Up to 2 pounds weekly. Unlimited length. Special 2-week *Superstart* program offers more rapid initial weight loss. Maintenance plan is 6 weeks.

#### Cost

$17–$20 to join; $10–$13 weekly. Fee entitles member to unlimited meetings for that week. Monthly meetings are free for Lifetime Members who have completed maintenance plan and maintain their weight goal within 2 pounds. *Personal Cuisine* prices vary, averaging about $70 weekly.

#### Healthy Lifestyle Components

Emphasizes making positive lifestyle changes, including regular exercise. Encourages daily minimum physical activity level.

#### Comments

Flexible program offering group support and well-balanced diet. Vegetarian plan available, plus healthy eating plans for pregnant and breastfeeding women. Encourages

**TABLE 3-1** Continued

long-term participation for members to attain their weight-loss goals. Lacks professional guidance at client level. No personalized counseling except in select markets.

### Availability

29,000 weekly meetings in 24 countries. Headquarters: Jericho, NY (516) 939-0400.

## CLINICAL PROGRAMS

### Health Management Resources (HMR)

#### Approach/Method

Medically supervised very-low-calorie diet (VLCD) of fortified, high-protein liquid meal replacements (520 to 800 kcal daily) or a low-calorie option consisting of liquid supplements and prepackaged HMR entrees (800 to 1,300 kcal daily). Dieters receive HMR Risk Factor Profile that measures and displays an individual's medical and lifestyle health risks. Mandatory weekly 90-minute group meetings. Maintenance meetings are 1 hour per week. One-to-one counseling. Need to have BMI >30 for VLCD.

#### Clients

Contraindications: pregnancy, lactation, and acute substance abuse. Require physician's written approval: some with acute psychiatric disorders, recent heart disease, cancer, renal or liver disease, insulin-dependent diabetes mellitus, and those who test positive for acquired immunodeficiency syndrome (AIDS).

#### Staff

Program developed by M.D.s, R.D.s, R.N.s, and psychologists. Each location has at least one M.D. and health educator on staff. Participants assigned "personal coaches" (R.D.s, exercise physiologists, health educators) who help dieters learn and practice weight-management skills. Dieters on VLCD see M.D. or R.N. weekly.

#### Expected Weight Loss/Length of Program

Averages 2 to 5 pounds weekly. Reducing phase varies according to weight-loss needs, but averages 12 weeks; refeeding phase (after liquids only) lasts about 6 weeks. Maintenance program recommended for up to 18 months.

#### Cost

Varies depending on diet chosen and medical conditions. Ranges from $80 to $130/week including medical visits. Cost may be covered by insurance. Maintenance is $60–$90/month.

#### Healthy Lifestyle Components

Recommends every client burn a minimum of 2,000 kcal in physical activity weekly.

## TABLE 3-1   Continued

Advocates consuming a diet with no more than 30 percent of calories from fat and at least 35 servings of fruits and vegetables per week. Emphasizes lifestyle issues in weekly classes and in personal coaching.

### Comments

Emphasizes exercise as a means for weight loss and control. Few decisions about what to eat. Supervised by a health professional. Requires a strong commitment to physical activity. Side effects of VLCD may include intolerance to cold, constipation, dizziness, dry skin, and headaches. All options include liquid supplement; diet is very high in protein, even at higher calorie levels.

### Availability

180 hospitals and medical settings nationwide. Headquarters: Boston, MA (617) 357-9876.

### Medifast

#### Approach/Method

Medifast is a physician-supervised very-low-calorie diet program of fortified meal replacements containing 450–500 kcal/day. *LifeStyles—The Medifast Program of Patient Support®* prepares patients to maintain their goal weight after completing the VLCD. Medifast also provides a low-calorie diet of approximately 860 kcal/day for those not indicated for the VLCD.

#### Clients

Contraindications: those who are not at least 30 percent above ideal body weight, those who have not reached sexual and physical maturation, pregnant and lactating women, those with a history of cerebrovascular accident, and those with conditions such as anorexia nervosa, bulimia, recent myocardial infarction, unstable angina, insulin-dependent diabetes, thrombophlebitis, active cancer, and uncompensated renal or hepatic disease.

#### Staff

Program supervised by a physician. At the corporate level, a medical advisory board of M.D.s, Ph.D.s, and R.D.s is consulted on program development.

#### Expected Weight Loss/Length of Program

Physician and patient arrive at an individualized goal weight. Metropolitan Life Insurance Company tables, Dietary Guidelines for Americans, and BMI charts used as guides. Weight loss varies with individual; average weight loss is 3–5 pounds/week. Weight Reduction Phase lasts 16 weeks and Realimentation Phase lasts 4–6 weeks. Maintenance strongly encouraged for up to 1 year.

## TABLE 3-1   Continued

### Cost

Cost for office visits, laboratory tests, and Medifast products vary by individual physician. The program ranges from $65 to $85/week. Costs may be covered by insurance.

### Healthy Lifestyle Components

The Medifast program includes a comprehensive education program called LifeStyles that includes behavior modification, recommended physical activity, and nutrition education. Instruction booklets and patient guides provided, including quarterly newsletter to patients.

### Comments

Close contact with one or more health professionals. Low calorie level promotes quick weight loss. Extensive product line. Company products and regular foods incorporated when VLCD not recommended. Must rely on company products during reducing phase. Maintenance program assists with transition to regular foods.

### Availability

15,000 physicians nationwide, primarily in office-based settings, and in six foreign countries. Headquarters: Jason Pharmaceuticals, Inc., Owings Mills, MD (410) 581-8042.

### New Direction

### Approach/Method

The New Direction System includes a medically supervised VLCD program of fortified meal replacements with 600–840 kcal/day. The OUTLook and ShapeWise programs are moderate-calorie programs of 1,000–1,500 kcal/day and include the use of regular food and fortified bars and beverages.

### Clients

Contraindications to VLCD: women with less than 40 pounds to lose and men with less than 50 pounds to lose (except in special cases), those less than 18 years of age, pregnant and lactating women, and those with conditions such as insulin-dependent (type I) diabetes, metastatic cancer, recent myocardial infarction, liver disease requiring protein restriction, and renal insufficiency.

### Staff

Weekly sessions in the New Direction and OUTLook programs are led by health professionals with degrees in dietetics, exercise physiology, behavioral counseling, or related fields. One-on-one counseling in each discipline is part of the program. Each program has a medical director.

**TABLE 3-1**  Continued

#### Expected Weight Loss/Length of Program

In the New Direction program, average weight losses of 3 pounds/week after the first few weeks are common. In the OUTLook and ShapeWise programs, losses greater than 2 pounds/week are grounds for concern (after the first 2 weeks). The Reducing Phase averages 12–16 weeks, the Adapting Phase (with transition to regular food) lasts 5 weeks, and the Sustaining Phase is a minimum of 6 months (12 months preferred). Ongoing continuing care is encouraged.

#### Cost

Varies with the program chosen, amount of weight to lose, and medical conditions. An approximate range is $40/week in the OUTLook and ShapeWise programs; $110–$120/week in the Reducing Phase of the VLCD and $0–$20/week in the later phases. Costs may be covered by insurance.

#### Healthy Lifestyle Components

Weekly classes have a strong behavioral component with an emphasis on problem-solving and lifestyle-skills development in nutrition and exercise.

#### Comments

Individualized care and close contact with health professionals. Must rely on company products during the Reducing Phase of VLCD program. Transition from VLCD to regular food requires supervision. Low calorie level promotes quick weight loss, most beneficial for people with certain health problems. Clients make few decisions about what to eat while on the VCLD. OUTLook and ShapeWise programs include regular food.

#### Availability

Headquarters: Ross Products Division, Abbott Laboratories, Columbus, OH (614) 624-7573.

#### Optifast

#### Approach/Method

Medically supervised program of fortified liquid meal replacements and/or fortified food bars, eventually including more regular foods. Dieters assigned an 800-, 950-, or 1,200-kcal plan. Weekly sessions on how to change eating behavior and one-to-one counseling.

#### Clients

Not allowed to join: individuals less than 30 percent or less than 50 pounds over desirable weight (corresponding to a BMI of approximately 30–32) and those less than 18 years of age. Contraindications for the low-calorie protocol include pregnant and

**TABLE 3-1** Continued

lactating women and individuals with recent acute myocardial infarction or unstable angina, insulin-dependent (type I) diabetes mellitus, and advanced liver or kidney disease.

### Staff

Dieters seen regularly by M.D.s, R.N.s, R.D.s, and psychologists at most locations; exercise physiologist used on consulting basis. Group meeting leaders are psychologists or dietitians. Meetings often include R.D.s. Clients assigned case manager who coordinates care.

### Expected Weight Loss/Length of Program

Program limits weight loss to 2 percent of body weight weekly. *Active Weight Loss Plan* lasts for about 13 weeks. Transition phase lasts for about 6 weeks. Maintenance, which begins at 20th week, is encouraged. No time limit on maintenance.

### Cost

Varies with type of diet and length of program. Costs range from $1,500 to $3,000, depending on health status and the amount of weight to lose. Price may include maintenance at some centers. Insurance may cover a portion of cost.

### Healthy Lifestyle Components

Emphasis on behavior modification and diet planning for "real food" in group and counseling sessions. Exercise physiologist available to help design personal exercise plan.

### Comments

Close contact with health professionals. Controlled calorie level promotes quick weight loss, most beneficial for people with certain health problems. Clients make few decisions about what to eat. Must rely on Optifast products during reducing phase.

### Availability

Numerous hospitals and clinics in U.S. and foreign countries. Headquarters: Sandoz Nutrition, Minneapolis, MN (800) 662-2540.

### Physicians in a Multidisciplinary Program

#### Approach/Method

Multidisciplinary programs may provide a program similar to HMR, New Direction, or Optifast. They may also provide food-based weight-loss programs or modifications of the two approaches. The multidisciplinary aspect implies the coordination of services, the availability of individual and/or group counseling, and comprehensive medical care.

## TABLE 3-1   Continued

### Staff

Typically physicians, dietitians, behavior therapists, exercise physiologists, psychologists, and counselors working individually and in group settings. Service providers should be licensed and regulated and should have their activities scrutinized by peers.

### Expected Weight Loss/Length of Program

Variable and adapted to the needs of patient. There should be a maintenance program with continuing patient access to services for sustaining care and reinforcement. Patient use of medications and consequences of surgery will be monitored.

### Cost

Varies with approach used and duration. Some programs will use a standard professional fee-for-service schedule of charges; others will use a single charge for a comprehensive set of services for a specified period of time. Potential for reimbursement from health-insurance plans. A packaged set of services may be substantially less expensive than the individual services in a fee-for-service arrangement.

### Health Lifestyle Components

Varies. All recognized factors in weight management will be considered.

### Comments

Similar to, but more extensive, services than physicians working alone. Professional staff coordinates all aspects of care and long-term management of obesity. Diverse staff is able to adapt care to the needs of patients, including the management of associated medical problems. These are often university-based programs, which have structured peer-review mechanisms and may conduct research. Costs for professional services tend to be high.

### Availability

Very limited.

## OTHERS

### Registered Dietitians (R.D.s)

### Approach/Method

Highly personalized approach to weight loss and maintenance.

### Clients

Those acceptable and not acceptable will vary with the R.D.

**TABLE 3-1** Continued

Staff

R.D.s have, at a minimum, baccalaureate degrees in nutrition or closely related field and have completed approved or accredited clinical training. Often have advanced degrees. R.D.s must pass a registration examination given by the Commission on Dietetic Registration of the American Dietetic Association and participate in continuing education.

Expected Weight Loss/Length of Program

Varies according to weight goal. Clients rarely encouraged to lose more than 2 pounds weekly.

Cost

Varies across the country, but can range from $35 to $150 per hour. Fees for weight-control groups may be substantially less than for individual counseling.

Healthy Lifestyle Components

Exercise encouraged as part of safe, sensible weight-control program. R.D.s help clients identify barriers to weight loss and maintenance, and provide education about healthy lifestyles.

Comments

Highly adaptable. Personalized approach to clients' health concerns. Trained health professionals who can address medical history and account for it in diet therapy, if necessary. Appropriate for any age group. Can be expensive.

Availability

Located in every state in private practice, outpatient hospital clinics, health maintenance organizations (HMOs), and in practice with M.D.s. For a free referral to a local R.D., call (800) 366-1655.

**Physicians Practicing Alone**

Approach/Method

Individualized approach to weight loss and maintenance. Patients able to coordinate the management of their weight with concurrent management of associated medical problems. Services can be adapted to specific needs. Options include medications and surgery to treat obesity.

**TABLE 3-1**   Continued

### Staff

Individual physicians possibly working with associates (e.g., nurses and physicians' assistants). Provision of services by licensed professional health-care providers.

### Expected Weight Loss/Length of Program

Varies with patient. Program may be of indefinite length and should be coordinated with care of related or unrelated medical issues.

### Cost

Varies. Fees will be comparable to those charged for comparable medical services. Cost may be reduced by reimbursement from health-insurance companies and avoidance of duplication of services in referrals for medical care by nonprofessional programs.

### Healthy Lifestyle Components

Varies with the physician and weight-loss approach. Should include exercise and nutrition counseling.

### Comments

Professional care. Coordination with other medical problems. Appropriate for patients with complex or serious associated medical problems. Long-term attention in the context of other medical care can be provided. The potential for using medications and/or surgery expands the opportunities for patients at varying stages of their disease. Individual physicians have the ability to vary the patient's care and intensity of the effort depending on the patient's life circumstances. Physicians often inadequately trained in nutrition and in low-calorie physiology. Cost for services can be high.

### Availability

Generally available, but many physicians are reluctant to treat obesity because of their lack of interest or training, recognition that support services that they cannot provide are needed, and concern for the limited usefulness of their intervention.

SOURCE: Ward, 1994. Copyright 1994 by Environmental Nutrition, Inc., 52 Riverside Drive, New York, NY 10024-6599. Adapted and expanded with permission. Descriptions reviewed by organizations for accuracy.

## APPROACHES TO TREATMENT

We have identified five broad approaches to treatment used by the do-it-yourself, nonclinical, and clinical programs: diet, physical activity, behavior modification, drug therapy, and gastric surgery. Not all approaches are used by, or available to, each category of programs. However, each program category uses one or more of these approaches.

### Diets

#### Balanced-Deficit Diets

Balanced-deficit diets provide 1,200 or more kcal/day and are usually nutritionally adequate, providing at least the minimum recommended number of servings from all major food groups. Many published diet books outline balanced-deficit diets, although not all are sensible (Dwyer and Lu, 1993). Balanced-deficit diets require little, if any, medical supervision except, for example, under circumstances in which the diet or resulting weight loss might alter a person's underlying medical condition and result in the need for management.

#### Low-Calorie Diets

Low-calorie diets provide approximately 800–1,200 kcal/day. Some of these diets utilize regular foods, while others are designed to use specially formulated or fortified products and prepackaged foods. A typical low-calorie diet is designed to provide no more than 25 percent of calories as fat, but many find it difficult to achieve and maintain such a low-fat intake. A low-calorie diet utilizing only regular foods may require vitamin-mineral supplementation to meet the nutritional needs of the client. Commercial low-calorie diet programs include Weight Watchers, Diet Workshop, Diet Center, Jenny Craig, and Nutri/System, all of which are based on the use of regular foods, prepackaged foods (which may be optional or required), and/or dietary supplements from the company. (These programs may provide balanced-deficit diets as well.) All of these programs use a multidisciplinary approach with combined diet, exercise, and behavior change.

Many low-calorie diets are also self-administered. Some over-the-counter diet products include Sweet Success (Nestlé) and Slim Fast. These diet products are specially formulated powders or foods designed as meal replacements. Weight loss with low-calorie diets averages approximately 0.5 to 1.5 kg/week (8.5 kg over 20 weeks) (NTF, 1993). Other low-calorie diets described in books range from low-fat, high-carbohydrate diets to nutritionally unbalanced diets void of any scientific basis (Dwyer and Lu, 1993).

Low-calorie diets are safe for patients who have comorbid conditions such as diabetes, hyperlipidemia, or hypertension. However, they should be followed only with physician approval and supervision by a health-care provider since the patient may become ketotic and dehydrated, especially if the diet is very low in carbohydrate (Dwyer and Lu, 1993). In addition, patients on medication (e.g., oral glucose-lowering agents) may require changes in their medication schedule or amount because of energy restriction and weight loss. The overwhelming majority of participants on low-calorie diets regain their weight lost within 5 years (NIH Technology Assessment Conference Panel, 1993), and the attrition rate in commercial programs is very high (e.g., more than 60 percent over 20 weeks) (Stunkard, 1992).

### Very-Low-Calorie Diets

Very-low-calorie diets (VLCDs) are modified fasts providing less than 800 kcal/day, and they replace usual food. Most VLCD programs are based in hospitals or clinics and include the commercial programs Optifast, Medifast, New Direction, and Health Management Resources (HMR) (Dwyer and Lu, 1993). They are medically supervised and administered by a multidisciplinary team including physicians, behavioral therapists, dietitians, exercise physiologists, and nurses. The most common VLCDs are formulations designed to supply 45–100 grams (0.8–1.5 g/kg of ideal body weight) per day of protein of high biological value (coming primarily from dairy sources, soy, or albumin); up to 100 grams of carbohydrate; a minimum of fat as essential fatty acids; and recommended allowances of vitamins, minerals, and electrolytes (NTF, 1993).

VLCDs are generally limited to moderately and severely obese individuals with a body mass index (BMI) of greater than 30 who have failed to lose weight by more conventional methods, but they may be appropriate for patients with a BMI of 27 to 30 who have a comorbid condition. Designed to generate a larger and more rapid weight loss than low-calorie diets, they are usually prescribed for 12 to 16 weeks (NTF, 1993). VLCDs have rapid, positive effects on the health of obese patients with comorbid conditions (Kanders and Blackburn, 1993). Improvements in glycemic control, decreases in systolic and diastolic blood pressure, and decreases in serum concentrations of total cholesterol, low-density-lipoprotein cholesterol, and triglycerides occur within 3 weeks.

In controlled clinical trials, VLCDs resulted in an average total loss of 20 kg over 12 weeks. In contrast, low-calorie diets combined with behavioral treatment produced an average loss of 8.5 kg over 20 to 24 weeks.

However, the vast majority of patients on VLCDs regain the weight within 5 years (Miura et al., 1989; Sikand et al., 1988; Wadden et al., 1989; Wing et al., 1991a). VLCDs are quite expensive compared to low-calorie diets; out-of-pocket expenses can exceed $3,500 for the diet itself, medical evaluation and monitoring, individual counseling, and group classes.

## Physical Activity

Although most of the do-it-yourself, nonclinical, and clinical programs mention physical activity, it frequently appears to be an afterthought, rather than an integral part of the intervention. Physical activity ranges in intensity from walking to vigorous activities, such as jogging and bicycling. The more vigorous the activity, the more the body's energy stores are utilized. Each individual should develop a realistic goal for increasing activity, starting with a low level that feels comfortable and progressing slowly to higher levels. One key to maintaining an increased level of physical activity is finding the kinds of activities that engage one's interests and can be fit into one's lifestyle and constraints on time. There are few studies of recidivism associated with exercise, though recidivism appears to be high (Dishman, 1988, 1991; Foreyt and Goodrick, 1994). Obesity treatment programs should include a systematically planned and integrated physical activity intervention in order to develop a lifestyle change associated with increased physical activity and thus energy expenditure.

## Behavior Modification

Behavior modification is a methodology aimed at helping individuals identify the idiosyncratic problems and barriers interfering with their weight loss and management. Specific behavioral principles are used to solve these problems. No obesity-treatment program can afford to ignore this treatment approach. The principles used in behavior modification typically include self-monitoring, stimulus control, contingency management, stress management, cognitive behavioral strategies, and social support.

*Self-monitoring* consists of two steps: self-observation and self-recording of those observations. Food and exercise diaries are used to assess the client's eating habits and activity levels. *Stimulus control* involves identifying the environmental cues associated with unhealthy eating and under-exercising. Modifying the cues often involves strategies such as limiting eating to specific times and places, buying food when not hungry, and laying out exercise clothing to encourage a regular habit of physical activity. *Contingency management* includes the use of rewards for appropriate behavior changes, such as reducing grams of fat in the diet and increasing minutes of daily exercise. *Stress management* involves the use of problem-solving strategies to reduce or cope with stressful events. Meditation, relaxation procedures, and regular exercise are examples of stress-reducing techniques. *Cognitive-behavioral strategies* are used to help change a client's attitudes and beliefs about unrealistic expectations, appropriate goals, and body image. Examples include the use of affirmations (positive self-statements) and visual imagery (seeing oneself eating and exercising appropriately). The principles and techniques are tailored to each person's specific problems. *Social support,* usually from the family or a group, is used to maintain motivation and provide reinforcement for appropriate behavior changes. All behavioral principles are used to help individuals adhere to a healthy diet and exercise program.

### Drug Therapy

There is increased interest in the use of medications to treat obesity, given the recent consensus that obesity is a chronic disease with biological and genetic bases that is affected by an environment promoting physical inactivity and consumption of energy-dense foods (Bouchard et al., 1990; Stunkard, 1990) (see Table 3-2). In reviews of short-term (<6 months), double-blind, placebo-controlled trials with 7,725 subjects, pharmacologic agents resulted in an average weight loss of 0.23 kg/week compared to placebo (Galloway et al., 1984; Goldstein and Potvin, 1994; Scoville, 1973).

In a review of 27 weight-reduction studies reported between 1967 and March 1992, Goldstein and Potvin (1994) examined the effect of drug therapy of at least 6 months' duration on weight loss and maintenance. The studies reviewed used a variety of agents, including dexfenfluramine, fluoxetine, mazindol, phentermine, and varied experimental designs. In those subjects who responded to drug therapy, weight loss leveled off after approximately 6 months. Goldstein and Potvin recommend that future research focus on identifying subgroups of individuals who are responsive and unresponsive to specific drugs.

If one compares obesity to other chronic diseases such as hypertension and non-insulin-dependent diabetes mellitus, obesity treatments should also include the option of using medication for periods longer than 6 months. However, few studies have investigated this option. In three studies, *d*-fenfluramine was studied for 52 weeks (Guy-Grand et al., 1989), fluoxetine for 52 weeks (Darga et al., 1991; Marcus et al., 1990), and the combination of phentermine and *d,l*-fenfluramine for 3.5 years (Weintraub et al., 1992a). In these studies, drugs helped to maintain lower body weight in a significant number of subjects without intolerable ad-

**TABLE 3-2**  Appetite-Suppressing Drugs

| Noradrenergic Agents | DEA[a] Schedule | Trade Name | Half-Life (hours) | Dosage Size (mg) | Daily Dose Range (mg) |
|---|---|---|---|---|---|
| Benzphetamine | III | Didrex | 6-12 | 25; 50 | 25-150 |
| Phendimetrazine | III | Anorex; Obalan; Phendiet; Plegine; Wehless; and others | 5-12 | 35 | 70-210 |
| Diethylpropion | IV | Tenuate; Tepanol | 4-6 | 25; 75 (slow release) | 75 |
| Mazindol | IV | Mazanor; Sanorex | 10 | 1 or 2 | 1-3 |
| Phentermine | IV | Fastin; Ionamin; Phentrol; Adipex-P; and others | 12-24 | 8; 15; 30 | 15-37.5 |
| Phenylpropanolamine | Over the counter | Dexatrim | 7-24 | 25 or 75 | 25-75 |
| Serotonergic agents | | | | | |
| Fenfluramine (d- or d-l) | IV | Pondimin | 11-30 | 20 | 60-120 |
| Fluoxetine | Not scheduled | Prozac; Lovan | 24-72 | 20; 60 | 60 |

[a]DEA = Drug Enforcement Agency. See box titled "Unreasonable Standards for Anti-Obesity Drugs?" for an explanation of the schedule classification.

SOURCE: Reproduced with permission, from G.A. Bray. Use and abuse of appetite-suppressant drugs in the treatment of obesity. Ann. Intern. Med. 1993;119:707–713.

## UNREASONABLE STANDARDS
## FOR ANTI-OBESITY DRUGS?

Do the standards used to evaluate drugs for the treatment of obesity differ from those applied to drugs to treat other chronic diseases? A drug for treating hypertension, for example, is considered efficacious if blood pressure decreases when the drug is taken. The drug is not required to continue to lower blood pressure further as therapy continues, nor is the patient judged to have failed when blood pressure increases after the medication is withdrawn. This is also the case for drugs used to treat diabetes, asthma, and schizophrenia or to lower blood cholesterol concentrations. For any specific drug, however, a patient may or may not respond in the desired manner.

In sharp contrast to antihypertensives and lipid-lowering drugs, anti-obesity drugs are expected to work for most obese patients independent of the etiology of the disease. Furthermore, there is an expectation that drugs will continue to lower body weight until a desirable weight is reached and will maintain the weight loss even after the drug is discontinued (Atkinson and Hubbard, 1994). One example of this expectation is the fact that medical practice review boards and/or state regulations in nearly all states prohibit prescribing anti-obesity drugs for longer than 3 months (personal communication, Richard L. Atkinson, M.D., Professor of Medicine and Nutritional Sciences, University of Wisconsin, Madison). These circumstances suggest that a double standard exists for the use of anti-obesity drugs. We suggest that these drugs be judged effective if they can produce small but medically significant weight losses and be used for maintenance of weight loss.

After evaluating the views of Pi-Sunyer and Campfield (personal communications at committee workshop, December 1993), we believe that anti-obesity drugs should be considered effective when their use in combination with a sound program of diet and exercise results in (1) achievement of weight loss of at least 5 percent of initial body weight and maintenance of that loss; (2) reduced body weight through a reduction of body fat with a sparing of body protein; (3) reduction of comorbidities; and (4) minimum or tolerable side effects and low abuse potential.

It should be noted that patients most appropriate for drug therapy include those with comorbidities (e.g., hypertension, hyperglycemia, dyslipidemias, and sleep apnea) that can be diminished with weight loss and those at high risk for obesity-related comorbidities. We recommend that the U.S. Food and Drug Administration (FDA), which must approve all prescription drugs, focus on the pathogenesis of obesity as a chronic disease and evaluate drugs for its treatment in that light.

Drugs either approved or in development for treating obesity may decrease energy intake (e.g., serotonin uptake inhibitors, peptide-based appetite suppressants), increase energy expenditure or thermogenesis (e.g., beta-adrenergic receptor agonists), stimulate lipolysis (e.g., alpha-adrenergic receptor antagonists), or decrease fat or other macronutrient absorption (e.g., pancreatic lipase inhibitors) (Bray, 1993c; Goldstein and Potvin, 1994).

A question arises as to why this country has lagged so far behind other countries in the approval and use of anti-obesity drugs. In the United States, no new drugs have been approved for the treatment of obesity since 1972 (Atkinson and Hubbard, 1994). For example, _d_-fenfluramine, approved in Europe and much of the rest of the world for some years, is still pending approval in this country. Furthermore, fluoxetine, approved in this country to treat depression and obsessive-compulsive disorder, has been under consideration by FDA for the treatment of obesity for more than 6 years (personal communication, Richard L. Atkinson, M.D.). Some of the barriers include a common view shared by the lay public, health-care providers, and government administrators that obesity is not a disease (Atkinson and Hubbard, 1994). Atkinson and Hubbard (1994) note that "obesity drugs are held to higher standards than drugs used for other diseases. Although it is generally agreed that obesity is a chronic disease, obesity drugs are limited to short-term use, no longer than a few weeks. Physicians who prescribe obesity drugs for longer periods are subject to scrutiny by State Medical Review Boards and may face loss of licensure." In contrast to current medical practice, Stallone and Stunkard (1992) have proposed that appetite-suppressant medication be used on a long-term basis or not at all.

Research on anti-obesity drugs has been hindered by fears of the abuse potential of these medications and previous indiscriminate prescription of these drugs by some physicians (Atkinson and Hubbard, 1994). This is also reflected in the Drug Enforcement Agency's classification of anti-obesity drugs. Schedule II drugs have a high abuse potential, Schedule III some abuse potential, and Schedule IV low abuse potential. The initial appetite-suppressant drugs (amphetamine, methamphetamine, and phenmetrazine), appropriately classified as Schedule II, are no longer in use. Other drugs in use, with little evidence of abuse potential, are still classified so that they are recommended for no more than a few weeks (personal communication, F. Xavier Pi-Sunyer, Chief, Division of Endocrinology, Diabetes, and Nutrition at St. Luke's/Roosevelt Hospital Center, New York City).

In three major studies of longer-term drug therapy (Darga et al., 1991; Marcus et al., 1990; Weintraub et al., 1992a, b), drugs helped some subjects maintain lower weights, and there is some indication the drugs may help change behavior. According to the work of Weintraub et al. (1992a, b), a combination of two types of drugs may be more effective for long-term weight loss and weight maintenance than either used alone. Because of regulation, use of medications is limited to the short term, no longer than a few weeks (Atkinson and Hubbard, 1994). Some physicians, however, may prescribe such drugs "off label," meaning not approved by FDA, for longer periods of time.

verse effects compared to controls. When medication was discontinued, weight was regained, and when medication was reintroduced, there was additional weight loss (Weintraub et al., 1992b). Not all individuals responded to drug treatment. As with other chronic diseases, it is unrealistic to expect that one therapeutic drug would be effective for all individuals.

Weintraub (1994) suggests that the standard crossover design in evaluating the effectiveness of a weight-management drug, in which subjects initially receive the drug and others the placebo and then at some point are switched to the other modality, is not appropriate. Subjects do not return to their baseline state before starting the next treatment. Weintraub believes that some of the variability in response to drug treatment can be reduced by a 3- to 6-week "run-in" period during which subjects are started on ancillary therapy, including calorie restriction, behavior modification, and exercise. One can then assess the degree of commitment of the subjects and their response to the ancillary therapy prior to drug treatment. Drug treatment is then added to the ancillary therapy. Weintraub encourages use of this approach when treating obese patients with drugs for weight management.

A National Institutes of Health workshop on the pharmacological treatment of obesity concluded that "obesity drugs produce short-term weight loss and may remain effective for extended periods of time in some patients" (Atkinson and Hubbard, 1994). Nevertheless, drugs should be used as only one component of a comprehensive weight-reduction program that includes attention to diet, activity, and behavior modification. According to Silverstone (1993), these drugs should be limited to patients who are medically at risk because of their condition, among which he includes those with a BMI of 30 or greater or those with a comorbid condition.

### Gastric Surgery

Because of its unique nature, the special requirements of participating patients, and the characteristics of the services implied in this type of program, the surgical treatment of obesity is a special subcategory of clinical programs. Two proven surgical procedures exist for the treatment of severe and very severe obesity: vertical banded gastroplasty and Roux-en-Y gastric bypass. Vertical banded gastroplasty consists of constructing a small pouch with a restricted outlet along the lesser curvature of the stomach. Roux-en-Y gastric bypass involves constructing a proximal gastric pouch whose outlet is a Y-shaped limb of small bowel of varying lengths (NIH, 1992). Vertical banded gastroplasty is less complex to perform and has fewer perioperative complications than gastric bypass, but produces less long-term weight loss (Sugerman et al., 1989). On the other hand, a higher risk of nutritional deficiencies exists following gastric bypass (NIH, 1992). Intestinal bypass surgery is no longer recommended as a surgical option to treat obesity (NIH, 1992).

The risk-benefit ratio must be evaluated for each patient when deciding if surgery should be utilized. Patients who have failed with nonsurgical measures and who are well informed and motivated may be considered. They must be able to participate in treatment and long-term follow-up. A BMI greater than 40 indicates the patient may be a potential candidate for surgical treatment (NIH, 1992). Patients with a BMI between 35 and 40 may be considered if they have high-risk comorbid conditions such as life-threatening cardiopulmonary problems or severe dia-

betes mellitus (NIH, 1992). Obesity-induced physical problems that interfere with lifestyle, for example, joint disease treatable but for obesity,
may also be an indication for surgery for patients with a BMI between 35
and 40 (NIH, 1992).

Substantial weight loss generally occurs within 12 months of the operation, with some of the weight being regained within 2 to 5 years. With
weight loss comes improvement in the comorbid conditions that often
accompany obesity. The risks associated with the surgical treatment of
obesity include postoperative complications, micronutrient deficiencies,
"dumping syndrome," and late postoperative depression (NIH, 1992).

There is compelling evidence that comorbidities are reduced in severely obese patients who have lost weight as a result of gastric surgery.
Therefore, it is puzzling that this treatment is not more widely used for
severely obese individuals at very high risk for obesity-related morbidity
and mortality. It is possible that health-care providers and individuals
alike fail to fully understand the severity and costs of obesity in terms of
both increased morbidity and mortality and its impact on the quality of
life. Perhaps there is also an intrinsic fear of the dangers of surgery due in
part to lack of knowledge. In fact, mortality associated with gastric surgery for obesity is less than 1 percent (Kral, 1992). It has been proposed
that most of the complications associated with this type of surgery, un-
like most other surgery, are modifiable by behavior. For example, Kral
(1994) notes that the vomiting seen in approximately 10 percent of patients after surgery is due more to eating behavior than to stenosis or
stricture of the gastroplasty stoma. Another reason for the limited use of
gastric surgery for obesity is that it is not always reimbursable (Chase,
1994). In the Swedish Obesity Study, patients in the surgical intervention
group reported marked improvements in health, mood, and obesity-specific problems compared to controls (Näslund, 1994). This same study
estimated that 7 percent of the costs to the work force of lost productivity
due to sick leave and disability pension are related to obesity. Obesity
surgery would profit from cost-benefit analyses that include the social
and psychological benefits that many experience from the procedure.

Weight-loss surgery clearly involves hospital care. Any surgical program should be supported by appropriate nutritional, medical, and psychological counseling for the long-term management of the patients enrolled, although some programs of this kind in fact have no such support
systems.

## CONCLUDING REMARKS

This chapter has provided an overview of the many weight-loss programs, which are organized for convenience into three major categories,

and the five broad approaches to treatment used by them. In most cases, do-it-yourself, nonclinical, and clinical programs may be appropriate for people at any level of overweight, and some are also applicable for people who are not overweight but who want to obtain information and learn skills to keep from developing a weight problem. Anti-obesity drugs produce short-term weight loss and may remain effective for extended periods, so regulatory policies at the state and federal levels may need to be modified to permit use of these agents by appropriate individuals for longer periods of time than often allowed at present. Surgery is an option only for individuals whose BMI exceeds 40 or for those with a BMI of 35–40 suffering from high-risk comorbid conditions. Recommended programs will almost always include a focus on improving diet, increasing physical activity, and modifying behaviors that lead to weight gain.

In the following section of this report, Chapters 4 through 8, we present a conceptual overview of decisionmaking and use it to develop criteria and a model for evaluating obesity-treatment programs. The *Weighing the Options* model presented in Chapter 8 provides a framework for the conduct of programs that should help consumers choose more wisely from among available programs and be more successful at long-term weight loss.

# 4

## Weighing the Options

Criteria for evaluating weight-management programs should relate to what the programs are attempting to achieve (i.e., their stated aims), what they might be expected to achieve (i.e., the standards to which they should be held), what impact they have on an individual's health and behavior in the short run (i.e., the process and short-term outcomes), and their ultimate long-term outcomes (i.e., their impact on the individual over time). We developed criteria by first studying a simple conceptual overview of decisionmaking and its consequences. In this overview, an individual decides to go with one of a number of options and, as a result, experiences a specific outcome (see Figure 4-1).

This conceptual overview is so basic that it can be applied widely to

**A simple conceptual overview for decisionmaking.**

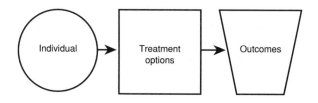

FIGURE 4-1

**TABLE 4-1**   Criteria for Evaluating Weight-Management Programs

---

**Criterion 1: The Match Between Program and Consumer**

| *Program* | *Person* |
|---|---|
| Who is appropriate for this program? | Should I be in this program, given my goals and characteristics? |

**Criterion 2: The Soundness and Safety of the Program**

| *Program* | *Person* |
|---|---|
| Is my program based on sound biological and behavioral principles, and is it safe for its intended participants? | Is the program safe and sound for me? |

**Criterion 3: Outcomes of the Program**

| *Program* | *Person* |
|---|---|
| What is the evidence for success of my program? | Are the benefits I am likely to achieve from the program worth the effort and cost? |

---

almost any situation requiring a decision, such as selecting a book at the library or choosing from among the many weight-loss options. Nevertheless, each of the three components of the overview suggests a criterion specific to evaluating obesity-treatment programs. Our three criteria for evaluating such programs are listed in Table 4-1, and their link with the conceptual overview is presented in Figure 4-2. We have presented each criterion from the point of view of the person (since it is the individual who is at the center of decisionmaking) and of the program (which can use the criteria, for example, to ensure quality control and conduct research on program effectiveness).

The following three chapters detail our three criteria. Chapter 5 focuses on Criterion 1, the match between the program and consumer. We present a number of published methods for matching in the obesity field and identify several factors that influence the decisions made by individuals. In Chapter 6, we focus on Criterion 2, the soundness and safety of the program, describing critical areas that need to be addressed by all obesity-treatment programs. Chapter 7, which addresses Criterion 3, outcomes of the program, provides a literature review on predictors of weight loss and maintenance. It also presents a new concept of weight that refocuses the goal of losing weight from weight loss alone to achieving and maintaining good health through weight management. In Chapter 8, we synthesize the information in this and the next three chapters to provide practical advice for programs and consumers to increase the probability of successful weight-management outcomes.

**Conceptual overview in choosing
and undertaking
an obesity-treatment program.**

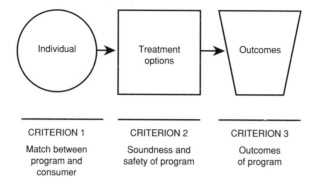

CRITERION 1

Match between
program and
consumer

CRITERION 2

Soundness and
safety of program

CRITERION 3

Outcomes
of program

**FIGURE 4-2**

# 5

## Criterion 1: The Match Between Program and Consumer

**O**ur first criterion for evaluating the outcomes of obesity treatments focuses on the issue of the match between person and treatment. That is, in seeking to establish criteria, we are faced with two questions: (1) How can we predict with any degree of precision which individuals will succeed in a given treatment program? (2) Are some programs suitable only for certain people, where suitability includes both the probability of success and the level of risk associated with undertaking the program? Answering these questions requires examining how individuals and treatments are matched, which is the subject of this chapter. We have deferred the issue of program safety, a critical component of matching, to the following chapter on the soundness and safety of weight-loss programs.

The issue of matching patients to treatment has long been a key aspect of medical treatment. This matching has traditionally been carried out by the practitioner, who follows his or her diagnosis with the treatment that he or she has found to be most specific and efficacious for the disorder under consideration and to have the fewest adverse effects. With the rise of specialization and the increase in available treatment options, the issue of matching has moved from the intuitions of the individual practitioner to systematic efforts at the level of theory and research to match disorders to treatments.

The field of alcoholism provides useful examples of matching patients to treatments (IOM, 1990). Recognizing that one uniform treatment program was unlikely to be appropriate for all patients, Bowman and

94

Jellinek as far back as 1941 advocated the matching of patients and treatment; by 1950, an experiment in matching patients to four treatment programs had been carried out (Wallerstein, 1956). Since then, research in treatment matching in alcoholism has accelerated, and several reports have defined many of the relevant matching variables (IOM, 1990). The field of obesity has lagged behind that of alcoholism in considering the matching of patients to treatments, probably as a reflection of the fact that self-treatment (i.e., voluntary dieting and exercise) is widely practiced and thought to be generally applicable to most obese people.

## SCHEMES FOR MATCHING IN THE OBESITY FIELD

It was not until the early 1980s that the first efforts at matching in obesity were reported. In 1981, Garrow proposed a system of classification of obesity as the necessary precondition for matching, together with treatments appropriate for the different "grades" of obesity. Garrow's classification was based on the body mass index (BMI) and divided obese persons into four groups: (1) Grade III, BMI > 40; (2) Grade II, BMI 30–40; (3) Grade I, BMI 25–29.9; and (4) Grade 0, BMI 20–24.9. Treatments were prescribed according to the grade of obesity, from surgery for Grade III, through dietary measures of greater or lesser stringency and the possible use of medication for intermediate grades, to reassurance about body weight for Grade 0.

Independent of Garrow, Stunkard (1984) proposed a similar matching scheme. His classification also divided obese persons on the basis of their weight, defining mild obesity as a percentage of overweight of less than 40, moderate obesity as 40–99 percent overweight, and severe obesity as 100 percent or more overweight. He matched these levels of obesity with treatment, recommending that severe obesity be treated with surgery, moderate obesity with diet and behavior modification under medical supervision, and mild obesity with behavior modification under lay auspices, as carried out by some commercial organizations.

A third effort at matching in obesity was published by Brownell and Wadden (1991). In this model, the authors divided obesity into four levels, once again assessed only in terms of percentage of overweight. The authors provided a greater number of treatment options, however, divided into five "steps" moving from self-directed diet programs and self-help groups for the thinnest persons (5–20 percent overweight) to, as in the earlier schemes, surgery for the most obese (at least 100 percent overweight). Furthermore, they provided a list of individual factors and program factors to be used in the matching decision. The model is shown in Figure 5-1.

## Three-stage process in selecting a treatment for an individual.

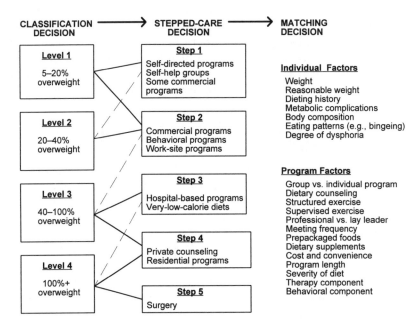

FIGURE 5-1   The classification decision divides individuals into four levels according to percentage of overweight. These levels dictate which of the five steps would be reasonable in the second stage, the stepped-care decision, on the principle that the least intensive, costly, and risky approach will be used from among alternative treatments. The third stage, the matching decision, is used to make the final selection of a program and is based on a combination of client and program variables. The dashed lines between the classification and stepped-care stages show the lowest level of treatment that may be beneficial, although more intensive treatment is usually necessary for people at the specified weight level. SOURCE: Adapted from Brownell and Wadden, 1991. Reprinted with permission of the Association for Advancement of Behavior Therapy.

Another approach to model construction was that of Bray, who added comorbidities to the degree of overweight in assessing the risks of obesity. In this model, an individual is placed in a risk category based on BMI and the presence or absence of "complicating factors," which include obesity-related comorbidities such as hypertension and hyperlipidemia as well as other factors indicating risk, such as a high waist-to-hip ratio and onset of obesity before 40 years of age. For ex-

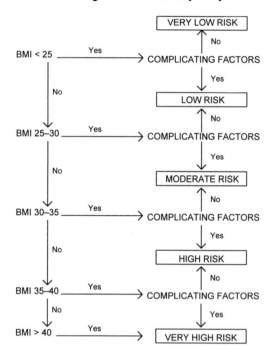

**Risk classification based on body mass index (BMI).**

FIGURE 5-2   The presence or absence of complicating factors determines the degree of health risk. Complicating factors include an elevated waist-hip ratio, non-insulin-dependent diabetes mellitus, hypertension, hyperlipidemia, male sex, and age younger than 40 years. Copyright 1987 by George A. Bray. Used with permission.

ample, an individual with a BMI of 34 is at "moderate risk" from his or her obesity without any complicating factors, and at "high risk" if one or more such factors are present. The Bray model is shown in Figure 5-2.

The evolution of matching schemes in the field of obesity has moved from the so-called static ones of Garrow, Stunkard, Brownell and Wadden, and Bray toward a more dynamic stepped-care model that prescribes the steps to be undertaken in arriving at a treatment decision. Stepped-care models are used in the treatment of hypertension (NHBPEP, 1993) and hypercholesterolemia (NCEP, 1993). They are based on the premise that the least invasive and costly treatments are applied during the earliest manifestations of progressive chronic conditions, especially when these conditions are not yet associated with any medical complications. Stepped care also assumes that treatment is cumulative or incremental—in other words, that nothing is lost by instituting a less aggressive or intensive treatment at an early stage and that, even if not sufficient, this treatment (e.g., diet therapy) can provide a foundation for therapies (e.g., use of drugs) that are added subsequently.

At our request, Dr. George Blackburn prepared a stepped-care model for obesity treatment that we hoped would help us in developing our criteria for the evaluation of weight-management programs. His model, shown in Figure 5-3, is based on one developed in 1978 (NAS, IOM Ad Hoc Advisory Group on Preventive Sciences, 1978) and includes a four-step treatment. In the model, all individuals assessed to be at risk participate in Step One over a 3- to 6-month treatment phase. Risk assessment involves identification of characteristics known to place individuals at increased risk for obesity-related morbidity and mortality. The goals in the Blackburn model include stopping weight gain and/or effecting a weight loss of 2 BMI units (approximately 10 pounds), while at the same time incorporating healthful lifestyle changes and improving the quality of life. This can be done largely through a self-help approach. Provisions are made for adjunctive therapy with "step-down" protocols to comply with a long-term program of nonpharmacologic, lifestyle treatment.

Participation in Step Two requires screening by the patient's primary-care physician. Patients are then referred to certified commercial weight-loss clinics (as defined by the New York City Division of Consumer Affairs in Winner [1991]) or support groups. Again, the goal is to stop weight gain and/or achieve a weight loss of 2 BMI units while incorporating healthy lifestyle changes and improving overall quality of life.

Step Three includes monitoring and supervision if the patient is at high risk for comorbid disease. Intervention is still via self-help, a commercial weight-loss clinic, or a primary-care physician. Additional goals include ameliorating obesity-related disease, achieving a 2–4-BMI-unit weight loss, and continuing weight loss until a healthy body weight is achieved.

Step Four is the most aggressive of the interventions. Intensive therapy can include the use of very-low-calorie diets (VLCDs), medication, surgery, and psychotherapy as necessary and appropriate. In addition to goals for Steps One through Four, an added goal is a 30–50 percent reduction of excess body fat with concomitant achievement of metabolic fitness.

# The Blackburn model.

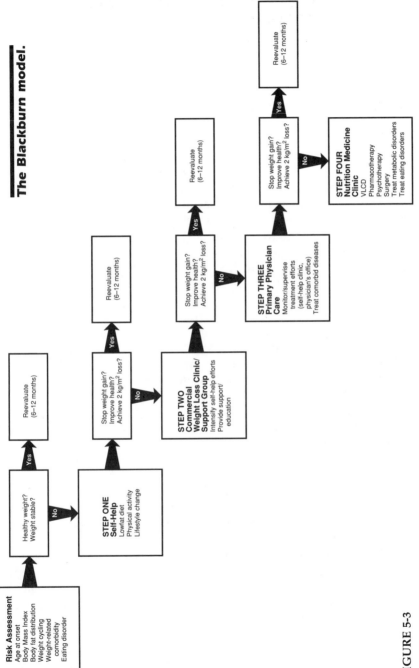

FIGURE 5-3

## THE INDIVIDUAL BASIS FOR MAKING DECISIONS

Another way to approach the matching of individuals with treatments is to identify important factors that may influence decisionmaking. We have identified three sets of such factors: (1) personal, situational, and global factors; (2) health status and weight-related risk factors; and (3) information and guidance.

*Personal factors* include demographic ones, such as age and gender, that cannot be changed, as well as psychosocial ones, such as motivation and readiness to change, that one can alter. *Situational factors* can be changed by the individual's actions; an example is using the stairs whenever appropriate rather than the elevator. Finally, *global factors* are those that influence the environment in which an individual lives, such as culture and views about weight; they typically change slowly over time from the efforts of large numbers of people. The ready availability and cost of a weight-loss program are two global factors that often influence a person's decision about whether or not to undertake a particular weight-loss program.

*Health status and weight-related risk factors* are factors that, as they worsen, may become an individual's primary motivation for losing weight. However, concerns about appearance are usually given by individuals seeking a weight-loss program, and these may conflict with actions taken on the basis of health-related considerations. For example, health considerations generally support small incremental weight losses to a level likely to be maintained over the long term, while appearance considerations predispose many to try repeatedly to achieve large weight losses at a rate requiring an unhealthy and ultimately unsustainable level of caloric restriction. Health considerations will argue against weight loss by those who consider themselves to be overweight but are not so by standards described in Chapter 2. There are strong reasons why health status should take precedence, especially in those at risk for comorbid conditions by family history or prior morbidity or those in whom comorbid conditions (e.g., diabetes, dyslipidemias, hypertension, sleep apnea, and osteoarthritis) are already present (see Chapter 2). Individuals should pay particular attention to their weight if they have a family history of premature comorbidities, increased visceral fat as indicated by waist-to-hip ratios in men of >1.0 and in women of >0.8, or BMIs associated with increased risk (>25 with one or more comorbid conditions and >27 without a comorbid condition).

*Information and guidance* come from a variety of sources, including the media (information and advertising); family, friends, and acquaintances (who relay their opinions and experiences with the various options); and health-care providers. The information and guidance may be sound or unsound, well intentioned or intended to deceive, and empowering or provoking inaction. They may also be incomplete or biased toward a particular program or approach that may not be suitable. Our recommendations for program disclosure presented in Chapter 8 are designed to increase the chances that individuals will receive a balanced and complete picture of the potential benefits and risks of each weight-loss option.

## CONCLUDING REMARKS

In some cases, it is possible to identify mismatches of individuals with weight-loss programs, at least in the sense of excluding people from particular options. For example, a healthy young woman with a BMI of 28 is no candidate for gastric surgery, while a very obese male with a BMI of 40 and hypertension—who has not lost weight despite many attempts—is not likely to be helped by a do-it-yourself diet book or exercise video. However, for most people who wish to lose weight, there is general agreement that it is not yet possible to match people with programs to significantly improve their chances of success. There has yet to be an empirical demonstration of the effectiveness of matching individuals with obesity treatments (Wilson, 1994b).

As the matching approaches described in this chapter indicate, we have some knowledge about components of the match and their association with successful weight management to make prudent recommendations. An individual with weight-related comorbidities, for example, should be encouraged either to choose a program with medical management or to be monitored by a physician throughout the program chosen. (See also Chapter 7 in which predictors for successful weight loss and maintenance are identified.) However, matching people to programs successfully will require a much better understanding of how individuals come to choose from among the options available and the characteristics of programs. This is a very important area for future research.

# 6

## Criterion 2: The Soundness and Safety of the Program

**O**ur second criterion for evaluating the outcomes of obesity treatments addresses the soundness and safety of the program. Insofar as the vast majority of dieters are self-helpers or joiners of weight-loss services, there is an almost total absence of controls for the efficacy and safety of weight-loss methods as actually practiced throughout the population. Because the personal choices that govern weight-loss efforts may be uninformed or misinformed about the health risks that attend obesity and the process of losing weight, we believe that all programs should meet some minimum expectations. Specifically, we recommend that four critical areas be addressed by all weight-loss and weight-management programs:

- assessment of physical health and psychological status of the client (including assessment of client's knowledge and attitudes related to weight and a periodic assessment to determine if the client is still committed to losing weight and learning the facts and skills to succeed);
- attention to diet;
- attention to physical activity; and
- ensuring program safety.

Issues and guidance within each of these four areas are discussed in this chapter.

## ASSESSMENT OF PHYSICAL HEALTH AND PSYCHOLOGICAL STATE

Individuals considering a do-it-yourself or nonclinical program to lose weight should have some basic knowledge about their overall state of health before they begin. This is important not only because we believe that all adults should assume some responsibility for their health care, but because this self-assessment should help them determine which programs might be best for them. Many nonclinical programs screen potential clients by measuring height and weight and asking questions about health status. Ideally, however, obese individuals should have a physician review their health history and provide a physical examination, with particular attention to obesity comorbidities prior to beginning a program. Individuals are almost always assessed by physicians as part of a clinical program. Since weight-management programs provide a service that can potentially improve or worsen the health of their clients, nonclinical or clinical programs that do not provide screenings of some kind should not be considered acceptable.

At a minimum, a person beginning a do-it-yourself program should measure body weight and height to calculate body mass index (BMI) and measure waist and hip circumference to obtain the waist-to-hip ratio. A nonclinical program should take these measurements and provide the client with the results. If a patient is being treated for obesity by a health-care provider, standards of acceptable medical practice should be followed. Weight-reduction efforts should not be made a prerequisite for treating a patient for conditions associated with obesity except for some types of elective surgery where obesity would compromise substantially the chance of success. A physical examination of the obese individual should include the standard components (e.g., measurements of weight and height; assessment of vital signs), as well as measurements of blood pressure and blood glucose and cholesterol concentrations, which indicate the status of comorbid conditions. The health-care provider should also conduct some type of psychological evaluation, perhaps using one or more of the scales, questionnaires, and other assessment instruments described in Appendix A. Screening for bulimia, binge eating, and depression is important because all require special attention if identified.

Certain questions should be posed by or to individuals before they begin any weight-management program. For a person interested in undertaking either a do-it-yourself or a nonclinical program, the answers will help him or her to determine which of the programs in these two categories are most likely to be successful or whether evaluation and advice from a health-care provider is called for first. A health-care provider should ask these questions as part of the patient assessment, and a "counselor" at a nonclinical program is likely to ask the potential client some of these questions as well. The questions include, but are not limited to, the following:

- What is my/your overall state of health?
- Do I/you have any weight-related comorbidities?
- Are there risk factors in my/your family history that would indicate high risk of obesity-associated problems and/or comorbidities in the future?
- Do I/you have any medical problems that should be resolved before attempting weight loss?
- Is it an appropriate time for me/you to lose weight (some contraindications include pregnancy, lactation, recent medical problems or surgery, and other significant issues in life that will interfere with the effort required for weight loss)?
- Do I/you have an eating disorder (e.g., binge eating or bulimia)? Am I/are you able to perform normal activities of daily living, including food selection and preparation and moderate exercise?
- What are my/your capacities and opportunities for restructuring my/your personal environment to succeed at weight loss?
- What are my/your short- and long-term weight-loss goals?
- Am I/are you ready to make a long-term commitment to a new lifestyle of healthful eating and regular physical activity?

Individuals will maximize their chances for success if conditions in their lives are right when they begin their obesity-treatment program. Readiness to change includes motivation, commitment, life circumstances, and other factors suggesting that this is or is not the time to start treatment. One useful instrument that individuals might complete before deciding their course of action is the Dieting Readiness Test (Brownell, 1990). This test can help individuals self-assess six areas associated with long-term success or failure: (1) their goals and attitudes, (2) hunger and eating cues, (3) control over eating, (4) binge eating and purging, (5) emotional eating, and (6) exercise patterns and attitudes. Although the test has not been validated and reliability has not been established, this tool can serve as a first step in assessing readiness to change.

We believe that physicians and other health-care providers should learn more about obesity and its treatment options. Although internists daily see patients whose medical care could be improved with weight reduction, little attention has been given to the education of physicians. One example of this lack of attention is found in the most recent edition of the American College of Physicians' Medical Knowledge Self-Assessment Program (MKSAP IX, 1991), which provides physicians with up to

144 Category 1 continuing medical education credits. MKSAP IX does not have a separate section on obesity. Fortunately, MKSAP X (1994) will contain a small section.

## DIET

How much one eats (and, to some extent, what one eats) is a major determinant of body weight. Therefore, food intake should play a central role in all weight-management efforts. The overall goal in obesity treatment is to obtain a negative energy balance, because this is the only way to lose weight and body fat (see box titled "Energy Balance"). Negative energy balance is established by reducing energy intake (i.e., eating less), increasing energy expenditure (i.e., performing more physical activity), or preferably both. All individuals need to alter their eating and activity patterns to lose weight. Programs that promise results without dieting and physical activity will surely be ineffective over the long term. This section focuses on diet, followed by a section on physical activity.

It is commonly believed that the obese overeat, but studies have not been able to make this connection consistently. Although obese subjects often underreport energy intake and overestimate physical activity (Lichtman et al., 1992), one cannot assume that all individuals with weight problems eat more than those of healthy weights. Energy requirements vary considerably among individuals, based on genetics, physiology, and metabolism, state of health, and, of course, factors such as level of physical activity, age, sex, body weight, and body composition. In experimental animals, genetically obese rodents have increased energy intake and decreased expenditure during development (Johnson et al., 1992). When obese rats (fafa) are pair-fed to their lean controls, weight gain is slower, but obese rats are still fatter than comparably fed lean rats (Cleary et al., 1980). At 6 months of age, obese rats (fafa) and lean rats have comparable energy intakes.

Although it is difficult to determine accurately an individual's food intake (from which the approximate energy and nutrient composition can be calculated), dietary assessment tools are available that can be self-administered or used by providers. These include diet histories, food records for varying lengths of time, repeated 24-hour recalls, food frequency questionnaires, and checklists. Many of these tools have been computerized for easy administration and more rapid interpretation. Appendix A discusses the major dietary assessment instruments used in obesity treatment.

A nutritionally adequate dietary pattern that provides all the essential nutrients and other important food constituents in the proper proportions and amounts is essential to good health. Today's dietary recom-

## ENERGY BALANCE

Energy balance refers to the difference between energy intake and expenditure. Both are usually measured in terms of kilocalories per day. Consistent with the principles of thermodynamics, loss of body-fat stores can be achieved only by establishing a negative energy balance (energy expenditure exceeds energy intake). Conversely, a positive energy balance (energy intake exceeds energy expenditure) will result in storage of energy in the body (accumulation of body fat). Individuals with the metabolic problems of a low rate of fat oxidation (Sheppard et al., 1991; Swinburn and Ravussin, 1993), and hyperinsulinemia (Bray, 1993b) and the metabolic and/or behavioral problems of low energy expenditure (Ravussin and Swinburn, 1992) are at special risk of weight gain and obesity.

Total energy intake is evaluated by adding the calorie content of all the food and drink consumed over the course of a day. Total energy expenditure (TEE) is evaluated by measuring three major components: (1) resting energy expenditure or REE (approximately 60–70 percent of TEE); (2) physical activity (15–20 percent of TEE, for a typical sedentary adult); and (3) the thermic effect of food (10 percent of TEE). REE varies among individuals according to age, sex, weight, genetics, and other factors. Control of REE is not well understood, but it is determined primarily by lean body mass. There seems to be little impact of physical activity or fitness level on REE. Other behaviors such as cigarette smoking may have a small effect on REE. However, small changes in REE, accumulated over time, can amount to a substantial number of calories and lead to alterations in body weight.

Energy expenditure due to voluntary physical activity is the most variable component of TEE. Whereas variations in REE are unlikely to account for more than about 200 kcal/day, energy expenditure from physical activity may range from a few hundred kilocalories per day in sedentary individuals to some 3,000 kcal/day for athletes in training or for workers engaged in heavy manual labor. Energy expenditure associated with voluntary physical activity thus has the potential to have the greatest impact on TEE. Simple questionnaires can be used to obtain a rough assessment of energy expended by being active. In contrast, assessing REE and the thermic effect of food requires relatively sophisticated laboratory measurements and is not feasible in most settings. However, formulas are available to predict REE, and the thermic effect of food can be approximated, as stated earlier, to be 10 percent of caloric intake.

Energy balance, while simple in concept, is a complex phenomenon, so the mathematical approach of estimating energy balance deficits often results in errors. Given that 1 pound of fat is equivalent to approximately 3,500 kcal, one can calculate that a caloric deficit of 500 kcal/day should result in a 1-pound loss of body weight per week. (However, one can lose a pound of water, which is equivalent to 0 kilocalories.) In fact, the predicted weight loss is often an overestimate of actual experience, owing to the influences of such subtle factors as changes in REE, hydration, and other metabolic and hormonal factors that may change with weight loss.

mendations emphasize eating a variety of foods from a relatively low-fat diet, including grain products, vegetables, legumes, fruits, low-fat dairy products, and, if desired, meat, poultry, and fish. The Food Guide Pyramid, the latest dietary guidance plan from the federal government, is considered by many to be one of the most useful educational tools for helping individuals meet dietary recommendations (see Figure 6-1). For each of the five basic food groups, the pyramid provides recommended numbers of servings. Individuals who follow these guidelines are likely to have a dietary pattern that meets or exceeds all nutrient requirements and over the long term reduces their risks of developing chronic degenerative diseases, such as cardiovascular disease and cancer. The Food Guide Pyramid is flexible enough for use by people of varied ethnic groups.

Other dietary guidance tools that complement the pyramid are the Recommended Dietary Allowances (RDAs) (NRC, 1989b) and one or more of several sets of dietary guidelines (e.g., those promulgated by the federal government [USDA/DHHS, 1990], the Institute of Medicine [IOM, 1992], and the National Cholesterol Education Program [NCEP, 1993]). The RDAs provide recommended intakes of vitamins, minerals, energy, and protein for population groups. The various sets of dietary guidelines advise that individual adults and children from age 2 consume a diet supplying no more than 30 percent of calories from fat and less than 10 percent from saturated fat; some (IOM, 1992; NCEP, 1993) also advise limiting cholesterol intake to no more than 300 mg/day.

Obese individuals using the Food Guide Pyramid should eat fewer servings from the food groups to reduce overall food (and therefore energy) intake. Table 6-1 provides recommendations for using the pyramid on a 1,200-kcal/day diet. Calories can be spared by even further limiting consumption of fats, simple sugars, and foods high in these components. Many dieting individuals can develop sound eating patterns with the help of the pyramid. In addition, a precalculated food exchange system developed by the American Diabetes Association and the American Dietetic Association (ADA and ADA, 1989) is a useful and practical tool that can help dieters eat a varied and nutritionally adequate diet while controlling energy intake.

## Effects of Diet Composition and Meal Size and Frequency

There is debate about the role of dietary fat in the development and maintenance of obesity and in weight loss. Some experimental studies, such as those by Miller et al. (1990), show that the obese eat a greater percentage of energy in the form of fat than the nonobese. When fat

**Food Guide Pyramid.**

# A Guide to Daily Food Choices

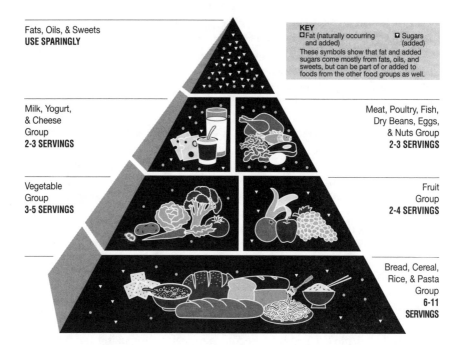

What Is a Serving?

*Bread Group:* 1 slice of bread; 1 ounce of ready-to-eat cereal; and 1/2 cup of cooked cereal, rice, or pasta.

*Vegetable Group:* 1 cup of raw leafy vegetables; 1/2 cup of other vegetables, cooked or chopped raw; and 3/4 cup of vegetable juice.

*Fruit Group:* 1 medium apple, banana, orange, etc.; 1/2 cup of chopped, cooked, or canned fruit; and 3/4 cup of fruit juice.

*Milk Group:* 1 cup of milk or yogurt; 1.5 ounces of natural cheese; and 2 ounces of processed cheese.

*Meat Group:* 2–3 ounces of cooked lean meat, poultry, or fish. Each 1/2 cup of cooked dry beans, 1 egg, or 2 tablespoons of peanut butter counts as 1 ounce of lean meat, poultry, or fish.

**FIGURE 6-1**    SOURCE: USDA, 1992.

**TABLE 6-1**   An Example of Modifying the Food
Guide Pyramid for Purposes of Weight Loss

| Food Group | Number of Servings for a 1,200-kcal Diet[a, b] |
|---|---|
| Bread group | 6[c] |
| Vegetable group | 3 |
| Fruit group | 2 |
| Milk group | 2[d] |
| Meat group (ounces) | 4[e] |

[a]Not recommended for pregnant or lactating women, children (depending on age), or those who have special dietary needs. At or below this low level of kilocalorie intake, it may not be possible to obtain recommended amounts of all nutrients from foods; therefore, it is important to make careful food choices, and the need for dietary supplements should be evaluated.

[b]This plan allows up to 1 teaspoon (4 grams) of added sugar and 5 grams of added fat.

[c]For maximum nutritional value, make whole-grain, high-fiber choices.

[d]Choose skim milk products. The discretionary 5 grams of added fat can be used here to select low- or reduced-fat dairy products.

[e]Select lean meat and use cooking methods that do not require added fat.

SOURCE: Adapted from USDA, 1992.

intake is increased or decreased, there are often comparable changes in body weight. However, not all obese individuals have an elevated fat intake. The evidence linking fat with increased weight gain and obesity is clearest in experimental animals where it is possible to control diet composition and measure food intake precisely. Under these conditions, a very-high-fat diet is associated with increased body fat, fat-cell size, and fat-cell number in normally lean rats (Faust et al., 1978). In one human study, male prisoners who were voluntarily overfed gained weight more readily when overfed a diet high in fat compared to a mixed diet (Danforth, 1985).

Studies on the amount of energy necessary to maintain body weight produce variable results. For example, Prewitt et al. (1991) reported that a lower energy intake was sufficient to maintain body weight over a 20-week period on a diet with 37 percent of energy from fat than with 21 percent of energy from fat. In contrast, Leibel et al. (1992) found no difference in the energy intake required to maintain body weight when fat in the diet was varied from 0 to 70 percent. The different results might be explained by the length of time each study was conducted. Leibel and colleagues studied their subjects for 15 to 56 days in a metabolic ward. Prewitt and colleagues, however, found that it took approximately 17 to 20 weeks for energy intakes to be significantly different in nonobese subjects between diets, whereas it took only 5 to 8 weeks in obese subjects. Studies demonstrating changes in nutrient oxidation rates in response to a high-carbohydrate diet (representing 60 percent of energy) compared to a high-fat diet (60 percent of energy) suggest that over long periods of time, the high-fat diet can be more energy efficient and facilitate increases in body fat. A fat-balance equation (rate of change of fat stores equals the rate of fat intake minus the rate of fat oxidation) has been developed to emphasize the importance that some place on utilizing low-fat diets for weight loss and more physical activity to increase fat oxidation (Swinburn and Ravussin, 1993).

The effect of the size and frequency of meals on adiposity is also important to consider. Isocaloric increases in meal frequency from one to two meals per day to four or more were correlated with lower cholesterol concentrations in a sample of 2,034 white men and women in California, aged 50–89 years (Edelstein et al., 1992). Similarly, increasing the frequency of feeding from three traditional meals to 17 eating occasions with similar macronutrient and energy content was associated with lower blood concentrations of cholesterol, apolipoprotein B, and insulin (Jenkins et al., 1989). These findings suggest that the efficiency of metabolism of food and its components varies on the basis of the amount consumed at one time and the frequency of consumption. These findings are important since they suggest that eating one major meal per day, which supplies the bulk of calories consumed, might increase the difficulties involved in losing weight. However, while it may be advantageous to consume smaller amounts of food more frequently, this approach can cause problems if the choices are not moderate or low in fat and energy content. It seems prudent to recommend that dieters try to consume at least three small meals per day. Breakfast in particular is an important meal for weight loss, as supported by observations showing that dieters who ate breakfast, compared to those who did not, had more healthful dietary patterns overall (Wingard et al., 1982).

### Dietary Recommendations

Dietary recommendations are similar for all healthy people, irrespective of weight. Those wishing to lose weight need to focus on creating an energy deficit by decreasing their total energy intake, utilizing, as much as possible, a variety of foods. Decreasing alcohol intake, foods of minimal nutritional value, and fats and simple sugars is a good strategy for reducing energy intake without eliminating essential nutrients. A weight-reduction diet should contain adequate protein to maintain nitrogen balance and limit the loss of lean body mass. Diets that avoid any major food group or that attribute special weight-loss benefits to a specific food, group of foods, or vitamin or mineral supplement are fundamentally unsound and may have undesirable long-term consequences to health.

Energy intakes of less than 1,200 kcal/day may not meet nutrient requirements, and a dietary supplement may be needed. Individuals consuming such low-calorie diets should seek the advice of a health-care provider (such as a physician or dietitian). A health-care provider knowledgeable about obesity and its treatment and the physiology of weight loss can help an individual develop a nutritionally adequate diet plan tailored to his or her weight-loss goals and appropriate to factors such as gender, age, dietary preferences, and level of physical activity (see box titled "Links Between Diet and Physical Activity").

Regarding dietary interventions, programs should (1) be held accountable for their claims about overall energy intake and predicted weight loss; (2) provide medical monitoring when appropriate (e.g., when using very-low-calorie diets [VLCDs]); (3) provide accurate descriptions of the composition of prescribed diets, with emphasis on their fat and carbohydrate content; (4) give attention to normalizing eating patterns in clients over the long term; and (5) ensure that the meal patterns and eating patterns promoted are sensitive to factors that affect individual success, such as age, gender, body weight, and ethnicity.

## PHYSICAL ACTIVITY

One's body weight is influenced to a substantial degree by the level of physical activity. Therefore, as with diet, activity level should play a central role in all weight-management efforts. As explained earlier, the goal in treating obesity is to obtain a negative energy balance because this is the only way to lose body fat (see box titled "Energy Balance"). Tools for assessing physical activity are described in Appendix A. Several simple questionnaires can provide helpful information on level of physical activity to individuals trying to lose weight.

Physical activity can lead to weight loss, but it is a slow process. One problem is that obese individuals are unable to expend many calories in an exercise session because they are not physically fit enough to sustain activity over several minutes. It may take several weeks or months of exercise training for these individuals to be able to increase their energy expenditure significantly. Nonetheless, controlled randomized clinical trials of the effect of exercise on weight loss show the benefits of increased activity (Wood et al., 1988, 1991).

## PHYSICAL ACTIVITY IN THE UNITED STATES

Approximately 25 percent of men and women in this country are essentially inactive (DHHS, 1991). These individuals have sedentary jobs, do no heavy house or yard work, do not participate in any sports or fitness programs, have no active recreational pursuits, and avoid physical activity during routine daily activities by taking elevators and escalators, driving short distances instead of walking, and searching for the closest parking place to their destination. Less than 20 percent of adults can be considered vigorously physically active (DHHS, 1991).

Data on physical activity habits from repeated surveys on representative samples of U.S. adults are available from the past 30 years. Unfortunately, variations in survey questions and the inherent difficulty of measuring physical activity habits limit conclusions that can be drawn regarding possible changes in physical activity levels over time. The most likely interpretation is that activity levels increased from about the late 1960s to the mid 1980s. There has apparently been little change since then (Stephens, 1987). It seems reasonable to assume that in the early part of the twentieth century, before automobiles came into common use and before the advent of the now ubiquitous labor-saving devices at home and at work, most adults had higher levels of total energy expenditure than they do today. The per-capita disappearance of calories from the food supply is lower today than in 1900, which supports the hypothesis that the population is less active now.

There are variations in activity levels across population subgroups. For example, younger individuals tend to be more active than older ones, men are more active than women, whites are more active than blacks and Hispanics, and those with higher levels of educational attainment are more active than the less well educated (Caspersen and Merritt, 1992; Caspersen et al., 1986, 1987; DiPietro and Caspersen, 1991; Schoenborn, 1986; Stephens et al., 1985). These variations are not large, however, and there is a high prevalence of inactivity in all population subgroups.

Physical activity may also be effective in preventing weight regain after a weight-loss program (Blair, 1993b). However, to provide additional support for this hypothesis, more studies are needed, especially those with randomized prospective designs. Studies suggest that individuals who have lost weight are much less likely to regain it if they are physically active (Kayman et al., 1990; Pavlou et al., 1989). Recommended programs should be safe and should identify the client for whom the program is intended. Restrictions or precautions, if any, and expected benefits in terms of weight loss and fitness should be addressed.

Physical activity has benefits for overweight individuals beyond the specific impact of energy expenditure during the activity. Overweight persons who are regularly physically active have better blood chemistry profiles (Tremblay et al., 1991) and a lower risk of morbidity and mortality (Blair et al., 1989b; Helmrich et al., 1991; Manson et al., 1991; Morris et al., 1990) than their overweight, sedentary peers. Other possible benefits of physical activity in obese individuals include increases in resting metabolic rate, fat oxidation, postexercise oxygen consumption, the thermic effect of food, and feelings of well-being. In addition, physical activity tends to preserve lean body mass during weight loss.

Physical activity is relatively safe for most individuals, and we do not recommend routine screening for most people before they begin a moderate exercise program. However, there is a transient increase in risk of cardiac arrest during the activity session, and this risk is higher for habitually sedentary individuals than for those who are regularly active. The absolute risk of cardiac arrest during exercise is small, and for those who establish a regular activity program, their overall mortality risk is substantially lower than that of sedentary people (Kohl et al., 1992).

There are few data on activity injury rates in the obese, but it seems reasonable to assume that these sedentary persons might be at a higher risk than comparable people of healthy weight. Overall injury rates in active individuals are somewhat higher than rates for those who are sedentary, but the difference is not as great as is commonly assumed. One population-based study reports that injuries severe enough to require a visit to a physician were only about 5 percent higher in active compared with sedentary individuals (Blair et al., 1987). Employees participating in a work-site health-promotion program had net injury rates of approximately 10 to 15 percent per year (Blair et al., 1987). Thus, some injuries can be expected with physical activity interventions, but most are not serious. Risk of orthopedic injury may be higher for obese individuals than for those of desirable weight, but no data are available for direct comparison. One study reports no difference in injury rates by body mass index, although there were few, if any, obese individuals in this population (Macera et al., 1989).

Dislike of vigorous exercise and lack of time are two key barriers to participation in physical activity for many people (see box titled "Physical Activity in the United States"). The traditional exercise prescription emphasizes a single exercise session per day at relatively high intensity. New evidence casts doubt on the validity of these recommendations. Three 10-minute exercise sessions per day appear to produce comparable changes in functional capacity as the same amount of exercise done in one 30-minute bout (Debusk et al., 1990). Recent exercise recommendations by groups such as the American Heart Association, the American College of Sports Medicine, and the Centers for Disease Control and Prevention stress the beneficial health and functional effects of the accumulation of moderate-intensity physical activity (Fletcher et al., 1992). These newer approaches to physical activity intervention may make increasing activity levels less intimidating and more inviting for sedentary persons.

## LINKS BETWEEN DIET AND PHYSICAL ACTIVITY

Recent reviews of studies that included both diet and exercise suggest that the combined interventions produce an approximately 2-kg greater weight loss compared to diet alone (King and Tribble, 1991). For example, Wood and colleagues (1991) studied the effect of a 1-year diet and activity intervention on weight in modestly overweight men and women. The interventions included diet alone and diet plus exercise. The men and women in the latter group sustained greater reductions of body weight, fat weight, and waist-to-hip ratio than those in the diet-only group. Recently, Bouchard et al. (1994) demonstrated in men that exercise is an efficient way to lose weight if subjects do not increase their food intake. The amount of energy necessary to maintain a stable body weight was determined in a group of young men isolated in a forestry camp. When the men consumed this amount of energy each day over 93 days but expended an additional 1,000 kcal/day in physical activity, they lost approximately 75 percent of the amount of weight predicted from the calculated energy deficit.

Unfortunately, energy intake and expenditure are difficult to measure with precision, which complicates assessment of energy balance in free-living individuals (see Appendix A). Consequently, several published studies show no relation of baseline energy intake (as estimated by a dietary assessment) or energy expenditure (as estimated by physical activity questionnaires) to subsequent weight change (Haffner et al., 1991; Klesges et al., 1992; Williamson et al., 1993). Some population-based studies show that increases in physical activity are associated with weight loss and decreases with weight gain (Klesges et al., 1992; Williamson et al., 1993). Interpreting these results is complicated by study designs in which activity and weight were measured at the same time, making it difficult to establish the temporal sequence of the changes. One recent report includes data from 530 women and 3,736 men who received three clinical examinations (Blair, 1993b). The average interval between the first and second examination was approximately 1.5 years, and the average interval between the second and third examination was approximately 4.5 years. Increases in fitness (assessed by a maximal exercise test) during the first interval were associated with decreases in body weight and skinfolds by the time of the third examination. Declines in fitness and reductions in self-reported physical activity from the first to the second examination were associated with weight gain at the third examination. These results held after multivariate adjustment for age and smoking habits.

Body-fat stores accumulate only as a result of a positive energy balance, and obesity usually develops from a small positive energy balance over the long term. Although programs may focus on diet or physical activity alone, emphasis should be placed on both energy expenditure and energy intake.

This may increase the probability that obese men and women can incorporate more activity into their lives, which is crucial for long-term success at weight management. Perhaps another barrier to exercise is the fact that many people believe myths about it, for example, that one needs to exercise hard or that a little bit of food more than makes up for the energy expenditure during exercise.

Because most obese persons are inactive, physical activity interventions in this group should be approached with low starting levels and slow progression to higher levels of activity. The ideal level of physical activity for a person is not known, but as a general rule, some activity is better than none at all and more is better than less. Therefore, we recommend that a gradual reshaping of a participant's physical activity pattern over time be the focus of intervention, rather than providing a strict, regimented, and specific dose of activity in an exercise prescription.

The most feasible mode of activity for most adults is walking. It can be done anywhere and requires no equipment other than a pair of comfortable shoes, and the intensity is not aversive for most obese persons. It is tempting to recommend a specific amount of activity for obese individuals, but we believe that it is better not to give a universal target for all. Each person should develop a realistic goal for increasing activity, perhaps with professional guidance, which can be modified over time as activity levels increase. It is reasonable to suggest a gradual progression up to 1 hour of moderate-intensity activity (such as brisk walking) each day (Bouchard et al., 1993). It is important to stress that this amount of activity does not need to be obtained in a single session, but can be accumulated over the course of a day. Those who cannot achieve this level of physical activity should remember that some activity is better than none at all. As participants become more physically fit, they will be capable of more activity; they may ultimately engage in more vigorous activities such as cycling, jogging, or other vigorous sports or recreational activities and thereby achieve their caloric-expenditure goals in a shorter period of time. Selection of activity goals and the type of activities to be used are highly individualized matters. Persons should be encouraged to find what works for them and should evaluate different approaches until a sustainable activity plan is developed.

## PROGRAM SAFETY

Generally, the more restrictive the diet, the greater are the risks of adverse effects associated with weight loss. Do-it-yourself and nonclinical programs must be safe for their clients. Clinical programs must also be as safe as reasonably possible, given that they are likely to be treating the very obese with comorbidities and health problems. Programs must insist that clients with one or more obesity-related comorbidities be monitored. A client should expect a program to provide detailed information about any potential risks that could occur. Special attention must be paid to the safety of programs for children, pregnant women, and the elderly. In general, no children or adolescents should be placed on a weight-management program without first consulting their pediatrician or family physician about the appropriateness of the program. Children or adolescents participating in a weight-management program should have their growth and development monitored by their physician.

There are a variety of minor and major risks associated with dieting. For example, there is an increase in the risk of gall bladder disease among people who lose weight rapidly. Two safety issues of interest in connection with weight loss—gallstones and psychological distress leading to depression or binge eating—are described below. Risks to health from weight loss vary with the individual and the type of program.

### Gallstones

Obese individuals produce bile with a higher concentration of cholesterol and are therefore at higher risk for gallstone formation. While their risk decreases after they reduce, it is highest during the period of weight loss, when the lithogenicity of their bile is increased further (Bennion and Grundy, 1975, 1978). Three-quarters of severely obese individuals who underwent gastric surgery had gallstones as determined by oral cholecystography an average of 1 year later (Wattchow et al., 1983). Several studies show that about 25 percent of patients on VLCDs have evidence of gallstones (Broomfield et al., 1988; Liddle et al., 1989). However, a study by Nunez and colleagues (1992) reported no increased incidence of gallstone formation among patients receiving a more liberal 1,200-kcal/day, 30 percent fat diet for 16 weeks. The prospective, longitudinal Nurses' Health Study found that the BMI-adjusted relative risk for cholecystectomy or unremoved gallstones was 1.27 to 1.66 among those who lost 4.0 to 9.9 kg in the previous 2 years and 1.57 to 2.4 in those losing 10 kg or more (Stampfer et al., 1992).

### Psychological Distress

Probably the best-studied psychological consequence of dieting is depression. As early as 1957, Stunkard reported on instances of "dieting depression" characterized by weakness, irritability, nervousness, and even psychotic manifestations occurring in obese persons in the course of their efforts at weight reduction (Stunkard, 1957). His review in 1974 summarized additional reports of depression during weight loss that had occurred during the intervening 17 years (Stunkard and Rush, 1974). In 1984, however, Wing and colleagues reported that, on average, obese individuals showed positive changes in mood during weight reduction programs (Wing et al., 1984), a finding confirmed by Wadden and Stunkard (1986) and Wadden et al. (1994).

The discrepancy in psychological state during weight loss depends in large part on the nature of the sample studied and the methods used to assess the psychological effects (Smoller et al., 1987). Early reports were based largely on observations by psychiatrists of obese patients undergoing psychodynamic psychotherapy; this sample of health-care providers was undoubtedly biased toward psychopathology. Furthermore, the psychiatrists' reports were based on observations made over the entire course of treatment. The later reports of positive changes in mood with weight loss were based largely on patients undergoing behavioral weight control. Also, these patients were assessed by paper-and-pencil tests usually administered only before and after treatment, so any shorter-term emotional disturbances would not be measured. Wadden et al. (1986) confirmed the hypothesis that the differences in reports were based on the method of assessment. In their study of 28 women who lost 19.2 kg, a significant decrease in pre- to post-measures of depression coexisted with a significant increase (often to clinically significant levels) in the level of depression during the course of treatment among half of the patients.

Dieting has been linked with the onset of binge eating, and anecdotal reports have linked rigid and restrictive VLCDs to an increased risk for binge eating (Spitzer et al., 1992; Wilson et al., 1993). The problem in validating this proposition is the very high prevalence of dieting, making it difficult to find people who binge who have not already dieted.

## CONCLUDING REMARKS

All weight-loss and weight-management programs should provide (or mandate or encourage) an assessment of the potential client's physical health and psychological status, attend to improvements in diet and increases in physical activity, and ensure that the program is at least reasonably safe. It is reasonable to expect that individuals have some basic knowledge about their overall state of physical health and psychological status that will help them determine if they are ready to try to lose weight and, if so, identify which programs might be best for them. Health-care providers as well should learn more about obesity and the treatment of this disease.

Because improvements in the quality of the diet and especially the amounts of food consumed are important to weight loss, as is modifying one's lifestyle to incorporate reasonable physical activity, any weight-loss program must attend to these two components, providing the participant with necessary information and, ideally, skills. Since dieting is not entirely risk free, programs must also make efforts to ensure that they are as safe as possible; this is of special importance to do-it-yourself and nonclinical programs where some participants may not be receiving any medical care or monitoring throughout the weight-loss attempt.

# 7

## Criterion 3: Outcomes of the Program

**T**his chapter focuses on our third criterion for evaluating the outcomes of obesity treatments: the nature of the outcomes themselves. Obesity treatment typically includes short-term efforts to reduce weight or curb weight gain. But because most people regain lost weight over time, true success must be based on long-term weight loss or weight control (i.e., maintained over 1 or more years). The weight range (expressed in pounds or a percentage of initial weight) considered to represent successful weight loss is variable. Chapter 2 provides several sets of recommendations for desirable weights.

Characterizations of weight-loss outcomes also differ, depending, for example, on the amount of total weight loss relative to initial weight, weight goals, and the time when weight maintenance actually begins (see Figure 7-1). Further, defining what constitutes successful weight loss in particular cases involves specifying time frames, individual characteristics, and any special conditions under which treatment was conducted. Since most individuals in the United States become heavier with age, considerations regarding whether the common tendency to gain weight has been affected should not be overlooked. The question of whether individuals who regain some or all of the weight lost in treatment would be considerably heavier had they not lost weight in the first place is of critical interest. These issues influence the definition of what specifically constitutes successful weight maintenance, and to the extent that they need further study and refinement, our discussion of predictors of successful weight loss and maintenance is limited.

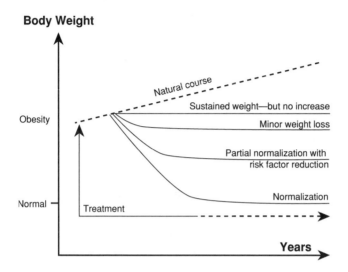

**Possible examples of success in obesity-treatment programs.**

**FIGURE 7-1** Adapted from Rössner, 1992.

This chapter summarizes the factors correlated with obesity-treatment outcomes. We discuss these factors in terms of providing recommendations for both obesity treatment and research, but for the reasons that follow, we have not incorporated them directly into our criteria for evaluating weight-management approaches.

Currently available obesity treatments are not producing the desired long-term outcomes for most dieters, so the predictors of favorable outcomes remain unknown. Most of the relevant information is based on results from clinical or research programs. Therefore, the available information on predictors of weight maintenance is most relevant to individuals who enroll in these programs, continue to attend the programs once enrolled (i.e., do not drop out after a few treatment sessions), and have follow-up assessments of weight change and associated variables. It is important to point out that such individuals probably do not represent those in the general population who are overweight or even those motivated to lose weight (Brownell, 1993), if only because they do not have access to such programs. More saliently, they may include a high proportion of persons who have failed on their own or in commercial programs and who thus may be less predisposed either physiologically or psychologically to achieve long-term weight maintenance (Brownell, 1993).

In addition to the limitation of using a database for a unique and poorly defined subset of the population, our understanding to date of successful weight management is further limited by its being based on studies in which the treatment approaches may have been less than ideal (e.g., separating weight management into discrete phases of weight loss and maintenance) and in which the outcomes used to evaluate success may not have been appropriate (e.g., reaching an ideal weight).

Predictors of successful weight management may differ in future studies that use different weight-management approaches, in particular, the components of the broader definition of success recommended toward the end of this chapter. The following review is limited by the existing literature, which has used the more narrow definition of success at weight management—simple weight loss.

## PREDICTORS OF WEIGHT LOSS

Factors that predict weight loss are shown in Table 7-1; these include personal, process, and treatment factors. Personal and process factors pertain to an individual; treatment factors pertain to a program.

### Personal Factors

Personal factors include initial weight or body mass index (BMI) and resting metabolic rate or resting energy expenditure (REE). The greater the initial BMI, the greater the initial weight loss. Additionally, although REE is most directly related to lean body mass, total weight affects REE as do age, gender, and height. Those with higher REE have higher energy requirements, facilitating more weight loss proportionate to intake. Adipose hypercellularity, usually associated with excessive deposition of fat cells in childhood, has been associated with greater weight loss. However, when the lower limit of adipose cell size is reached, further weight loss is difficult, often leaving the person still obese. Another problem is that the smaller fat cells may produce more lipoprotein lipase, which may stimulate hunger and facilitate increased fat deposition (Kern et al., 1990). Because it is difficult to measure fat cell number, estimates of percentage of total body fat and body-fat distribution are more useful measures for assessing progress (Perri et al., 1992). Although body-fat distribution is not a clear predictor of weight loss, women with upper-body obesity may be more likely to improve their waist-to-hip ratio (WHR) with weight loss, while the WHR for women with lower-body obesity tends to remain constant with weight loss (Wadden et al., 1988).

Self-efficacy is a person's confidence in his or her ability to perform a given task or achieve a certain goal. Higher perceived self-efficacy in

**TABLE 7-1**  Predictors of Weight Loss

POSITIVE PREDICTORS
> *Personal Factors*
> High initial body weight or body mass index
> High resting metabolic rate or resting energy expenditure
> High perceived self-efficacy
>
> *Process Factors*
> Attendance at program
> Experiencing weight loss early in program
>
> *Treatment Factors*
> Increased length of treatment
> Having social support
> Engaging in physical activity
> Incorporation of behavior modification techniques
> > Self-monitoring
> > Goal setting
> > Slowing rate of eating

NEGATIVE PREDICTORS
> Repeated attempts at weight loss
> Experiencing perceived stress
> (Others include the opposites of the positive indicators)

NONPREDICTORS
> Total body fat, fat distribution, and body composition
> Personality/psychopathology test results
> Dietary restraint
> Binge eating

NOTE:  With the exception of resting metabolic rate, the absence of metabolic and physiological factors as predictors of weight loss is not an oversight. The measurement of metabolic factors is beyond the practice of the vast majority of obesity-treatment programs, and it is not surprising that data are not available. It is likely that with additional research, some factors can be identified. For example, although adipose tissue lipoprotein lipase (LPL) activity is increased in obesity, there are no studies identifying LPL activity as a predictor of weight loss. Future studies are needed to identify metabolic and physiologic predictors of weight loss (see Chapter 10).

SOURCES:  Brownell and Wadden, 1992; Foreyt and Goodrick, 1991, 1994; O'Neil and Jarrell, 1992; Perri et al., 1992; and Wadden and Letizia, 1992.

weight management has been found to predict greater weight loss (Oettingen and Wadden, 1991). Assessing self-efficacy before weight-loss treatment begins and applying cognitive-behavioral methods to increase low levels may increase overall response to treatment.

Further research is needed to determine how apparent self-regulatory deficits in eating control and dieting behaviors affect success in weight management (Wilson, 1993). Although dietary restraint and binge eating have been reported as factors that reduce success in weight-loss programs, results are conflicting (Wadden and Letizia, 1992).

### Process Factors

Process factors include attendance and early weight loss. Attending intervention classes has consistently been shown to be related to weight loss. Early weight loss in programs is related to final weight loss as well as to attendance (Wadden and Bell, 1990). However, some speculate that a higher level of early weight loss, especially if the final attained weight is too low, may increase the likelihood of relapse. Alternatively, smaller changes in weight reflecting gradual changes in eating and exercise habits may ensure better maintenance (Goodrick and Foreyt, 1991). Small initial weight losses have been related to early dropout for females in very-low-calorie programs (Wadden et al., 1991). A client may leave a program out of frustration, or leaving may reflect insufficient motivation. Counseling clients to accept a slower rate of weight loss may result in better treatment retention. Some believe that large changes in lifestyle lead to better success at long-term weight management (see, for example, Ornish, 1993), but there are no studies to support this view.

The correlation between attendance and weight loss seems obvious, but both factors may be influenced by a third one, such as increased motivation or fear. Table 7-2 lists those factors that have been reported to be correlated with attendance in weight-management programs. Age, weight, percentage of body fat, mood, and age of onset of obesity have not been linked with attendance. Excessive stress from life difficulties predicts early dropout and weight regain (Wadden and Letizia, 1992).

A feeling of lethargy is associated with obesity (Sims, 1988; Thompson et al., 1982). This lack of energy is expected to be related to poorer attendance at, and adherence to, a weight-loss program, and this has been found in one study (Pekarik et al., 1984). Excessive use of caffeine to feel more energetic while on restrictive diets has been observed. Future research should evaluate the efficacy of monitoring perceived energy level while paying special attention to behaviors that affect energy expenditure (e.g., sleeping patterns, physical activity, and intake of specific foods and beverages). A gradual approach to exercise or increasing physical activity focused on boosting perceived energy could prove to be efficacious.

Most behavioral treatment programs use closed groups (i.e., groups that form at the beginning of a program and stay together throughout treatment without new members joining). Attrition rates in such pro-

**TABLE 7-2** Predictors of Attendance in Weight-Management Programs

POSITIVE PREDICTORS
Closed-group classes
Use of refundable deposits
Perceived health improvement

NEGATIVE PREDICTORS
Stress
Small initial loss
Low perceived energy

NONPREDICTORS
Age
Beginning weight
Percentage of body fat
Mood
Age of onset of obesity
Hunger susceptibility

SOURCES: Foreyt and Goodrick, 1991, 1994; Perri et al., 1992; Rössner, 1992; and Wadden and Letizia, 1992.

grams average about 13 percent, compared to dropout rates of up to 70 percent in some commercial programs using open groups (i.e., groups that allow participants to attend any time during treatment) (Volkmar et al., 1981). Closed groups may help build group cohesiveness and may allow for a scheduled treatment protocol. In addition, open groups tend to be larger than the 8- to 12-member classes in typical behavioral treatments.

Weight loss and attendance can be improved through the use of refundable deposits. Several studies evaluating the effectiveness of programs requiring strong monetary contracts for weight loss or dietary compliance have shown that these procedures enhance weight loss compared to programs that have similar educational content, but in which participants are encouraged to develop contracts on their own (Jeffery et al., 1978, 1983, 1984a). Similarly, attendance and attrition can be improved by having the participants deposit money that is refundable upon completing treatment. Use of such deposits can keep attrition rates below 10 percent (Wilson and Brownell, 1980).

As described in Chapter 2, small weight losses can lead to improvements in health risks. Perceived benefits of this type have been observed to improve the motivation and attendance of those whose rate of weight loss is not as fast as expected (Foreyt, 1987).

## Treatment Factors

The numerous aspects of provider behavior and program content and process that may influence both the enrollment of clients (i.e., which kinds are attracted to the program) and the outcomes of treatment have not been well studied (Blackburn, 1993; Wadden, 1993). However, some program variables are consistently related to outcomes. Length of treatment predicts weight loss. This is shown, for example, in a study where increasing the treatment length from 20 to 40 weeks increased weight loss from 10.5 kg at week 20 to 13.5 kg at week 40 (Perri et al., 1989). Social influences from therapist contact and peer support may be partly responsible for this result, apart from the effect of the client's receiving extended training in behavioral self-management methods. Control over eating and exercise may be improved when individuals rely on peers to get them through situations involving temptations (Goodrick and Foreyt, 1991). Using peer-influence processes such as group problem solving and telephone contacts improves long-term weight management (Perri et al., 1992).

Studies investigating the effect of exercise on weight loss have reported mixed results (Wadden and Letizia, 1992). However, exercise has been shown to be one of the best predictors of maintenance, so it makes sense to emphasize its importance during treatment and follow-up. Exercise may improve body composition and blood lipid profiles (Blair, 1993a; Uchino et al., 1991) as well as reduce stress and improve well-being. These health factors should be further researched and promoted for successful weight management.

Self-monitoring (i.e., the recording of dietary intake and exercise) is the cornerstone of behavioral treatment and has been correlated with success (Perrri et al., 1989). While the information feedback from this process appears to be highly useful in treatment, it is difficult to determine whether self-monitoring is a cause or correlate of good results.

Goal setting in terms of eating, exercise, and weight goals has also been correlated with success at weight loss (Bandura and Simon, 1977; Dubbert and Wilson, 1938). This activity goes together with the concept of making gradual, incremental changes to ensure success. Slowing the rate of eating is also correlated with successful weight management (Speigel et al., 1991).

## PREDICTORS OF WEIGHT-LOSS MAINTENANCE

Maintenance of reduced weight is the most difficult aspect of long-term treatment. Interventions that provide clients with a "maintenance" program produce better maintenance of weight loss than those without a follow-up program (Björvell and Rössner, 1992; Perri et al., 1988). The expectation of the client, and often the claim of weight-loss programs, is that all excess weight will be lost and the new weight maintained. The reality is that most treated individuals gradually return to their original weight following treatment. Keesey (1989) has argued that just as a thermostat maintains room temperature, a person's metabolism maintains body weight at a set level. In this "set-point" theory, obesity is seen as a normal state for some individuals, and lowered weight gradually returns to its natural level through metabolic regulation. For persons with naturally high set-points, successful maintenance probably requires them to commit to a diet that supplies less than needed to satisfy hunger. We believe that goals for weight maintenance should also include delaying weight regain or maintenance of smaller weight losses.

Regain is a complex phenomenon and may be facilitated by biological factors causing a disorder of energy metabolism (Hirsch and Leibel, 1991), by psychological factors such as interpersonal problems leading to uncontrolled eating (Grilo et al., 1989; O'Neil and Jarrell, 1992), by family dysfunction (Fischman-Havstad and Marston, 1984), or by other problems (see Table 7-3). For many people, life in this country is conducive to obesity and to regain after treatment, given the abundance of food, wide availability of high-fat products, and limited opportunities for exercise (Brownell, 1991b; Brownell and Wadden, 1991; Rodin, 1993).

Physical activity is a strong predictor of maintenance of weight loss.

**TABLE 7-3**  Predictors of Maintenance of Weight Loss

POSITIVE PREDICTORS
   Physical activity
   Self-monitoring
   Positive coping style
   Continued contact
   Normalization of eating
   Reduction of comorbidities

NEGATIVE PREDICTORS
   Negative life events
   Family dysfunction

NOTE: As with Table 7-1, there are no physiological and metabolic factors listed as predictors of maintenance of weight loss. There are not sufficient data to include these factors, making this a future research need (see Chapter 10).

SOURCES: Foreyt and Goodrick, 1991, 1994; Perri et al., 1992; and Wadden and Letizia, 1992.

For example, one study of municipal employees in a supervised exercise program consisting of three weekly 90-minute aerobic sessions found that subjects who stopped exercising began to regain lost weight, while other subjects who had not been exercising began to lose weight when they joined the exercise program (Pavlou et al., 1989). Several positive psychological effects of exercise may have implications for long-term adherence and weight maintenance in the obese. Inferences drawn from clinical experience and data from several studies support the conclusion that the psychological effects of exercise may be the important mechanism, although physiological mechanisms linking exercise to weight control are certainly significant (Grilo et al., 1993a). Higher levels of physical fitness predict more positive mental health, with enhanced self-concept and general self-efficacy and reduced anxiety, stress, and depression (Grilo et al., 1993b). If subjects perceive that these benefits are caused by exercise, they may be more likely to continue physical activity and thus have better weight control. Research is needed to discover ways to increase exercise itself and adherence to physical activity in the obese, and to study how exercise and its psychological effects interact to promote a more physically active lifestyle. One promising approach that might appeal to the obese is home-based exercise programs that can generate adherence rates equal to or better than group exercise classes (King et al., 1993).

Individuals who confront life stressors with a positive, problem-solving attitude are more likely to have greater success in any endeavor, including weight management (Kayman et al., 1990). Self-monitoring and continued contact with therapists and peers are also correlated with successful maintenance (Perri, 1992).

## POPULATION CHARACTERISTICS AS
## PREDICTORS OF WEIGHT MANAGEMENT

Many of the predictive factors in Tables 7-1, 7-2, and 7-3 vary by population characteristics. This variability can account for differences in rates of successful weight management across population subgroups. However, as pointed out earlier, data based on clinical or research programs may not describe the situation in the general population, because only a small percentage of the population enrolls in formal programs (Jeffery et al., 1984a; Levy and Heaton, 1993). Weight management in the general population may be better than one would expect on the basis of the obesity-treatment literature. The high and increasing prevalence of obesity, however, argues against the assertion that successful weight management is widespread in this country. In any case, the characteristics of individuals that identify groups having a higher- or lower-than-average tendency to gain weight or a greater difficulty in losing weight may be useful for general guidance in designing programs for various population subgroups. These variables may also provide a basis for identifying the mechanisms that predispose individuals in these groups to a given weight-gain profile.

### Gender

Gender is the population variable most strongly associated with weight maintenance. Women enter adulthood smaller than men but have a greater predisposition to weight gain and more variability in their adult weight status compared to men (Williamson, 1993; Williamson et al., 1993). Female reproductive variables are among the obvious potential candidates for causes of weight gain in young adult women. Menopause does not appear to be associated with weight gain independent of the age differences between pre- and postmenopausal women, although hormone replacement therapy may be linked to greater weight gain (Wing et al., 1991b).

Several lines of evidence indicate that weight-loss motivations for men and women differ in their nature and intensity. Dieting is more prevalent among women than among men, and more women enroll in obesity-treatment programs. Women are more motivated to diet to improve their appearance, while men are motivated more by health and fitness concerns. However, many studies find that success rates in weight-loss programs vary by gender, with women experiencing smaller weight losses than men (Adams et al., 1986; Kramer et al., 1989; Kumanyika et al., 1991; Lavery and Loewy, 1993; O'Neil et al., 1979; Stevens et al., 1993; Wing et al., 1987). National survey data suggest that men and women use different weight-loss strategies when dieting (Levy and Heaton, 1993), and abnormal-eating behaviors, which may be causes or consequences of unsuccessful dieting, are more prevalent in women (Connors and Johnson, 1987; Rand and Kuldau, 1992). Gender differences in exercise patterns may also affect success. Rössner (1992) suggests that the higher lean body mass of men, overall and at any given body weight, could be one factor in men's greater weight loss. The predominance of easier-to-mobilize abdominal, compared to gluteal-femoral, fat could be another factor. Men also have higher energy requirements and could, theoretically, undertake caloric restriction over a wide range of intakes. Overall, whether gender differences in obesity treatment outcomes can be explained by careful adjustment of known determinants of weight loss is unclear. This is an important area for future research.

## Age

Several weight-loss predictors are associated with age or aging. Age, therefore, potentially confounds many associations of other population characteristics with weight-management variables. The average pattern of weight change shifts from a tendency to gain weight in youth and middle age to a net loss of weight after age 50 or 60 (Williamson et al., 1990). However, decreases in lean body mass and metabolic rate that occur with aging in most older adults may decrease their ability to lose weight when they attempt it (Tzankoff and Norris, 1977; Vaughn et al., 1991). The prevalence of dieting decreases as age increases (Piani and Schoenborn, 1993; Schoenborn, 1988), but at least two surveys indicate that the duration of dieting among persons trying to lose weight is longer in older persons (Levy and Heaton, 1993; Williamson et al., 1992). Sedentary behavior, health problems, and functional limitations increase with aging (King et al., 1992). Thus, older persons who enroll in treatment programs may be less likely to adopt or adhere to exercise regimens. Motivations for weight loss at older ages may shift more toward concerns for health instead of appearance (Hayes and Ross, 1987).

### Race, Ethnicity, and Socioeconomic Status

Although obesity among whites varies with demographic categories and may be related to ethnic origins, the high prevalence of obesity in several racial/ethnic minority populations in the United States is striking, especially among women (Kumanyika, 1994). Obesity affects up to 80 percent of adults in some age groups among black, Hispanic, Native American, and Pacific Islander populations. The high prevalence of obesity in these populations, compared to less overweight populations, may reflect greater problems with avoiding weight gain or with losing weight. Associations of race/ethnicity with weight may include the effects of low socioeconomic status (which predisposes females to obesity) (Sobal and Stunkard, 1989), pregnancy-related weight gains (Dawson and Thompson, 1990), dieting motivations and practices, lower levels of leisure-time physical activity (King et al., 1992), and residence in the southern United States (Piani and Schoenborn, 1993; Schoenborn, 1988).

Stress, which was noted earlier in this chapter as a negative predictor of weight loss, may predispose susceptible individuals to abdominal obesity through negative health-related behaviors and neuroendocrine disturbances (Björntorp, 1993). Race, ethnicity, and low socioeconomic status are associated with numerous potential sources of stress (e.g., discrimination, living in substandard housing, and being unable to afford basic necessities). However, whether excess stress is a mediator of these demographic factors on weight management is not known. The subjective elements of perceived stress (i.e., the threshold above which stress is perceived or the importance assigned to a given stress) are influenced by culture (Dohrenwend et al., 1978). This complicates cross-cultural comparisons of the prevalence of stress or of its effects.

Studies that provide a randomized, controlled comparison suggest that black women or black participants in the United States lose less weight than whites under the same conditions of behavioral treatment (Kumanyika et al., 1991; Wylie-Rosett et al., 1993). Observational follow-up data from a national survey also indicate that black women are less likely than white women to lose weight during adulthood (Kahn et al., 1991). Behavioral factors that could predispose black women and men to have a relatively greater difficulty with weight loss are easier to identify than metabolic variables that may be operating, although the latter are not precluded. Attitudes indicating a more multidimensional and less uniformly negative view of obesity among blacks than among whites have been documented as indirect evidence that the motivation for weight reduction is lower in black women (Allan et al., 1993; Kumanyika et al., 1992). Black women responding to a survey were more likely than white women to agree with the statement that there is little people can do to change their body weight (IBNMRR, 1993).

Survey data on self-reported weight-loss practices suggest that differences in weight management between black and white women are influenced primarily by factors relating to differences in the duration of adherence to weight-control regimens rather than to the level of adherence while on the regimen. Williamson et al. (1992) reported that black women were less likely than white women to be involved in long-duration weight-loss attempts ($\geq 1$ year), but that race was not related to the rate of weight loss and to weight losses achieved among the subset of women who remained on diets. A report of a work-site lifestyle change program also provides evidence consistent with this finding (Brill et al., 1991). Blacks were significantly less likely to enroll in the program, and those who enrolled were significantly less likely to remain in the program. However, among those who did not drop out, weight losses among blacks were similar to those of whites.

The national survey data analyzed by Williamson et al. (1992) showed a higher starting weight for the current weight-loss attempts in blacks compared to whites. This may reflect the common finding that, compared to white women, fewer black women who are not overweight are dieting. A survey of weight-control practices of blacks and whites shows differences in dieting strategies, with black dieters reporting more practices defined as questionable (Levy and Heaton, 1993). One study has found that blacks lose less weight than whites from gastric surgery

(Sugerman et al., 1989). Although differences in response to surgery may imply biological differences, behavioral differences influence the ultimate weight loss following obesity surgery and may explain the racial difference (Sugerman et al., 1989).

Most potential associations between race/ethnicity and weight have been clearly documented for black women; relatively fewer data exist for black men or for men or women in other ethnic groups. Data on Hispanic men and women, often not subdivided by specific Hispanic ethnicity, in some cases show patterns that are intermediate between those of blacks and whites and in other cases more similar to those of whites (Brill et al., 1991; Piani and Schoenborn, 1993; Schoenborn, 1988; Serdula et al., 1993; Williamson et al., 1992). One older study indicated a lower level of concern about weight among Mexican-Americans compared to whites from the same region, although this difference was not present in the group with a higher socioeconomic status (Stern et al., 1982).

Education is strongly associated with several weight-management variables. The prevalence of dieting increases with education, even among those who are not overweight (Levy and Heaton, 1993; Piani and Schoenborn, 1993; Schoenborn, 1988). Education is positively related to level of leisure-time physical activity, although negatively associated with occupational activity (King et al., 1992). The work-site study reported by Brill et al. (1991) noted that persons with advanced degrees were more likely to enroll in and less likely to drop out of the program. It has been suggested that one mechanism for a favorable effect of education on weight management may be through increased self-efficacy (Leigh et al., 1992). Dieting prevalence also increases with income (Piani and Schoenborn, 1993; Schoenborn, 1988). Low social class has been associated with poor exercise program adherence in some studies (King et al., 1992).

## A NEW PERSPECTIVE ON WEIGHT-MANAGEMENT OUTCOMES

The signs are clear that a different perspective on obesity-treatment outcomes is needed. The prevalence of obesity in this country is increasing despite the spending of more than $33 billion per year on weight-loss products and services (U.S. Congress, 1990). Although some evidence shows improvements in several risk factors for chronic degenerative diseases related in part to obesity, the economic, medical, and social costs of obesity in this country are still enormous. Many people are obsessed with their weight in a culture that encourages one both subtly and overtly to equate thinness with beauty and obesity with sloth.

We recommend that the definition of success that is applied in evaluating weight-loss programs be broadened and made more realistic based on the research summarized in Chapter 2 documenting that small weight losses can reduce the risks of developing chronic diseases. Specifically, the goal of obesity treatment should be refocused from weight loss alone to *weight management*, achieving the best weight possible in the context of overall health. In contrast to weight loss, the primary purpose of weight management is to achieve and maintain good health. This concept includes weight loss but is not limited to it. We recommend that weight-loss programs be judged more by their effects on the overall health of participants than by their effects on weight alone. The criteria set forth in this report are framed around weight management.

We have identified four components of successful weight management: (1) long-term weight loss, (2) improvement in obesity-related comorbidities, (3) improved health practices, and (4) monitoring of adverse effects that might result from the program. To assess objectively whether successful weight management has been achieved, it is necessary to provide guidance on assessing each component.

### Long-Term Weight Loss

Long-term weight loss is often referred to as maintenance, as in maintenance of lost weight. As described earlier in this chapter, most people in weight-loss programs lose weight but fail to maintain the loss. The amount of weight lost is, of course, easy to measure objectively. However, defining what is meant by long-term weight loss is a subjective matter. For practical purposes, we will define long-term as meaning 1 year or more, and weight loss of any significance as the loss of $\geq 5$ percent of body weight and/or a reduction in BMI by 1 or more units. Successful long-term weight loss by our definition means losing at least 5 percent of body weight (or reducing BMI) by the completion of a weight-loss program or the weight-loss portion of a weight-management program, and keeping it below our definition of significant weight loss for at least 1 year. It can still be achieved even though some weight is regained, as long as the net weight loss stays significant as defined.

### Improvement in Obesity-Related Comorbidities

As described in Chapter 2, comorbidities associated with obesity include high blood pressure (>140/90), elevated lipid concentrations (cholesterol >200 mg/dl or triglycerides >225 mg/dl), and the presence of non-insulin-dependent diabetes mellitus, osteoarthritis of weight-bearing joints, and sleep apnea. Each comorbidity can be objectively determined or evaluated by a health-care provider. Successful weight management should include improvement in one or more of these comorbidities if present to a degree considered clinically significant by a health-care provider.

### Improved Health Practices

Improved health practices include obtaining health-related knowledge; engaging in good eating habits and regular physical activity; obtaining regular medical attention, particularly regular screening if one has not achieved a healthy weight (to identify as early as possible the presence of comorbid conditions); and improving self-esteem and attitudes about self-care. Such practices help to maximize one's chances for successful weight management, decrease the risks of developing a variety of degenerative chronic diseases, and enable many major medical problems to be caught at an early stage.

Obese individuals, as they go through treatment, should develop a reasonable understanding of the disease, including its causes and treatments, the benefits of diet and exercise, the effects of excess weight on the body over time, and the benefits to health from weight loss. Short of giving individuals tests as they begin and complete a program to see if knowledge of obesity has increased, this component can be assessed indirectly by evaluating whether basic information about obesity is presented by the option (e.g., discussed prominently in a diet book or as part of the classes and counseling sessions in a commercial program) and whether the individual reads or hears it (e.g., reads the book in its entirety or attends most of the classes and counseling sessions of the program).

Eating habits can be assessed by using one of the dietary assessment tools in Appendix A. For practical purposes, we define a good dietary pattern as one where the individual meets the recommendations of the Food Guide Pyramid on at least 4 of 7 days. (Such a dietary pattern might be inappropriate during the treatment phase of a clinical program where specially formulated products are used. During this period, the standard of nutritional adequacy should be meeting the Recommended Dietary Allowances for all nutrients except energy over the course of a week.) Again for practical purposes, we define regular physical activity as the accumulation of one-half hour or more of moderate-intensity activity (such as brisk walking) four or more times a week, and preferably daily. We believe it prudent for an obese individual to see a physician at yearly intervals for a physical examination and appropriate follow-up. Individuals who have not achieved a healthy weight (such as a BMI of less than 25 through age 34 and less than 27 beyond age 34; see Chapter 2) either have obesity-related comorbidities or are at risk of developing them at some future point. Regular screening of these individuals by a health-care provider will help to identify as early as possible the presence of comorbid conditions and lead to the initiation of appropriate treatment or continuation of it. Dietary patterns and physical activity are difficult to measure objectively since they usually depend on the individual's own characterization of these factors. In contrast, medical visits can be documented with the individual's physician.

Improved well-being is a positive subjective feeling by the individual that includes feeling good about oneself (positive self-esteem) and healthy attitudes about self-care with a desire to practice it. These feelings can be assessed by available questionnaires (see Appendix A), but most of these tools are best used by health-care providers trained in their use and interpretation. We recommend that all programs administer a test such as the Dieting Readiness Test to assess how well equipped a person is to undertake a weight-management program; individuals in a do-it-yourself program will need to self-administer and score the test. Clinical programs, in addition to using the Dieting Readiness Test or a similar test, should administer a test such as the General Well-Being Schedule, which provides a useful evaluation of the psychological health of the client and can help uncover potential psychological pathologies. Both of these tests are provided in Appendix B.

### Monitoring of Adverse Effects That Might Result from Program

As described in Chapter 6, weight loss poses potential risks to health. The more restrictive the diet, the greater are the risks of adverse effects. All clinical and nonclinical programs should periodically question their clients about any changes in health while on the program and should encourage them to volunteer such information if changes in health, particularly negative ones, occur. Consumers undertaking a do-it-yourself program should be particularly aware of the fact that their efforts may have adverse effects and should pay attention to any changes in their health. Experiencing an adverse effect while on a weight-management program may or may not be related to the program (it may be a worsening of health as a result of the obesity), but it should be evaluated. Depending on the nature of the problem, in some cases the program will need to be modified for the individual and in other cases it should be discontinued.

We believe that weight-loss programs should be judged by how well individuals do in these four areas, and potential clients should expect that a high-quality program will attend to, or urge attention be paid to (since most of these components are not under the direct control of the program), each of these areas. In Chapter 8, we provide recommendations on how these components might be addressed by programs.

## CONCLUDING REMARKS

Life in the United States is conducive to obesity. Easy availability of an energy-rich diet and limited opportunities for exercise set the stage for a nation of overweight "couch potatoes." Available data suggest that most obese individuals who try to lose weight in intervention programs do not maintain the losses they achieve during treatment. For the small numbers of people who do maintain their losses without drugs or surgery, the most important factors associated with long-term success include a regular habit of exercise, continued contact with the treatment program, normalization of eating patterns with continued control of energy intake, continued self-monitoring of diet and exercise, and a positive, problem-solving attitude toward life's stressors. Family dysfunction and negative life events are associated strongly with weight rebound.

Given the experiences of dieters and the research demonstrating that relatively small weight losses can reduce the prevalence and severity of comorbid conditions associated with obesity, we recommend that obesity-treatment programs focus more on weight management than on weight loss and broaden the definition of success to include, for example, better health, improved health practices, more and better health-related knowledge, and improved well-being. The next chapter suggests how this broader definition of success and the current knowledge of predictors of success can be used along with recommendations in Chapters 5 and 6 to facilitate the process of decisionmaking about program appropriateness, soundness, safety, and outcomes.

# 8

## Weighing the Options: Application of Committee's Criteria

$\mathbf{C}$hapters 4 through 7 present and expand upon a decisionmaking framework to describe the thought processes of an individual embarking on and evaluating a weight-management program. This chapter summarizes that information in a model we call *Weighing the Options* (see Figure 8-1). It is a conceptual model of the decisionmaking process leading to treatment and outcome. Outcome, in turn, leads to evaluation or reevaluation of the choice of program, whereby one returns to the beginning of the model. It is our attempt to combine, in graphic form, consumer choice with program options and evaluations.

### DERIVATION OF THE MODEL

The *Weighing the Options* model emphasizes implicitly that weight management for obese individuals requires a *lifelong* plan. It shows explicitly that the individual is at the center of decisionmaking, with input received from a variety of sources. A central feature of the model is that it broadens the definition of a successful outcome. The model emphasizes that weight management is a dynamic process in which both individuals and programs set and evaluate goals periodically and employ a variety of strategies for attaining these goals. It is meant to be used by both a program and an individual.

Our recommendations for evaluating weight-management outcomes (Criterion 3) include both specific (quantitative) and more general (qualitative) ones. We have identified common goals for all weight-manage-

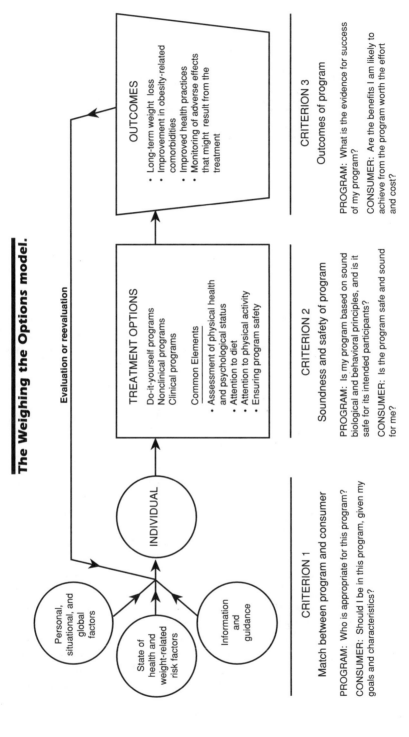

**The Weighing the Options model.**

FIGURE 8-1

---

**CHOOSING A WEIGHT-MANAGEMENT OPTION:**
**AN ANALOGY**

Perhaps a helpful analogy to choosing a weight-management option is deciding how to approach financial planning. An individual may not want to have a financial plan, may have a variety of specific financial goals, or may wish simply to achieve financial security but have no strategy for doing so. He or she initiates the process by deciding what techniques to use to manage assets. An individual may choose to manage them personally with help from articles, books, or self-help groups; with others by joining an investment club or taking a class in financial planning; or by going to a professional for help. Two or more options might be combined. And, for some individuals, life circumstances force them to react to financial issues as they arise, when planning is not a realistic option.

An individual meeting with a financial planner is often asked to complete a questionnaire that helps the planner to evaluate the client's assets, past history, and projected gain, and to identify appropriate long- and short-term goals. Since there is the implicit assumption that financial management also requires lifelong planning, some individuals work in partnership with financial planners, and goals are reviewed and redefined periodically as circumstances and income change.

---

ment efforts. The means of evaluating these outcomes will vary depending on the type of program (do-it-yourself, nonclinical, or clinical) and the claims it makes for success.

Three criteria, introduced in Chapter 4, are used to structure the evaluation of weight-management programs: Criterion 1, the match between the program and consumer; Criterion 2, the soundness and safety of the program; and Criterion 3, the outcomes of the program. The programs themselves are characterized as do-it-yourself, nonclinical, and clinical (see Chapter 3). The recommendations presented in the next section are both quantitative and qualitative, depending on the information base pertaining to each criterion, and may vary with the type of program. Generally, conservative treatments should be used for mildly obese individuals without comorbidities, whereas more aggressive treatments such as surgery should be reserved for those at high or very high risk. For example, a person with a body mass index (BMI) greater than 40 who has hypertension and has failed in attempts at weight loss might be a potential candidate for gastric surgery. Surgery would not be an option for an individual with a BMI of 28, even with obesity-related comorbidities. Readers should not interpret these remarks as an endorsement of a stepped-care approach to weight management. We do not, for example, recommend that individuals try a clinical program only after they fail at do-it-yourself or nonclinical programs.

We are well aware that the recommendations in this chapter will elicit a variety of reactions. Some will consider them to be overly general and not providing sufficiently detailed guidance to consumers for selecting a program and to programs for improving the quality of their services. Others will see the recommendations as being too prescriptive—too much like implicit standards of care that regulatory agencies or consumer-protection bodies at the national, state, or local levels might turn into regulations resulting in potentially onerous and expensive limitations on the conduct of major commercial weight-loss programs. We developed our recommendations without engaging in this debate and based them on the scientific research available and the deliberative judgment of the committee. As one expert committee, we think it likely that implementing the recommendations in this chapter will help more people to lose weight successfully, improve overall health, and keep off excess weight over the long term. How they are implemented, however, should be decided not by us but by broad constituencies through an interactive process of public discussion. Consumers, weight-management programs, and regulatory agencies should all find these recommendations of use in somewhat different ways.

Our recommendations are meant to apply to the weight-management programs that use data or testimonials in their advertising and promotional activities to suggest that weight loss is likely to be successful with them or that they are more effective than competing programs. Programs that engage in these activities should be held to some level of proof of their contentions, so they must be encouraged to collect certain types of information in standardized ways and to provide certain kinds of information to potential clients. Potential clients, in turn, should be encouraged to expect this information from programs, so that programs that do not comply may be put at a competitive disadvantage and thereby become motivated to rethink their position. This information is needed so that consumers can make informed choices and there can be reasonable oversight of programs by regulatory agencies such as the Federal Trade Commission, the Food and Drug Administration, and state medical practice review boards, as well as by interested biomedical scientists. Weight-management programs that do not make claims of success—such as classes provided by a community YMCA or YWCA, counseling by dietitians at a local hospital, or meetings of a local chapter of Overeaters Anonymous—should not be required to assume the data-collection burdens and expense of meeting our recommendations, but should endeavor to do so if resources permit. Given that the loss of even a small amount of weight may benefit health, we want interested clients to have many options in their communities to receive help in achieving a healthful lifestyle.

We are, as some critics would assert, singling out weight-loss programs for special attention in contrast to, for example, smoking-cessation or alcohol treatment programs. We believe strongly that weight-loss programs require special attention. Unfortunately, our health-care system has not treated obesity as a chronic disease requiring long-term management, even as the prevalence of this disease continues to increase. We believe that a new concept of obesity treatment is needed, and this report represents a first effort by a group of multidisciplinary biomedical experts convened by the Food and Nutrition Board of the Institute of Medicine to stimulate this process. As detailed in Chapter 7, we have proposed expanding the concept of weight loss to include long-term weight management with the ultimate goal of improved health. This report provides clients, obesity-management programs, researchers, and policy-makers with recommendations by which to evaluate programs and outcomes. Although there will undoubtedly be discussion about the specific details of our recommendations, we believe that consensus exists about the need for them.

## APPLICATION OF OUR CRITERIA

This section describes our recommendations for satisfying the three criteria described in Chapters 4–7 and illustrated in Figure 8-1. Programs could use these criteria to enhance quality control; monitor adherence to national, state, or local regulations; and conduct research and market analyses (or permit them to be conducted by outside scientists) on their effectiveness. Individuals would use these criteria to help them select a program and to evaluate periodically whether the program meets their changing needs.

### Criterion 1: Match Between Program and Consumer

Weight-loss programs attempt to meet consumer needs and desires, and consumers determine their goals for weight loss partly on the basis of program claims. In Chapter 5, we describe three sets of factors that influence an individual's choice of programs: (1) personal, situational, and global factors (e.g., age, gender, motivation, readiness to change, views about weight and appearance, and the cost and ready availability of a program); (2) health status and weight-related risk factors (e.g., presence or absence of hypertension, dyslipidemias, and diabetes and family history or other comorbidities); and (3) information and guidance (e.g., from family, friends, books, magazines, advertising, and health-care professionals). Consumers choose a program based on some combination of these factors. In Chapter 7, we identify factors most frequently linked with success at weight loss and maintenance of that loss. These include a habit of regular exercise, continued contact with the treatment program, reasonable and nutritious eating patterns, continued self-monitoring of diet and exercise, a positive problem-solving attitude toward life's stressors, and positive changes in physiological factors that are often adversely affected by obesity.

Given that the goal in matching consumers with programs is to maximize the chances of achieving long-term weight loss, it is unfortunate that the ability of consumers and health-care providers to make successful matches is limited at present. The complex interactions that occur between an individual and the many factors that influence program choice are beyond the current ability of biomedical science to explain, much less predict. Clearly, there is a need for future research to reduce the chances of mismatches. Nevertheless, it is possible to make some prudent qualitative recommendations to increase the likelihood of a successful match.

### Program's Perspective: Who Is Appropriate for This Program?

Each program decides what types of clients are appropriate and inappropriate given its specific philosophies, protocols, and treatment approaches. Pregnant women and individuals who are underweight or anorectic are inappropriate candidates for any weight-loss program. Nonclinical programs should require (and do-it-yourself programs should advise) that lactating women, children, and adolescents, as well as those with bulimia; significant cardiovascular, renal, or psychiatric disease; diabetes; or other significant medical problems undertake weight loss only under medical supervision. Nonclinical programs should encourage clients with obesity-related comorbidities or other health problems to maintain contact with their health-care provider for the duration of the program. Both nonclinical and clinical programs should obtain some information on the state of health and weight-loss goals of potential clients to determine if they are appropriate for a specific program and what types of individualized attention they may require.

Do-it-yourself programs such as those provided in diet books, diet plans in magazines, or over-the-counter weight-loss devices or products should provide information in the text or other instructional materials on who might and who should not use the program. Since there is usually no legal obligation that this information be provided or that it be true and complete, it is the responsibility of the publisher or manufacturer of the program to provide it voluntarily. In general, the lack of such information or the suggestion that the program is for anyone who wishes to lose weight (no matter how much one desires or needs to lose or one's age, state of health, or stage of life) should arouse suspicion that the program might not be sound.

### Consumer's Perspective: Should I Be in This Program, Given My Goals and Characteristics?

Because consumers decide on their own or with the help of others (e.g., family, friends, or health-care providers) whether to enter a weight-loss program and which one to choose, they must consider carefully their weight-loss goals and whether they are appropriate candidates for weight loss, and decide whether the time is right for them to devote the considerable attention and effort required to succeed. It is important that consumers commit time and energy to losing weight and maintaining the weight loss; they will fail if they do not make sincere efforts, no matter how good the program.

We believe that individuals should have the right to select the therapeutic modality they believe to be most suited to their needs or to select no treatment—although we hope they will seek guidance from health-care providers in making their decision. Some individuals may find treatment too onerous or otherwise unsuitable. In this case, they should expect that the provider will not withhold medical assistance required to treat any medical problems that might be related to their weight or hold them accountable for those problems.

Individuals should expect a program to provide them with sufficient information to help assess whether they are appropriate or inappropriate potential candidates. We strongly recommend that those contemplating a do-it-yourself or nonclinical program be evaluated first by a health-care provider (or have been assessed in the recent past) before proceeding. They should discuss the program or product with their health-care provider to determine whether it is sound and appropriate. Individuals who are extremely obese (i.e., BMI >40) and have failed at attempts to lose weight should discuss with their health-care provider the risks they face and the options available to them, such as gastric surgery and medications. These two options should be used as appropriate with a program of diet, physical activity, and behavior modification.

### Criterion 2: Soundness and Safety of the Program

Weight-management programs should be based on sound biological and behavioral principles and should be relatively safe for their intended participants. Each of the following components is essential to address in applying the criterion.

**Health and Weight Status** Healthy weights are generally associated with a BMI of 19–25 in those 19–34 years of age and 21–27 in those 35 years of age and older (USDA and DHHS, 1990). However, individuals with a BMI of 25–27 are at slight risk from obesity if they have no comorbidities and at moderate risk if they do (see Figure 2-6). Beyond these ranges, health risks increase as BMI increases. Health risks also increase with excess visceral fat (waist-to-hip ratio [WHR] >1.0 for males and >0.8 for females), high blood pressure (>140/90), dyslipidemias (total cholesterol and triglyceride concentrations of >200 and >225 mg/dl, respectively), non-insulin-dependent diabetes mellitus, and a family history of premature death due to cardiovascular disease (e.g., parent, grandparent, sibling, uncle, or aunt dying before age 50). Weight loss usually improves the management of obesity-related comorbidities or decreases the risks of their development.

**Psychological Status** Psychological status can be assessed by using the tools listed in Appendix A. At this time, we recommend that prior to beginning a weight-management program, all individuals take the Dieting Readiness Test (discussed in Chapter 6 and presented in Appendix B) or some comparable test, which can be administered and scored by the individual or appropriate staff at a nonclinical program. Such a test helps to point out potential problems with motivation and attitudes toward dieting and exercise. Clinical programs should also administer the General Well-Being Schedule (also discussed in Chapter 6 and presented in Appendix B) or a comparable test to identify frank psychological pathologies (e.g., depression) and determine whether an individual should be referred for more in-depth psychological assessment before beginning the program.

**Diet** Consumption of a calorically modified diet containing a variety of foods is required for long-term weight management in individuals with or tending toward obesity. For practical purposes, we define a good dietary pattern as one in which the individual meets the Food Guide Pyramid guidelines on at least 4 of 7 days. A few nonclinical but many clinical programs put their clients on diets that are based on the use of special nutritional products and dietary supplements; this is generally appropriate during the treatment phase but is often difficult to sustain for long periods of time. Decreasing total energy intake and the consumption of dietary fat, sugar, and alcohol, while providing adequate nutrients, dietary fiber, and protein to maintain nitrogen balance and limit the loss of lean body mass, is a time-tested way to lose weight safely.

Although we do not prescribe a minimal level of energy intake for safe weight loss, clients should be made aware that energy intakes of less than 1,200 kcal/day will usually not meet nutrient requirements and that a vitamin-mineral supplement will be needed. Diets of less than 800 kcal/day should not be used except under a physician's supervision.

**Physical Activity** Regular physical activity is also essential for long-term weight management because it helps to promote weight loss and decrease regain, reduce obesity-related risk factors, and decrease morbidity and mortality. For practical purposes, we define a minimal level of physical activity as the accumulation of one-half hour or more of moderate-intensity activity (such as brisk walking) four or more times a week.

**Safety** All programs should be reasonably safe and pose minimal untoward health risks to clients. Risks vary by program. Generally, approaches that require oversight by physicians (e.g., use of drugs and surgery) or special diets that deviate substantially from healthy eating patterns, or are very low in energy content, pose the most risk. The nature of complications varies with the weight-loss method used. Diets that are not nutritionally adequate in protein, vitamins, minerals, and dietary fiber should be used only for compelling reasons—on a temporary basis and with appropriate supplementation—during the treatment phase of weight loss.

### Program's Perspective: Is My Program Based on Sound Biological and Behavioral Principles, and Is It Safe for Its Intended Participants?

All providers should take steps to ensure that their programs are safe and sound. Nonclinical and clinical programs can provide information about the qualifications and training of staff as well as appropriate corporate managers and, if desired, consultants involved in developing the program. Authors and other originators of do-it-yourself programs should cite their credentials, qualifications, and experiences in managing obesity.

Clinical programs should be able to assess the physical and psychological health of their patients. Nonclinical and do-it-yourself programs, in contrast, can only encourage clients to have such an assessment conducted by their health-care providers. All programs should encourage individuals to know their blood pressure and blood lipid concentrations; whether or not they have diabetes, osteoarthritis in weight-bearing joints, or sleep apnea; and whether a family member has died prematurely from coronary heart disease. Do-it-yourself and nonclinical programs should strongly encourage individuals who have one or more of these risk factors to be under the care of a health-care provider. These programs should develop simple checklists for clients to highlight the importance of routinely monitoring health status. Clinical programs should assess all clients for these risk factors.

Nonclinical and clinical programs should measure the height and weight of clients and calculate their BMI and WHR, providing both the results and the information to interpret those results. Do-it-yourself programs should encourage their clients to take these measurements and make these calculations, instruct them how to do so, and explain the results.

Clients in nonclinical and clinical programs should have their diets and physical activity patterns evaluated at least at the beginning and end of the treatment phase of the program and every 6 months during any maintenance phase (see Appendix A for various assessment tools). Nonclinical programs should assess the psychological status of clients with the Dieting Readiness Test; clinical programs should use it along with the General Well-Being Schedule (see Appendix B; however, comparable assessment tools are appropriate). Do-it-yourself programs should inform clients about the importance of attention to diet, physical activity, and psychological assessment (by providing, for example, the Dieting Readiness Test), and give explicit guidance in how to do so (as discussed above and in earlier chapters).

Since no weight-loss attempt is risk free, it is incumbent on each program to inform potential clients about the known and hypothetical risks of that program. Clinical programs have special responsibilities to assess and manage potential risks, especially when special diets (such as very-low-calorie diets), drugs, or surgery are used as part of the treatment. For example, if a diet is not nutritionally adequate, clients should be given or advised to take dietary supplements. Potential side effects of the dietary program and of specific drugs used for treating obesity should be explained, including the potential for drug-drug interactions. Patients considering gastric surgery should be counseled on the operative and perioperative surgical risks (NIH, 1992).

### Consumer's Perspective: Is the Program Safe and Sound for Me?

Given the limitations of do-it-yourself and nonclinical programs to assess health compared to clinical programs, consumers choosing the former have a greater responsibility for self-monitoring their health. Consumers should have a good understanding of the program of interest and what they can expect from it throughout the treatment and any maintenance phase. They should have access to information about the qualifications and training of staff in nonclinical and clinical programs and the credentials and qualifications of the author/originator of a do-it-yourself program.

Clients should expect that the program of interest will be a safe and sound one (by meeting our recommendations for them as detailed above). We recommend that they monitor their weight weekly and continue to assess (or have assessed) their diet and physical activity patterns at 6-month intervals or more frequently after the weight-loss phase of a program. This will act as a useful periodic check on these two major influences of weight and will help to maintain weight loss.

### Criterion 3: Outcomes of the Program

In Chapter 7, we recommend that weight-loss programs be judged by how well individuals do in four areas: (1) long-term weight loss, (2) improvement in obesity-related comorbidities, (3) improved health practices, and (4) monitoring of adverse effects that might result from the program. We note that potential clients should expect that a high-quality program will attend to, or urge attention be paid to (since most of these components are not under the direct control of the program), each of these areas. For practical purposes, we have developed qualitative and quantitative measures for each of these components of successful weight management (see box titled "Measures of Successful Weight Management").

Achieving these outcomes is a joint responsibility of the program and the individual. A program, for example, can provide exemplary information and guidance on healthful eating, incorporating more activity into one's life, and enhancing self-esteem, but it is the individual's responsibility to put this into practice. Also, do-it-yourself and nonclinical programs can encourage an individual to be screened by a health-care provider, but they may not be able to provide such screening nor should they be expected to find a provider for someone without medical insurance.

### Program's Perspective: What Is the Evidence for Success of My Program?

It is not cost effective or practical for most do-it-yourself programs to evaluate their outcomes. Nevertheless, they can make sure that they cover the importance of long-term weight loss and the reduction of obesity-related comorbidities, provide information and guidance on improving health behaviors, and discuss in detail the potential health risks from weight loss in general and their program in particular.

Because clients come physically to nonclinical and clinical programs,

## MEASURES OF SUCCESSFUL WEIGHT MANAGEMENT

**Long-Term Weight Loss** Long term means 1 year or more, and weight loss of any significance is the loss of ≥5 percent of body weight or a reduction in BMI by 1 or more units.

**Improvement in Obesity-Related Comorbidities** One or more associated risk factors (e.g., high blood pressure; elevated blood concentrations of cholesterol, triglycerides, or glucose; and non-insulin-dependent diabetes mellitus), if present, should be improved to a degree considered clinically significant.

**Improved Health Practices** Obtaining health-related knowledge may be assessed indirectly by evaluating whether basic information about obesity is presented by the program and whether the individual reads or hears it. Engaging in good eating habits may be assessed by using a dietary assessment tool such as those cited in Appendix A or evidence that the individual meets the recommendations of the Food Guide Pyramid on at least 4 of 7 days. Engaging in regular physical activity involves one-half hour or more of moderate-intensity activity (such as brisk walking) four or more times a week and preferably daily. Obtaining regular medical attention includes seeing a physician at yearly intervals, particularly if the individual has not achieved a healthy weight. Regular screening of these individuals by a health-care provider will help to identify as early as possible the presence of comorbid conditions and lead to the initiation or continuation of appropriate treatment. Improved well-being can be assessed through questionnaires described in Appendix A. For all programs, we recommend a test such as the Dieting Readiness Test and, in addition, for clinical programs only, the General Well-Being Schedule (see Appendix B).

**Monitoring of Adverse Effects That Might Result from Program** Clinical and nonclinical programs should question their clients periodically about any changes in health while on the program and should encourage them to volunteer such information if changes do occur. A do-it-yourself program should inform consumers that because the program may potentially have adverse health effects, they should be attentive to any changes in their health while on it.

the programs can monitor and document their weight loss over time. Such programs should have quality control procedures in place to ensure that protocols are adhered to by staff and to modify those protocols as warranted given the experiences and feedback of clients. They should also have mechanisms to evaluate the success of their programs. If the company is organized as a franchise, mechanisms should be available to evaluate the program as a whole and at individual sites.

All programs should also provide information and guidance on improving health behaviors and should discuss the potential risks of dieting, including those from their programs. Do-it-yourself and nonclinical programs should encourage clients (and strongly encourage those with obesity-related comorbidities) to have regular contact with a health-care provider throughout the treatment and maintenance phases of their weight loss so that their overall health can be monitored as well as the disposition of any comorbidities. Clinical programs should be expected to provide this medical assessment and monitoring.

It is appropriate that weight-management programs continue to be judged primarily on their success in achieving long-term weight loss (including small weight losses that are maintained). However, in addition, programs should be judged on their ability to empower their clients to eat a healthful diet and become more active, reduce obesity-related comorbidities, improve the objective and subjective measures of their quality of life, and make desired changes in health-related knowledge and attitudes.

### Consumer's Perspective: Are the Benefits I Am Likely to Achieve from the Program Worth the Effort and Cost?

When they begin a weight-management program, consumers must recognize that they and the program have responsibilities for the final outcome. To improve their chances for success, consumers should choose programs that focus on long-term weight management; provide instruction in healthful eating, increasing activity, and improving self-esteem; and explain thoroughly the potential health risks from weight loss. Individuals interested in a specific do-it-yourself program should search in the program literature for evidence that the program is successful; if information on success is absent or consists primarily of testimonials or other anecdotal evidence (including, in the case of programs by health-care providers, only their own clients or patients), the program should be viewed with suspicion.

Consumers should look for programs that devote considerable effort to helping people change their behaviors through information, guidance, and skill training. To make the most of the weight-management effort, however, consumers should have realistic expectations of a program and be willing to devote the time and effort required. Those in do-it-yourself and nonclinical programs should be in touch with a health-care provider who can monitor the status of any obesity-related comorbidities and changes in health.

When an individual chooses a program, it should be in light of his or her short- and long-term goals for weight management. Our *Weighing the Options* model (see Figure 8-1) is a dynamic one that incorporates periodic reevaluation by the client and program to assess whether an individual and a program are meeting these goals and whether the goals or the treatment should be modified. We recommend these evaluations every 3 to 6 months.

## TRUTH AND FULL DISCLOSURE

This section describes the nature and amount of information to be disclosed to individuals considering a weight-management program. Information on program disclosure should be sufficient to enable the client to make informed choices among the program options and, we hope, decrease unrealistic expectations. Our recommendations, if put into practice, should also lead to decreases in unsubstantiated claims and thus highlight unethical behavior by the programs themselves. The background for these recommendations is the extensive literature on informed voluntary consent that has become a key element in research on human subjects (Faden et al., 1986). This section builds on several sets of guidelines: those of the National Institutes of Health (NIH) Technology Assessment Conference Panel (1993) on methods for voluntary weight loss and control, the weight-loss guidelines for Michigan (Drewnowski, 1990; Petersmarck, 1992), the truth-in-dieting regulation in New York City (Winner, 1991), and rules developed by the Federal Trade Commission for use by commercial programs in making specific claims (see Chapter 1).

Any weight-management program has a responsibility to prospective clients to provide truthful and unambiguous information that is not misleading or subject to misinterpretation. This includes a written (and, for nonclinical and clinical programs, oral) description of the risks and benefits of treatment and the opportunity to ask questions. To assist individuals in making informed choices from the many nonclinical and clinical programs, information made available should include the nature of a given program, its structure and management, and a description of its staff, including training; all costs, including effort and time; the type of client typically served by the program; and the short- and long-term treatment outcomes. Key elements of these recommendations are provided in Table 8-1. Obviously there can be no such standardization for do-it-yourself programs, given the nature of the individual's interaction with these programs, the wide variety of approaches that they encompass (e.g., books, devices, products, and dietary supplements), and their almost unlimited freedom to make statements and claims.

To facilitate comparisons between programs, we recommend that obesity management programs collect the data summarized in Table 8-2. At the current time, it is difficult to compare different programs, in part because of differences in the clients selected and in the data collected and reported.

**TABLE 8-1** Program Disclosure of Information

---

All potential clients of weight-management programs should receive information such as the following:

- A truthful, unambiguous, and nonmisleading statement of the approach and goals of the program. Part of such a statement might read, for example, "We are a program that emphasizes changes in lifestyle, with group instruction in diet and physical activity."
- A brief description of the credentials of staff, with more detailed information available on request. For example, "Our staff is composed of one physician (M.D.), two registered nurses (R.N.s), three registered dietitians (R.D.s), one master's-level exercise physiologist, and one Ph.D.-level psychologist. At your first visit, you will be seen by the physician. At each visit you will be seen by a dietitian and exercise physiologist and after every five visits by the psychologist. Résumés of our staff are available on request."
- A statement of the client population and experiences over a period of 9 months or more. For example, "To date, we have seen 823 clients for at least three visits each. Although only 26 clients have participated in this program for more than 1 year, they have maintained an average weight loss of 12 pounds."
- A full disclosure of costs. For example, "If you avail yourself of all our facilities with one weekly visit for a period of 1 year, the total cost to you will be between $2,000 and $2,500." Costs should include the initial cost; ongoing costs and additional cost of extra products, services, supplements, and laboratory tests; and costs paid by the average client. Programs may also wish to provide information on the experiences clients have had in recovering their costs from third-party payers.
- A statement of procedures recommended for clients. For example, "We urge that each of our clients see a physician before joining our program. If you have high blood pressure or diabetes, you should see your physician at intervals of his or her choosing while with our program."

---

If programs make claims for long-term maintenance of weight loss, the percentage of clients who have lost weight and maintained it for 1 and 2 years should be provided (along with the percentage of clients for whom the information is available) as well as the average weight loss. Many companies use testimonials, often from prominent people, to show a program's success at achieving weight loss. In these cases, they should also cite the experience of their clients in general (as noted above) or cite the general experience of similar dieters taken from reports in the scientific literature.

Scholarly research using data collected from weight-management companies should be conducted according to generally accepted protocols for approval and consent. We also endorse guidelines prepared by Apfelbaum et al. (1987) on information to include in scientific papers on the results of obesity treatments. The guidelines are intended to help investigators compare the results of different programs reported in the literature, which is often impossible to do now given the differences in

**TABLE 8-2**  Collection of Data by Weight-Management Programs

---

1.  The number of people attending the first treatment session. (This is the group of potential clients and those who will become actual clients.)

2.  Number of clients attending their first two treatment sessions (a gauge of those who have really begun a program) and percentage continuing to participate in the program at 1, 3, 6, and 12 months. (These timepoints seem reasonable but are selected somewhat arbitrarily, for while there is no set of ideal timepoints, it is important to have a set for standardization and comparison among programs. Programs may, of course, use additional timepoints.)

3.  Average weight, height, BMI, and WHR of clients attending the first two sessions and appropriate measures of change in these variables at 1, 3, 6, and 12 months in the program. (These data should be assembled by gender and, if possible, by race, age, and starting weight or BMI.)

4.  The percentage of actual clients who complete each of the stages of the treatment program. This means either the number of clients that complete the program's prescribed number of sessions (e.g., 8 weeks for an 8-week program) or the number of clients in treatment at 3 months.

5.  The percentage of actual clients who re-enroll in the same program for further treatment. (This figure should not necessarily be interpreted as a measure of client failure in a program; it may indicate satisfaction with the program.)

---

kinds of data reported. Apfelbaum et al. recommend that reports of research should include (1) the number of patients (or clients) considered for treatment; (2) number of patients accepted for treatment; (3) number of patients dropping out of treatment; (4) gender and age distribution of patients; (5) BMI of patients, including mean, standard deviation, median range, and interquartile range; (6) duration of treatment; (7) duration of follow-up (a minimum of 1 year strongly recommended); (8) number of patients in follow-up; (9) weight changes during follow-up, and how obtained (e.g., self-report or actual measurement); (10) waist and hip measurements before and after treatment; and (11) costs of the treatment.

## CONCLUDING REMARKS

This chapter has provided a variety of qualitative and quantitative recommendations that, if implemented, will lead to weight-management programs' being evaluated in a more comprehensive and systematic manner than is possible today. Their implementation will also help consumers choose from among the programs in a more informed manner. These recommendations are meant to apply to programs that advertise their success at helping people lose weight and often promote their superiority over competing programs. We are aware that they will elicit both supportive and critical reactions, but we believe there is consensus that recommendations are needed and will serve a useful purpose. They are the product of our expert committee based on the scientific research available and collective judgment, and we put them forward to generate discussion and action. It is our hope and expectation that the recommendations in this chapter will evolve and be acted upon based on such discussions, on assessment of the outcomes of the activities they generate, and on future research.

# 9

## Prevention of Obesity

The prevention of obesity is a topic that must be considered given the major increases both in the prevalence of obesity and in the mean body weights of people in the United States over the past decade (see Chapter 2). Despite the appeal of prevention as an ideal, it appears that this country as a whole has been unable to prevent obesity. The results of more limited and focused efforts at prevention, described later in this chapter, have hardly been more successful. These facts led a recent review to conclude that "we have not been able to prevent obesity in the past and we do not have the tools to do better in the future" (Stunkard, in press).

It has been proposed that genetic vulnerability may lie at the root of the current epidemic of obesity and the problem of controlling, let alone preventing, obesity (Bouchard, 1994). However, there has been no real change in the gene pool during this period of increasing obesity. The root of the problem, rather, must lie in the powerful social and cultural forces that promote an energy-rich diet and a sedentary lifestyle. But if social and cultural forces can promote obesity, these same forces should be able to control it. Therein lies the still unrealized potential for preventing obesity.

There is some ambiguity of terminology in the prevention literature. The verb *prevent* implies taking an action or interposing an impediment to stop or keep something from happening. Different ideas about what it is that should be stopped or kept from happening have been suggested in terms of obesity prevention. Is it the incidence of obesity itself? Is it preventing weight gain among those treated for obesity to prevent progression from a moderate to more severe levels? Does the success of prevention efforts depend upon the effect on comorbid medical disabilities (e.g., diabetes or hypertension)? Is what should be stopped or kept from happening an underlying risk condition or predisposition factor for obesity development?

A recent Institute of Medicine (IOM) report recommends an approach to clarifying definitions of prevention that, although developed in relation to mental disorders, apply to obesity (IOM, 1994). This IOM report reviews existing classification systems for preventive interventions for physical illness. The familiar public health classification system designates three types of prevention: *primary*, *secondary*, and *tertiary*. The goal of primary prevention is to decrease the number of new cases (incidence) of a disorder. In secondary prevention, the goal is to lower the rate of established cases of the disorder in the population (prevalence). Tertiary prevention seeks to stabilize or decrease the amount of disability associated with an existing disorder. For obesity, tertiary prevention could refer to decreasing the progression to more severe obesity or decreasing the likelihood of associated musculoskeletal, metabolic, or vascular disorders (e.g., osteoarthritis, diabetes, or cardiovascular disease).

When this prevention classification system was introduced more than 25 years ago, the implicit disease model was one of an acute condition with a specific and unifactorial cause. It was assumed that mechanisms linking the cause of a specific disease to its subsequent occurrence could be identified. In the intervening years, many chronic diseases prevalent in this country have been recognized as having multifactorial etiologies. Research on these diseases has advanced our knowledge about the complicated relations that exist between risk factors and protective factors for disease and the outcomes of preventive interventions. But this knowledge can breed the pessimistic view that prevention efforts will be futile until the etiologies of diseases are better understood (IOM, 1994).

According to this analysis, the concept of *risk reduction* is critical to prevention programs and research. Addressing the degrees of risk for a condition supplants the more simplistic concept of prevention in which a disease is simply present or absent. Risk factors refer to those characteristics that, if present for a particular individual, make it more likely that this person (compared to someone selected from the general population) will develop a disorder (Werner and Smith, 1992). Both risk and protective factors are included here. Research also shows that many at-risk individuals have factors in their background or environment that protect against the development of a disorder (Garmezy, 1983).

In furthering the establishment of successful preventive intervention programs, the IOM report recommends instituting a "preventive intervention research cycle." This research cycle consists of, first, description of the interplay between risk and protective factors; next, identification of causal risk factors that may be alterable through interventions; finally, systematic, empirical, and rigorous testing of these interventions, most often in preventive intervention trials.

At the current stage of research into preventing obesity, work is still in the first two phases of this research cycle: identifying high-risk and protective factors for the development of obesity, and determining which factors are malleable and can be altered by preventive interventions. We recommend continuing this early research on the determinants of obesity and pilot-testing promising interventions before funds are allocated for large-scale community prevention trials. Promising research studies that have already appeared in the scientific literature are reviewed later in this chapter.

The recent IOM report also recommended an alternative terminology for physical disease prevention, proposed by Gordon (1987), and we adopt it here (see Figure 9-1). This terminology identifies three types of prevention: *universal, selective,* and *indicated* prevention. Each category represents a population group, rather than a disorder or disease state, to whom preventive interventions are directed. *Universal* preventive measures or interventions are designed for everyone in the eligible population. *Selective* preventive measures are directed toward a *subgroup* of the

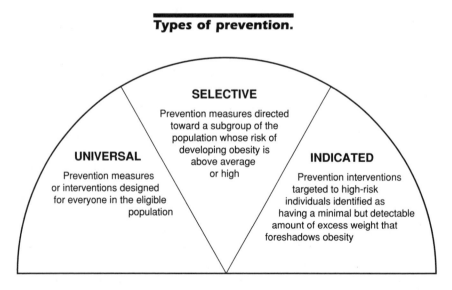

**Types of prevention.**

FIGURE 9-1    Adapted from IOM, 1994.

population whose risk of developing the disorder is above average or high. *Indicated* preventive interventions are targeted to high-risk *individuals* identified as having minimal but detectable signs or symptoms that foreshadow the disorder, or exhibiting biological markers indicating predisposition, who do not meet the full diagnostic criteria for the disorder itself.

The earlier IOM report reserves the term *prevention* for those interventions that occur *before* the onset of a diagnosed disorder. What was previously known as *tertiary prevention* is redefined as *maintenance intervention*, whose aim is to reduce the disability associated with an ongoing disorder. Maintenance interventions, which can be supportive, educational, and/or pharmacological, are provided on a long-term basis to reduce relapse and recurrence. Consistent with the IOM definition of prevention (i.e., interventions that occur before onset), we do not include here a discussion of *maintenance* of weight to prevent the exacerbation of obesity or its complications in those in whom the condition is established. Factors affecting long-term weight management in the obese are discussed in Chapter 7.

The primary aim of obesity prevention is to reduce the number of new cases of obesity. This can be accomplished by means of a risk-reduction model. Even if the obesity outcomes are in the distant future, the decrease in risk factors and increase in protective factors for obesity can be identified. An important secondary aim is to delay the onset of obesity. The goals of indicated prevention programs are harder to define than those of universal and selective prevention programs. They might be framed in terms of reducing the length of time initial weight gain persists beyond certain pre-obese limits and halting its progression before diagnostic criteria for obesity are met. Even if the individual does eventually develop obesity, the prior preventive intervention may still have had an effect by reducing the duration or severity of the disorder.

The remainder of the chapter describes all three areas of prevention with reference to the prevention of obesity. Each area is described with respect to rationale, outcome measures, specific examples of programs, and criteria for evaluating prevention outcomes.

## UNIVERSAL PREVENTION

In accord with the traditional concept of primary prevention, universal prevention programs are geared to the general public and all members of specific eligible groups, such as children, the elderly, or pregnant women. Examples of universal prevention measures (which can often be applied without professional assistance) include prenatal care, use of seat belts, prevention of smoking, and consuming a nutritionally adequate diet (IOM, 1994). Such programs have advantages when their cost per person is low and the intervention is acceptable, low risk, and effective for the population involved. It is important to note that the target population (e.g., the general public) often includes individuals who have already developed the designated disorder.

As discussed in Chapter 2, obesity is becoming more rather than less prevalent in the United States. Universal prevention programs may help stabilize or even reverse the trend toward increased obesity in the general population. Universal programs can be classified into two broad categories: (1) preventive education and skills targeted toward individuals (e.g., programs in various settings designed to enhance nutritional knowledge and increase physical activity, thereby informing the public about the nature of weight change so that uninvolved and unaffected people can avoid negative or adverse consequences); and (2) modification of social and economic policies in an attempt to reduce the population's exposure to the environmental causes of obesity (e.g., mandated changes in food composition, regulation of food advertising, and food labeling). Programs in the first category often are derived from an individual clinical treatment model and evaluated in terms of weight change and the health habits of individual participants. Programs in the second category often are linked with a public health model, and results can be evaluated in terms of changes in the population distribution of body mass index (BMI).

### Outcome Measures for Universal Prevention

Six outcome measures for this type of prevention can be identified:

1.   reduction in the prevalence of obesity in the general population (this is a logical outcome to use when evaluating universal prevention programs; however, it must be noted that what counts as a reduction in the prevalence of obesity will share in the same arbitrariness as the definition of obesity used [see Stunkard, in press]);

2.   an overall reduction in average weight of the U.S. population;

3.   improvements in nutritional intake, eating habits, exercise, and other health-related activities;

4.   improved knowledge, attitudes, and norms regarding nutrition, weight, eating habits, and exercise;

5.   decreased rates of comorbidity problems (e.g., hypertension and diabetes); and

6.   public policy and environmental change indices (e.g., regulations concerning food labeling and label claims).

## Examples of Universal Prevention Programs

### Family-Based Programs

The family context can influence children's eating behavior and risk for obesity in several ways, including parental verbal prompts at mealtime, nonverbal influences such as food purchases and food presentation, modeling influences of adult eating behaviors, and use of food for nonnutritious purposes (Ray and Klesges, 1993). In one study, Pisacano et al. (1978) gave instruction in health education to parents of infants, emphasizing a low-fat, prudent diet. Compared with a usual-care control group, the prevalence of obesity was significantly reduced for intervention group children for a period ranging from 3 months to 3 years. Nader (1993) proposes that the family be an essential part of programs designed to prevent and treat obesity. An example of this type of program, in which overweight children are treated in the family context (Epstein et al., 1990b), is described later in this chapter in the section on indicated prevention.

### School-Based Programs

In a recent review of school-based obesity prevention programs, Resnicow (1993) emphasizes the importance of the school environment, pointing out that more than 95 percent of American youth aged 5–17 are enrolled in school and that children eat one to two meals per day there. Most school-based prevention programs include nutrition education and exercise components. Resnicow (1993) reviews six studies showing significant benefits of intervention. Other studies that evaluated the effects of physical education on childhood adiposity show less promise. In an evaluation of one such study, Project SPARK, Sallis et al. (1993) report that children did not significantly reduce their BMI or adiposity after 2 years of participating in a physical activity promotion program.

### Work-Site-Based Programs

After completing school, employed people spend more time at work than any other activity. Health-promotion programs at the work site provide access to large numbers of persons who can be reached at relatively low cost. Despite the promise of such programs, a general review of studies in this area is not encouraging. Work-site programs designed to control problems such as hypertension and smoking have been highly successful. By contrast, the results of weight-control programs at the work site have been consistently disappointing (Taylor and Stunkard, 1993).

## Community-Wide Programs

Another approach to preventing and reducing the prevalence of obesity is to focus on the entire population within a specified community. Community-based approaches to weight reduction are typically part of broader educational programs focused on cardiovascular risk reduction and helping individuals adopt a healthier lifestyle. The goal of such programs is to achieve at least small changes in most people who live in a particular geographic area. The results of four such projects have been reported: the Stanford Three-Community Study (Farquhar et al., 1977), Stanford Five-City Study (Farquhar et al., 1990), Minnesota Heart Health Program (Luepker et al., 1994), and North Karelia (Finland) Project (Puska et al., 1983).

All four programs were devoted to cardiovascular risk reduction and thus provided the opportunity to compare efforts to control obesity with those to control smoking, hypertension, and blood cholesterol concentrations. Obesity turned out to be far harder to control than the other coronary risk factors. In contrast to the reasonable effectiveness of the other risk-factor reduction efforts, no program interrupted the increase in the prevalence of obesity. The Minnesota and North Karelia projects showed no difference between the experimental and contrast communities in the rate of increase in obesity. In the Stanford Three Community Study, weight did not increase in the experimental community, while it rose 0.45 kg in the contrast community. In the Stanford Five-City Study, the comparable values were increases of 0.54 and 1.25 kg.

## Environmental-Change Programs

Any review of universal prevention methods would be incomplete without a brief description of environmental-change programs, some of which touch on public-policy issues. In this approach to universal prevention, the goal is to modify social and economic policies so as to reduce the population's exposure to environmental causes of obesity. Among the prevention strategies that have been proposed or implemented are (1) regulating the abuse potential of food products (e.g., specifying a maximum caloric density and fat or sugar content in processed foods); (2) regulating advertising and other promotional practices for food (e.g., controlling advertising of sugared cereals to children); and (3) modifying economic policies related to food (e.g., increasing excise taxes based on the fat and sugar content of food products). Environmental changes to encourage physical activity include the development of safe bicycle lanes in urban areas, as well as safe and inviting places to walk, and the provision of well-maintained stairwells as options to elevators. Unfortunately, little or no research has been conducted to document the effects of such changes, so the potential of environmental change from these and related public health approaches to modify individual behaviors remains unknown.

## SELECTIVE PREVENTION

High-risk subgroups may be distinguished by age, gender, occupation, family history, and other characteristics. The risk may be imminent or occur over a lifetime; risk groups are identified on the basis of biological, psychological, or social/cultural risk factors that are known to be associated with the onset of the disorder. Examples of interventions for target groups include annual mammograms for women with a positive family history of breast cancer, special immunizations (e.g., yellow fever) for groups who travel in high-risk areas where the disease is still prevalent, preschool programs for all children from poor neighborhoods, and support groups for elderly widows. Obesity prevention programs that target entire high-risk groups (e.g., black adolescent females, children of obese parents, and Native American children living in impoverished communities) meet the definition of selective prevention.

Selective prevention programs and policies are designed for groups at high risk for obesity or already overweight but not yet obese. Treatment programs for children diagnosed as obese are not included, since this represents treatment of an already developed condition (although it is recognized that the treatment of childhood obesity may affect that proportion of adult obesity that is carried over from childhood). Programs that target high-risk but still nonobese children or adolescents in order to develop lifetime behavioral patterns protecting against obesity would qualify.

Personal high-risk factors for obesity include predispositional factors at the individual level (e.g., family history of obesity or non-insulin-dependent diabetes mellitus and low resting metabolic rate), personal eating habits and physical activity (e.g., a high-fat diet coupled with a sedentary lifestyle), developmental periods associated with weight gain (e.g., early childhood, prepuberty, ages 25–34, and late adulthood), and critical life events (e.g., pregnancy and menopause). Other demographic risk factors include gender (women are heavier than men, particularly those with lower education and socioeconomic status) and minority status (e.g., overweight is more common in black and Hispanic females) (Sobal and Stunkard, 1989).

Many commercial weight-loss programs and diets are geared to the general population, including a majority of people who are overweight but not necessarily obese. Since studies show that even a relatively small loss of weight can provide health benefits (see Chapter 2), this large population of dieters may benefit from prevention-based programs (e.g., by developing a healthier lifestyle).

### Outcome Measures for Selective Prevention

Selective prevention has three outcome measures:

1. prevention of weight gain in high-risk individuals and groups;
2. decreased excessive dieting among dieters; and
3. improved lifestyle patterns (better nutrition, more exercise, and decreased eating disorders).

### Examples of Selective Prevention Programs

#### Programs That Target Overweight Adolescents in High-Risk Groups

Some school-based programs target populations that are at high risk for obesity. Examples include minority school populations such as Native American and Mexican-American school children. Davis et al. (1993b) describe a school-based program for Navajo and Pueblo children from rural elementary schools in New Mexico. Foreyt and Cousins (1993) describe school-based programs for Mexican-American children. Both studies are in progress and no results have been published.

#### Commercial Weight-Loss Programs and Diets

As described in Chapters 1 and 2, weight loss is big business. However, since not everyone who diets or attends a commercial program is obese, many overweight, nonobese people are involved in these programs. In the face of data showing high relapse rates in follow-ups of commercial diet programs, some programs now deemphasize fixed dietary weight-loss goals in favor of a more balanced, lifestyle-change program focusing, for example, on healthier eating habits, exercise, and maintenance of weight loss (see Table 3-1). These programs may be effective in the selective prevention of obesity among high-risk groups.

### INDICATED PREVENTION

In the past, indicated prevention has sometimes been referred to as *secondary prevention* or *early intervention*. With regard to obesity prevention, indicated preventive methods or programs can be designed for individuals (in contrast to entire groups, as in selective prevention) who show biological markers for obesity or who are already overweight but do not meet the diagnostic criteria for obesity. Risk factors for such individuals include a family history of obesity as well as biological markers and the development of early symptoms of the disorder. Although research is still in the preliminary stages of identifying reliable biological markers, programs that target individuals who are already overweight (or whose health risks are increased owing to their weight and/or a sedentary lifestyle) may prove effective.

### Outcome Measures for Indicated Prevention Programs

There are two outcome measures for indicated prevention programs:

1.   reduction in the number of obese people who go on to develop obesity-related comorbidities (e.g., reduced adult obesity among overweight children receiving intervention in childhood); and
2.   increase in the number of obese people who are successful in attaining and maintaining relatively small weight losses (e.g., 10 percent of initial body weight) and a decrease in the number who gain a small amount of weight (e.g., 2 kg).

### Examples of Indicated Prevention

Promising results have been reported by Epstein et al. (1990c). Although this study could also be considered a treatment program for obese children (since subjects had to be $\geq 20$ percent over ideal body weight for age, height, and sex), its goal was to prevent adult obesity. We include this study as an example because the same approach could be adopted with children who are overweight but not obese. In the study, Epstein and colleagues used a prospective, randomized design to examine the effects of behavioral, family-based treatment on percent overweight and growth over 10 years in obese 6- to 12-year-old children. Obese children with their parents were randomized to three groups that were provided similar diet, exercise, and behavior-management training, but differed in the way in which behavioral reinforcement was provided. In one group, both parent and child were reinforced; in the second only the child was reinforced. The third group was a nonspecific control group in which families were reinforced for attendance only. Children in the first group showed significantly greater decreases in percent overweight after 5 and 10 years (–11.2 and –7.5 percent, respectively) than children in the nonspecific control group (+7.9 and +14.3 percent, respectively). Results of children in the second group were midway between the other two groups, but not significantly different from either.

This study has been replicated in three additional randomized treatment studies designed to change the diet and exercise behaviors of obese children treated with behavioral family therapy (Epstein et al., 1994). Averaging across all four studies, Epstein and colleagues note that over a 10-year period, 34 percent of their subjects decreased their percent overweight by ≥20 percent, and 30 percent were no longer obese. The children did best when both they and their parents were targeted and reinforced for weight loss and when the children were treated with aerobic exercise and exercise was incorporated into their lifestyle. This 10-year success in the treatment of childhood obesity stands in marked contrast to the disappointing long-term results in treating adult obesity (Wilson, 1994a).

## CONCLUDING REMARKS

Many approaches to prevent obesity appear promising, though few studies are available to document long-term positive outcomes. Since success in prevention programs is often equated with the absence of future problems, the impact of universal prevention programs that target education and behavior change (e.g., in diet or exercise patterns) is difficult to evaluate except through longitudinal population studies. The recent literature in prevention has focused more on working with groups or individuals who are known to be at risk for a particular disorder. The emphasis on working with high-risk individuals with interventions that are matched or targeted to specific risk factors (as in selective and indicated prevention strategies) appears to have considerable merit. Only a few studies of this type have been conducted in obesity prevention. Future research on the development of prevention programs targeted to those at high risk for obesity is necessary before any conclusions can be drawn concerning this promising new approach.

# 10

## Research and Policy
## Recommendations

There is an epidemic of obesity in the United States among both adults and children that shows no signs of abating. In Chapter 2, we estimate the economic costs of obesity to exceed $100 billion per year, counting the costs of illness resulting from this disease and the money spent on weight-reduction products and services. Given that obesity is one of the most important public health problems, it is perhaps both surprising and unfortunate that the causes of obesity and its management remain poorly understood and that research into preventing and treating it has not yielded more promising results. The National Institutes of Health (NIH) spent approximately $35 million in fiscal year 1992 on direct research in obesity, representing about 10 percent of total NIH obligations in biomedical nutrition research and training that year, or 0.4 percent of total NIH research and training expenditures (NIH, 1994). Given the magnitude of the problem of obesity in this country, we agree with a recent recommendation of the National Task Force on Prevention and Treatment of Obesity of NIH to double the current NIH expenditures on direct obesity research in real dollars over the next five years (NTF, 1994a).

Several publications have provided well-considered recommendations for further research to better understand, prevent, and treat obesity. These include *The Surgeon General's Report on Nutrition and Health* (DHHS, 1988), the National Academy of Sciences report *Diet and Health* (NRC, 1989a), and *Opportunities in the Nutrition and Food Sciences* by the Institute of Medicine (IOM, 1993). Most recently, the National Task Force on Prevention and Treatment of Obesity of NIH has published a comprehensive report on research needs in obesity (NTF, 1994a). The report presents research recommendations in the following areas: genetic and environmental determinants of obesity, the role of obesity in the pathogenesis of chronic diseases, treatment of obesity, prevention of obesity, and communicating research findings to the lay public and health-care providers. The interested reader should refer to these publications, which, taken together, set forth a comprehensive set of needs in obesity research. The research and policy recommendations discussed below are focused more directly on the contents of this report.

## CAUSES OF OBESITY AND ASSOCIATED COMORBIDITIES

One of the more perplexing aspects of obesity treatment is why the vast majority of individuals are largely unsuccessful at long-term management of their weight. We believe that it is because the symptoms of obesity are treated rather than its fundamental causes. It is clear that obesity in many individuals involves an interaction between genes and the environment. Until the fundamental causes of this disease with multiple etiologies are understood—its pathophysiology and development at the genetic, molecular, and cellular levels and its interactions with relevant environmental factors—obesity will be extremely difficult to prevent and cure.

An analogy that may prove helpful is that of the evolution of therapy for cystic fibrosis (CF). The treatment of this debilitating disease has traditionally focused on relieving the symptoms (i.e., the pulmonary infections), improving bronchial draining, and improving nutrition. Though conventional treatments have improved incrementally over time, they provide only short-term improvements in the quality and quantity of life, and more than 90 percent of individuals with CF die at an average age of 29 years (Fuchs et al., 1994). Recent genetic and molecular studies on CF have uncovered the structural defects that lead to pathogenesis. For example, it was discovered that the accumulation of secretions that block the airways is a result of the release of extracellular DNA by leukocytes. In addition, advances in molecular genetics have led to an understanding of the fundamental genetic defect in CF to the extent that gene-replacement therapy is being studied (Zabner et al., 1993). One of the clinical benefits to date of this research into the molecular and genetic underpinnings of CF has been the development of aerosolized recombinant human DNAse, which is now used to make the secretions easier to expectorate (Davis, 1994; Fuchs et al., 1994).

Using the exciting tools of biotechnology to prevent or cure obesity is undoubtedly distant. However, some tools already exist that can be applied to understanding the causes, pathophysiology, and development of obesity at the genetic, molecular, and cellular levels. Research approaches to identify and assess the multigenic components of obesity include the use of animal models and, in humans, studying twins and families. Further characterization of the human genome should aid in identification of the genetic components of human obesity, particularly as variable phenotypic expressions of obesity are better delineated. Special emphasis should be placed on obtaining a fundamental understanding of the events that contribute to the development of comorbidities. This understanding can ultimately be applied to the development of more effective treatment strategies, including more effective drugs designed to modify specific defects.

Much also remains to be learned about the behavioral and environmental influences on the expression of obesity. The fact that genetic and environmental determinants of obesity vary among population groups makes this variation and the reasons for it important areas of research.

## TREATMENT OF OBESITY AND MAINTENANCE OF WEIGHT LOSS

There is general agreement that the basic elements of obesity treatment should include self-monitoring, goal setting, exercise, nutrition education, stress management, and social support. However, there is a great need for research in these areas. Among them, though not listed in any priority order, are the following:

- Determine the physiological, biochemical, molecular, and behavioral mechanisms by which antiobesity drugs and gastric surgery promote long-term weight loss.
- Determine whether a gradual fat-reduction method is more effective than restrictive dieting for long-term weight maintenance and improvement in health.
- Uncover the physiological and psychological mechanisms responsible for loss and regain of eating control (e.g., avoidance of excessive restrictions and binges) with various eating patterns.
- Show how counselors may be more successful at persuading and empowering those individuals focused on becoming thin to set realistic goal weights for themselves and become more focused on improving their dietary patterns and level of fitness.
- Identify the period of attendance required to produce group cohesion and effective peer-support networks. Because longer treatments have produced greater weight losses, there is a need to discover optimal

treatment length and methods, while taking cost effectiveness into account.

• Determine factors that can predict an individual's success with different types of diet and activity interventions.

• Identify program components that constitute successful weight maintenance through diet and activity without inducing undesirable consequences (e.g., harm to psychological well-being and overcompensation).

• Explore the use of self-help groups to enhance and maintain long-term healthy eating and exercise behaviors.

• Understand the development or etiological significance of eating disorders in obese individuals.

• Define the determinants of physical activity and healthy dietary patterns and how to initiate and maintain them in various population subgroups.

• Determine the effects of various environmental and situational factors on food selection and the initiation of physical activity. Are individuals who exercise more or less likely to be sedentary the rest of the day?

• Understand temporal trends in natural weight changes and develop strategies for individuals to identify, desire, achieve, and maintain healthy weights.

• Describe the long-term effects of various eating patterns (e.g., meals versus snacks and night eating) as they might affect the development of obesity.

• Determine how nutrients and activity patterns may affect genetic potential in regard to fat distribution patterns, eating habits, and food cravings.

• Elucidate the roles of diet and activity in the prevention of weight gain.

• Investigate the relative importance of how one loses weight (e.g., through diet or a combination of methods) to the risk of obesity-related diseases.

• Study whether rate of weight loss affects one's ability to keep weight off in the long run and whether it is easier to maintain lower or higher levels of weight loss.

• Investigate how individuals make decisions about which weight-loss method or program to select and which to reject.

## PREVENTION OF OBESITY

The prevention of obesity should be given a high priority in any rational system of health care. However, given the very limited success of efforts at prevention, the pressing need is for more research. We consider the prevention of obesity from the point of view of (1) preventing obesity from occurring, (2) preventing weight gain following weight reduction, and (3) preventing further weight gain among obese persons who cannot lose weight. Of these three, a large amount of research has been devoted to item 2 with, as yet, disappointing results. This research has been conducted within the framework of treatment. It will undoubtedly continue within this framework and thus is less relevant in terms of prevention than the other two items.

Preventing obesity from occurring is, of course, highly desirable and often the object of enthusiastic advocacy. It is therefore important to keep in mind the disappointing results of universal prevention as shown in the carefully conducted community risk-factor-reduction trials (see Chapter 9). It may be that more tightly focused programs of prevention will be more effective. Such programs might reasonably be focused on a particular stage in life (e.g., childhood, adolescence, early middle age, or pregnancy), on particular locations (e.g., school, work site, or community center), or on special circumstances (e.g., smoking cessation or pregnancy). The prevention of further weight gain in persons who cannot lose weight is an area that has been largely neglected in the past and one that could conceivably yield substantial health benefits.

Additional research needs in the area of obesity prevention are as follows:

- Studies are needed to assess the usefulness of medication(s), including combinations of drugs, in the prevention of both further weight gain and regain of weight following treatment. Recent studies of long-term use of medication, refuting the belief that tolerance develops to its effects, clear the way for more aggressive use of this therapy.
- Studies should be designed to assess the applicability of a "harm-reduction" approach to prevention. Developed originally as an approach to substance abuse prevention and treatment (Marlatt and Tapert, 1993; Marlatt et al., 1993), harm reduction is based on a continuum model, with incremental changes encouraged (e.g., encouragement of proximal goals of gradual weight loss over time in contrast to traditional programs with their emphasis on distal goals of ideal weight loss). The harm-reduction model is consistent with a stepped-care approach that begins with the least intensive intervention before proceeding to more intensive and expensive steps.
- Studies are needed that compare the impact of prevention programs designed for specific weight-loss goals with others designed to (1) affect personal beliefs in ideal body image, (2) decrease reliance on exag-

gerated dietary behaviors, and (3) treat associated eating disorders (e.g., binge and purge cycling).

• Studies should be conducted to investigate the effects of prevention programs representing either (1) individual clinic-based intervention programs designed to modify personal behavior; (2) community-based public health programs, including public policy and regulatory policy change; or (3) a combination of both clinical and public health approaches.

• Research on unaided weight management is necessary, for example, natural-history studies of formerly obese people who learned to manage their weight successfully by themselves and investigations of people who are at risk for obesity but who nonetheless maintain healthy weights. We recommend that, where possible, such long-term studies be included as part of ongoing long-term clinical and observational trials (e.g., the NIH Women's Health Initiative).

## POLICY RECOMMENDATIONS

While we are optimistic that research will eventually uncover the causes of obesity and lead to better management, prevention, and treatment of this disease, the application of scientific findings alone is rarely enough to resolve public health problems. Public policies are needed to translate the research findings into usable information for the public and health-care providers and to create an environment that encourages the attainment and maintenance of healthy weight, healthful dietary patterns, and regular physical activity.

As described throughout this report, obesity is a major public health problem and is arguably the main nutritional and metabolic disease in this country. However, scientists are quite ignorant about the causes of obesity as well as its prevention and treatment. Therefore, it is best that priority be given to research to understand its causes, rather than spending substantial amounts of money on major new large-scale efforts to prevent and treat this disease given the inadequate tools we have at present.

Our first policy recommendation is that there be a change in thinking in this country by the public and health-care providers alike to treat obesity as an important chronic, degenerative disease that debilitates individuals and kills prematurely. Obesity is a disease that has fundamental genetic and cellular components as well as social and behavioral components. Recognizing obesity as one of this country's most important nutrition-related diseases has important consequences for the funding of research by government, foundations, and private agencies; for health-care reform; and for oversight of the weight-loss industry by regulatory agencies.

Our second policy recommendation concerns the need for increased recognition and support for research in genetics and molecular and cellular biology to aid in understanding the causes of obesity and its associated comorbidities. Research in these areas should be greatly expanded to take advantage of the new knowledge and techniques in molecular genetics and cell physiology that are contributing to substantial advances in the treatment of numerous other diseases. Expanding and coordinating this important research effort will require a greater organizational emphasis both within NIH itself and in other agencies. Developing a research work force that can make the necessary discoveries and applications is going to require careful reevaluation of current training patterns and enhancement of training with a very strong interdisciplinary flavor. Research into the causes and, ultimately, the prevention of obesity requires people trained in the basic sciences as well as dietetics and the social sciences.

Our third policy recommendation is that there be developed a more aggressive policy of informing the public and health-care providers about the nature of obesity, the difficulties inherent in treating this disease, and the need for susceptible individuals to take steps to prevent its occurrence or minimize its development. The techniques to be utilized are those suggested for informing the public of methods to be used in the evaluation of obesity treatment (Chapter 8). Health-care providers could be encouraged to discuss obesity with their obese clients and with those who are beginning to gain excess weight. What is needed are simple messages and communications between the provider and the person at the very early stages of weight gain as well as when the person is obese.

Other important policy recommendations include the following:

• One set of definitions and standards should be developed for defining and measuring obesity. The current variation in terminology used to describe excess weight leads to difficulties in identifying precisely the extent of obesity and in trying to compare the results of different studies. Not only are terms such as *overweight* and *obesity* used interchangeably, there is considerable disagreement concerning how to identify those at increased risk from excess weight. Disagreement also exists about the body mass index (BMI) cutoff between a "healthy" and an "unhealthy" weight.

• To enable more individuals who would like to lose weight to take advantage of the many programs that currently exist, study is needed on payment models and how cost affects the entry of people into programs, their participation in them, and the long-term outcomes for the participants. As this country debates health-care reform, attention should be paid to reimbursement mechanisms for nutrition services generally and for obesity treatment programs—certainly the clinical programs and some of the appropriate nonclinical programs as well.

•   Initiatives should be developed that will motivate more people to become physically active. While physical activity enhances health and helps to prevent and treat obesity, people must believe they can fit it into their lives and think of it as an enjoyable way to spend time before they will make the effort. To encourage activity, communities should consider developing innovative social-marketing campaigns, more safe and well-lighted walking and bicycle paths and playgrounds, and low- or no-cost recreation centers supporting a variety of activities. At the national level, the U.S. Public Health Service should continue to expand its efforts to become a more visible advocate of the pleasures and health benefits of an active lifestyle, particularly to children, adolescents, the elderly, and those in lower socioeconomic groups.

•   Investigations should be conducted to determine what methods are most likely to be productive in increasing physician training in the management of obesity.

•   The potential impacts of modifying health insurance reimbursement systems on the treatment and long-term management of obesity should be examined.

### CONCLUDING REMARKS

The epidemic of obesity in the United States is increasing at a cost to this country of more than $100 billion per year, yet research to understand the causes of this disease and how to more effectively prevent and treat it is seriously underfunded. This chapter has identified some important research needs that offer the hope of substantially reducing the prevalence of this important public health problem, thereby decreasing health-care costs and improving the overall health of the U.S. population. We urge NIH in particular to increase its funding of investigator-initiated research to answer fundamental questions, such as those presented in this chapter, pertaining to the treatment and prevention of obesity.

# Appendixes

# A

Assessment Instruments of
Relevance to Obesity
Treatment

$\mathbf{A}$ppendix A discusses instruments assessing psychological and behavioral factors, diet, and physical activity. Most of these
instruments are not meant to be used in weight-management programs
because they are impractical for such purposes or are geared towards use
in clinical and field settings by researchers familiar with their proper
administration. In particular, the wide variety of assessment instruments
for psychological and behavioral factors and for physical activity are published here for the first time. As researchers and policy developers work
towards providing weight-management programs with more practical
tools to assess the psychosocial health, diet, and activity patterns of their
clients and potential clients, the tools presented here should provide a
useful starting point.

## ASSESSING PSYCHOSOCIAL AND BEHAVIORAL
## ASPECTS OF OBESITY AND WEIGHT LOSS

Regardless of the genetic and environmental factors that cause obesity, the psychological significance of this disease is important. Obese
individuals who join comprehensive weight-loss programs experience
major physiological changes, undertake major changes in lifestyle, and
attempt to curtail a strongly appetitive behavior. Therefore, the psychological consequences of dieting and weight loss are important to examine
(O'Neil and Jarrell, 1992). This section of Appendix A describes assessment instruments used in the related areas of obesity and psychopathol-

ogy, behavioral factors in dieting, and psychological effects of dieting and weight regain. These instruments are for use by health-care providers with appropriate training in psychometric assessment and familiarity with a particular test being administered.

## Obesity and Psychopathology

For many years, obesity was considered a disorder with pronounced psychological underpinnings. The obese were considered to overeat in response to negative feelings such as insecurity, sadness, and frustration, or more particularly because of their inability to establish positive interpersonal relationships. More recently this traditional view has changed dramatically on the basis of new research findings. If obesity were caused by psychological dysfunction, one would expect to find a higher incidence of psychopathology among obese individuals compared to nonobese controls. Population-based studies have not found this to be the case (Wadden and Stunkard, 1985). These results do not show that obese patients have greater problems than any other medical or surgical patients. In addition, there do not appear to be personality characteristics unique to obese individuals (Leon and Roth, 1977).

Rather than a cause, psychopathology in the obese is now seen as a consequence of the prejudice and discrimination they face because of their weight (Wadden and Stunkard, 1993). This social stigmatization and discrimination experienced by obese individuals often leads to negative self-esteem and an unfavorable body image. Although enhanced self-esteem and a more positive body image may result from weight loss, these same factors may keep some people from entering treatment in the first place. Thus, two general psychological factors appear to be important in the assessment of obese individuals before treatment: self-esteem and body image.

### Self-Esteem

In one longitudinal study of obese and nonobese children, Klesges (in press) reported that physical self-esteem was consistently related to the development of obesity, although it accounted for less than 5 percent of the variance in changes in body fat. Wadden and Foster (1992) note that feelings of guilt and shame over one's inability to control weight are likely to diminish the self-esteem of some obese persons. Patients losing weight, on the other hand, often display increased self-confidence and self-esteem. According to O'Neil and Jarrell (1992), increased self-esteem and reduced social discrimination may lead to more assertiveness and optimism and a willingness to make other life changes, even those that involve some personal risk. Two measures of self-esteem include the Tennessee Self-Concept Scale and the Rosenberg Self-Esteem Scale. One measure of well-being is the Well-Being General Schedule.

Tennessee Self-Concept Scale   This scale is self-administered and contains 100 items, each of which is rated on a 5-point Likert scale ranging from "completely false" to "completely true" (Fitts, 1964). It measures three internal dimensions (Identity, Self-Satisfaction, and Behavior) and five external dimensions (Physical Self, Moral-Ethical Self, Personal Self, Family Self, and Social Self) of self-concept. This scale takes about 25 minutes to complete. Reliability coefficients range from 0.66 to 0.94. Test-retest reliabilities are reported from 0.60 to 0.92. Concerning validity, correlations with the Coopersmith Self-Esteem Inventory range between 0.64 and 0.75 (Archaumbault, 1992; Dowd, 1992).

Rosenberg Self-Esteem Scale   The Rosenberg Scale provides a global measure of self-esteem (Goldman and Osborne, 1985; Rosenberg, 1965, 1979). Subjects indicate their agreement with statements about their perceived worth and confidence. The scale consists of 10 items, each of which is rated on a 4-point Likert scale ranging from "strongly agree" to "strongly disagree." The reliability coefficient alpha has been reported at 0.75, with a test-retest reliability of 0.85 (Goldman and Mitchell, 1990).

General Well-Being Schedule   This schedule measures subjective well-being and distress in the previous month (McDowell and Newell, 1987; NCHS, 1977). The self-report scale assesses how the subject feels about his inner personal state rather than about external conditions. The six dimensions covered are Anxiety, Depression, General Health, Positive Well-Being, Self-Control, and Vitality. The scale consists of 18 items. Fourteen items have 6-point responses that vary by item content; four items on different feeling dimensions have an 11-point response format. Higher scores indicate that the person does not have a sense of well-being. The reliability alpha coefficient ranges from 0.91 to 0.95. Test-retest reliability coefficients range from 0.68 to 0.85. Correlations among the subscale dimensions range from 0.16 to 0.72. The scale also shows good correlational validity with interviewer's ratings of depression and other depression and anxiety scales (Fazio, 1977). See Appendix B for the full test.

### Body Image

Some obese people suffer intense negative feelings about their bodies. Stunkard and Mendelson (1967) point to a pattern sometimes found in childhood or adolescent obesity in which subjects view their bodies as grotesque or loathsome, believing that others look at them with horror and contempt. The problem of body image disparagement is particularly striking in young Caucasian women of upper-middle socioeconomic status, in which the prevalence of obesity is very low but the sanctions against it are very high (Sobal and Stunkard, 1989). Body image represents the cognitive perception of one's body size and appearance along with the emotional response to these perceptions. Four measures of body image include the Body-Cathexis and Self-Cathexis Scale, Body Satisfaction Scale, Body Shape Questionnaire, and the Body Parts Satisfaction Scale.

*Body-Cathexis and Self-Cathexis Scale*   This is a self-administered scale that consists of two parts (Secord and Jourard, 1953). The first asks subjects to rate 46 body parts and functions on a 5-point scale ranging from "Have strong feelings and wish change could somehow be made" to "Consider myself fortunate." The second part concerns self cathexis and lists 55 items that represent conceptual aspects of the self, which are rated on the same scale as the first part. Three scores are obtained: Total Body Cathexis (BC), Total Self Cathexis (SC), and an Anxiety Indicator score based on the BC items most negatively perceived by each sex. Reliability on the BC is given at 0.81, on the SC at 0.90, and on the Anxiety Indicator at 0.72. Intercorrelations between the BC and SC scores are significant, and the scale as a whole has been shown to be a stable measure, with a test-retest reliability coefficient of 0.87 (Tucker, 1981).

*Body Satisfaction Scale*   The Body Satisfaction Scale (Slade et al., 1990) is based on the Body Cathexis Scale (Secord and Jourard, 1953). This simple self-administered scale assesses satisfaction/dissatisfaction with 16 body parts and is sensitive to eating disorders and obesity. The items are rated on a 7-point scale ranging from "very satisfied" to "very unsatisfied." Higher ratings indicate greater body dissatisfaction. Three summative scales (General, Head Parts [above the neck], and Body Parts [below the head]) are derived from the scale. It takes 2–3 minutes to complete. Internal consistency alpha coefficients for the three summative scales range from 0.79 to 0.89. The Body Satisfaction Scale has been shown to correlate positively with the Body Shape Questionnaire (Cooper et al., 1987).

*Body Shape Questionnaire*   This questionnaire is a self-report instrument that measures concerns about body shape, particularly the experience of feeling fat (Cooper et al., 1987). A total score is calculated from its 34 items, which are rated on a 6-point Likert scale ranging from "never" to "always." The scale refers to the subject's state over the previous four weeks. The questionnaire is simple to complete (about 10 minutes). Both concurrent and discriminant validity have been shown to be good.

Body Parts Satisfaction Scale This scale, which assesses satisfaction with the body, consists of 24 items on body parts as well as an overall appearance item (Berscheid et al., 1973). The items are rated on a 6-point Likert scale from "extremely dissatisfied" to "extremely satisfied." The reliability alpha coefficient has been reported as 0.89 (Noles et al., 1985).

### Behavioral Factors in Dieting

Disordered eating behavior is sometimes associated with dieting and weight loss. Although no evidence supports an "obese eating style" (O'Neil and Jarrell, 1992), there is increasing evidence to suggest that dieting may increase the incidence of eating disorders, particularly binge eating. First identified by Stunkard (1959), binge eating is characterized by eating a large amount of food in a short period of time, followed by severe discomfort and self-condemnation. Binge eating appears to be prevalent among the obese: estimates among obese individuals seeking treatment range from 23 percent to 82 percent (Loro and Orleans, 1981). We describe seven different measures of disordered eating (Eating Disorders Inventory, Eating Inventory/Three-Factor Eating Questionnaire, Eating Attitudes Test, Eating Disorder Examination, Questionnaire on Eating and Weight Patterns, and the Stanford Eating Behavior Questionnaire), including one designed specifically to assess binge eating (Binge Eating Scale).

Eating Disorders Inventory The Eating Disorders Inventory (Garner, 1991) is a 64-item self-report test to measure cognitive and behavioral characteristics of anorexia and bulimia nervosa. It consists of eight subscales: Drive for Thinness, Bulimia, Body Dissatisfaction, Ineffectiveness, Perfectionism, Interpersonal Distrust, Interceptive Awareness, and Maturity Fears. The items are rated on a 6-point scale from "always" to "never," and subscale scores are the total of all item scores for that particular subscale. Reliability coefficients for the subscales range from 0.65 to 0.91, and convergent and discriminant validity are established in subjects with anorexia and bulimia. The validity of the scale in an obese population has not been established, but it may help to identify characteristics associated with binge eating in the obese (Lowe and Caputo, 1991).

Eating Inventory/Three-Factor Eating Questionnaire This self-report questionnaire yields three dimensions of eating behavior: cognitive control of eating behavior, disinhibition of control, and susceptibility to hunger (Stunkard and Messick, 1985). The questionnaire is divided into two parts, with the first consisting of 36 true-false items and the second consisting of 15 rated items. The Eating Inventory takes approximately 15 minutes to complete. Reliability alpha coefficients for the three factors range from 0.85 to 0.93.

*Eating Attitudes Test (EAT)*  The EAT (Garner and Garfinkel, 1979; Garner et al., 1982) is available as both a 40-item and 26-item measure of the symptoms of eating disorders. It can be used to identify subjects who are experiencing abnormal eating patterns that interfere with normal psychosocial functioning. The multifactorial 26-item, 6-point Likert scale correlates highly with the original 40-item scale ($r = 0.98$). Three factors, or clusters of items, arise from the EAT: Dieting (avoidance of fattening foods and preoccupations with shape), Bulimia and Food Preoccupation, and Oral Control (items reflecting self-control about food and social pressure regarding weight). Reliability correlation alpha for the EAT-26 is 0.90. The EAT displays acceptable criterion-related validity.

*Eating Disorder Examination (EDE)*  The EDE (Cooper and Fairburn, 1987) is a 62-item semistructured clinical interview for assessing the specific psychopathology of eating disorders, including concerns about shape and weight. The exam is designed to assess the present state of patients, and all questions refer to the previous four-week period of time. Each item has at least one mandatory probe question and optional subsidiary questions. Most ratings are made on a 7-point scale, either in terms of severity or in terms of frequency of occurrence at a defined level of severity. The interview takes between 30 minutes and one hour to complete. Interrater reliability of all EDE items is uniformly high. The interview is not intended for use as a diagnostic instrument but as a research measure providing a comprehensive profile of the characteristic psychopathological features of patients with eating disorders.

*Questionnaire on Eating and Weight Patterns (QEWP)*  The QEWP was developed to assess binge eating disorder in large study groups and was used in two multisite field trials establishing the prevalence of binge eating disorder (Spitzer et al., 1992, 1993). The questionnaire contains items regarding demographics, frequency and duration of binge eating, compensatory behaviors for weight control, degree of distress regarding binge eating, and the presence of accompanying behavioral indicators of loss of control. All questions about current functioning and eating behavior focus on the previous six months. Higher scores on the GEWP are correlated with binge eating and a higher prevalence of psychiatric comorbidity (Yanovski et al., 1992, 1993).

*Stanford Eating Behavior Questionnaire*  This is an extensive self-report questionnaire used to collect information on subjects' demographics, weight history, eating patterns, medical history, psychiatric history, and family history (Agras, 1987). It also contains 10 items that specifically address binge eating behavior.

*Binge Eating Scale*  This scale is a 16-item, self-report questionnaire that identifies individuals with a spectrum of binge eating difficulties (Gormally et al., 1982). The scale describes both behavioral manifestations (e.g., eating large amounts of food) and feelings surrounding a binge episode (e.g., guilt, fear of being unable to control what or how much one is eating). It is scored by summing the individual weights for each item, with high scores indicating more severe binge-eating problems. The scale is useful in distinguishing levels of binge-eating severity and appears to have high internal consistency. It also correlates well with clinical interviews for diagnosing disordered eating behaviors.

### Psychological Effects of Dieting

Psychological factors contribute to dieting behavior in several ways. First, variables such as dieting readiness and self-efficacy may be important in terms of whether or not an obese individual will seek treatment to lose weight. Second, dieting itself may affect mood, and mood in turn may influence dieting efforts. Third, factors such as stress and social support may have an impact on dieting behavior. Finally, dieting programs should also affect the participant's cognitive knowledge base about obesity, nutrition, exercise, and the pros and cons of dieting.

### Dieting Readiness and Self-Efficacy

Scales have been developed to assess a patient's readiness for embarking on a weight-loss program; they assess items such as goals and attitudes, exercise patterns and attitudes, and hunger and eating cues. One scale, the Restraint Scale, has been proposed as a measure of unsuccessful attempts at dieting (Herman and Polivy, 1984). It is a 10-item scale that addresses two factors, weight fluctuation and dietary restraint (the latter concept first proposed by Herman and Mack [1975]). A more widely used measure of readiness for dieting is the Dieting Readiness Scale described below.

Self-efficacy is a concept closely related to diet readiness. It refers to an individual's subjective estimate of his or her ability or capacity to engage in specific dieting behaviors and exercise, or to cope with high-risk situations for relapse or weight regain. Such measures are important for measuring change over treatment (e.g., does treatment enhance self-efficacy and thereby increase success at long-term weight loss?) and to implement treatment matching or relapse prevention. Five measures of self-efficacy for eating behaviors and exercise are the Dieter's Inventory of Eating Temptations, Self-Efficacy for Eating Behaviors Scale, Self-Efficacy for Exercise Behaviors Scale, Physical Self-Efficacy Scale, and the Exercise Specific Self-Efficacy Scale.

*Dieting Readiness Scale*  This scale assesses whether a person is prepared to undertake a diet at the point when they decide to begin a new attempt at weight loss (Brownell, 1990). The scale is divided into six sections that assess attitudes toward weight loss: Goals and Attitudes, Hunger and Eating Cues, Control Over Eating, Binge Eating and Purging, Emotional Eating, and Exercise Patterns and Attitudes. Each section contains its own questions, which are rated on a 5-point Likert scale, and its own scoring key. Since each section is scored separately, the individual sections may help subjects identify strengths and weaknesses in their weight-loss attitudes that could affect success. Because the scale is fairly new, reliability and validity have not been established. See Appendix B for the full test.

*Dieter's Inventory of Eating Temptations (DIET)*  This self-report inventory is designed to assess behavioral competence in six situations related to weight control: Overeating, Negative Emotions, Exercise, Resisting Temptation, Positive Social, and Food Choice (Schlundt and Zimering, 1988). Low competence in these situations indicates a lack of self-control. Obese subjects rate themselves as less competent than normal-weight subjects in the overeating, negative emotions, and exercise situations. The inventory correlates with self-reported eating and control behaviors. Reliability coefficient alphas for the six DIET scales range from 0.68 to 0.93. Test-retest reliability correlations for the scales range from 0.81 to 0.96.

*Self-Efficacy for Eating Behaviors Scale*  This scale consists of 89 items and asks the subject to "please rate how confident you are that you could really motivate yourself to do things like these consistently, for at least six months" (Sallis et al., 1987). Ratings are made on a 5-point Likert scale, with responses ranging from "Sure I could not do it" to "Sure I could do it," with a response option for "does not apply." The scale has five subscales: Resisting Relapse, Reducing Calories, Reducing Salt, Reducing Fat, and Behavioral Skills. The alpha coefficients for internal consistency on the subscales range from 0.85 to 0.93. Test-retest reliabilities ranged from 0.43 to 0.64. All self-efficacy for eating factors are correlated significantly with reported "heart-healthy" health habits.

**Self-Efficacy for Exercise Behaviors Scale** The scale consists of 49 items and asks the subject to "please rate how confident you are that you could really motivate yourself to do things like these consistently, for at least six months" (Sallis et al., 1987). Ratings are made on a 5-point Likert scale, with responses ranging from "Sure I could not do it" to "Sure I could do it," with a response option for "does not apply." The scale has two subscales: Resisting Relapse and Making Time for Exercise. The alpha coefficients for internal consistency on the subscales range from 0.83 to 0.85. Test-retest reliability is 0.68 for both subscales. Both exercise self-efficacy factors are correlated significantly with reported participation in vigorous activity.

**Physical Self-Efficacy Scale** The Physical Self-Efficacy Scale consists of a 10-item Perceived Physical Ability (PPA) subscale and a 12-item Physical Self-Presentation Confidence (PSPC) subscale (Ryckman et al., 1982). Higher scores on the PPA indicate higher perceived physical ability, and higher scores on the PSPC reflect greater confidence in presentation of physical skills. The scores on the two subscales can be summed into an overall Physical Self-Efficacy (PSE) score. Higher values on the PSE indicate a stronger sense of physical self-efficacy. Reliability alphas are 0.84 for the PPA, 0.74 for the PSPC, and 0.81 for the PSE. Test-retest reliability and convergent, concurrent, discriminant, and predictive validity on the PSE and its subscales are good.

**Exercise Specific Self-Efficacy Scale** This scale assesses perceived capabilities to exercise three times per week in the face of barriers to participation (McAuley, 1992; McAuley and Jacobson, 1991). These barriers were determined through an attributional analysis of reasons for dropping out of exercise. Sample items include the subjects' belief in ability to exercise regularly if they failed to make progress quickly enough, exercise conflicting with other activities such as work, being bored with the exercise activity, and feeling self-conscious about their appearance. The reliability alpha coefficient for the scale is 0.88. The scale helps to identify possible psychological mechanisms influencing the adoption and maintenance of exercise behavior.

### Dieting and Mood

Although one early review examining mood changes during weight reduction noted a high incidence of negative emotional responses

(Stunkard and Rush, 1974), more recent reviews (Wing et al., 1984) do not find increases in measures of depression or anxiety as a result of weight loss. Perhaps this is because later studies are often more group-oriented and provide emotional buffers or social support. Nonetheless, some patients may experience problem mood states, such as depression, that need to be assessed. Although few studies have examined the psychological consequences of regaining weight, Brownell and Stunkard (1981) found that although patients' depression scores decreased as they lost weight, depression levels rose for those patients who regained weight during a one-year follow-up period. The Beck Depression Inventory and the Hamilton Psychiatric Rating Scale for Depression are two frequently used measures of depression.

Beck Depression Inventory (BDI)  BDI is used to detect possible depression and to assess its severity (Beck et al., 1961, 1988). It measures cognitive, affective, somatic, and performance-related symptoms of depression. BDI can be self-administered or administered orally and takes 5–15 minutes to complete. The scale consists of a total score of 21 items, or sets of statements, answered on a 0-to-3 scale of severity of depressive problems. The possible score range is from 0 to 63, with higher scores indicating greater severity of depression. The subject is asked to consider feelings in the last week. The internal consistency coefficient alpha for the BDI ranges from 0.73 to 0.95. Test-retest correlations range from 0.48 to 0.86. Discriminant validity has been reported to be fairly strong, and the scale has been shown to correlate well with biological and somatological issues, suicidal behaviors, alcoholism, adjustment, and life crisis. Concurrent validity studies show correlations between 0.60 and 0.76 with clinical ratings and other depression scales (Conoley, 1992; Sundberg, 1992).

Hamilton Psychiatric Rating Scale for Depression  This scale consists of 17 items presented by an interviewer in a semistructured interview (Hamilton, 1960). Items are scored 0–2 or 0–4 to reflect increasing severity of the symptom. Scores are totaled, and higher scores indicate more severe depression. Inter-rater reliability has ranged between 0.80 and 0.90 (Goldman and Mitchell, 1990).

### Stress and Social Support

Untoward life events often have a substantial impact on obese patients' psychosocial functioning and their ability to control weight. Such events include loss of a family member and work, financial, or health problems. Four examples of measures designed to assess major life events and social readjustment are the Social Readjustment Rating Scale, Life

Experiences Survey, Recent Life Changes Questionnaire, and the Life Events Checklist.

*Social Readjustment Rating Scale* This is a self-administered scale that rates the number, type, and magnitude of stressful life events and determines relationships between life stress and indices of health and adjustment (Holmes and Rahe, 1967). Each of the 43 items was constructed to contain life events whose occurrence either indicates or requires a major change in the life pattern of the individual.

*Life Experiences Survey* This survey (Heilbrun, 1984; Johnson and Sarason, 1979) evolved from the Social Readjustment Rating Scale but offers two new features. It allows for separate positive and negative stress scores and requires the subject to rate the degree of impact of any relevant event on a 4-point scale from "no impact" to "extremely negative or positive." The survey includes 57 items: 47 specific events for all respondents and 10 items designed primarily for students. The scale inquires about events experienced during the previous year. The negative stress score is the sum of ratings for all events identified as involving undesirable stress. The positive stress score is calculated in the same way for events perceived as having positive impact. Test-retest correlations show moderate reliability (0.56 to 0.88) for the negative stress score but lower reliability (0.19 to 0.53) for the positive stress score.

*Recent Life Changes Questionnaire* This questionnaire is a 55-item scale that provides a method of measuring life change (Rahe, 1975). The questionnaire includes the five categories of Health, Work, Home and Family, Personal-Social, and Financial. Subjects indicate whether they experienced various life changes over the previous two years and when these changes occurred. Reliability has been given as 0.84 and correlation with a schedule of recent experiences was 0.67 (Goldman and Mitchell, 1990).

*Life Events Checklist* The Life Events Checklist (Bhagat et al., 1985) measures total life stress. It consists of 83 items, and subjects use a 7-point scale from –3 to +3 to rate the degree of positive or negative impact that each event had on their life in the previous three years. Seventy-eight events are listed on the scale, and five items are left blank so that the subject can fill in unique events not included in the checklist. The areas covered by the checklist include work, finances, legal matters, social activities, residence, children, family, health, love, and marriage. Reliability alpha coefficients range from 0.53 to 0.77 (Goldman and Mitchell, 1990).

The impact of stress may be moderated by the patient's access to significant social support in the environment. Social support may be derived from participation in group weight-loss programs (particularly if they allow time to process personal problems), or may come from friends or family members. O'Reilly and Thomas (1989) have reviewed social support measures in health behavior research. They synthesized a measure derived from previous research that is specific to risk-reduction efforts. Results show their measure predicts health behavior maintenance. This questionnaire takes about 10–20 minutes to complete.

Sallis et al. (1987) have developed scales for measuring social support for diet and exercise. Two diet support scales (Family Support for Eating Scale and Friend Support for Eating Scale) and two exercise support scales (Family Support for Exercise Scale and Friend Support for Exercise Scale) are available. Subjects rate the frequency with which both family and friends had said or done what was described in the item during the previous three months. Items are rated on a 5-point scale, ranging from "none" to "very often." These scales have good reliability and are correlated with self-reported exercise and diet habits, providing evidence of concurrent criterion-related and construct validity.

### Knowledge Assessment

In addition to the goal of weight loss itself, programs can be designed to teach patients more about the nature of obesity, nutrition, exercise, health risks, and the pros and cons of dieting. Such knowledge may have beneficial long-term effects on maintenance of weight loss and future attempts to lose weight. An example is the Adult and Child Behavior Knowledge Scales.

*Adult and Child Behavior Knowledge Scales*  These scales measure knowledge of health behaviors related to cardiovascular disease (Vega et al., 1987). They focus on behavioral capability rather than on the link between behavior and disease. The subscales assess knowledge of dietary sodium, dietary fat, and exercise. The Adult Knowledge Scale consists of 18 multiple-choice and true-false items (six in each of the three subscales) and has a reliability alpha coefficient of 0.80. Test-retest reliability for the total score is also acceptable at 0.76. The Child Knowledge Scale consists of nine multiple-choice and true-false items (three in each of the three subscales) and has a reliability alpha coefficient of 0.51. Test-retest reliability for the total score is 0.73. The Health Behavior Knowledge Scales are useful in assessing differences in knowledge levels among adults and children of differing cultural and language groups.

## ASSESSING DIET

There are several dietary assessment tools for quantitating energy and nutrient intakes. These include repeated 24-hour dietary recalls with trained interviewers, food records for varying lengths of time, diet histories, food frequency questionnaires and checklists, calorie counters, and forms for monitoring intake of various food groups. Recently, computerized programs have been developed to greatly expedite data analysis and provide immediate feedback.

In general, dietary assessment methods can be differentiated between those needed for research purposes to survey a population and those used in clinical settings for assessing usual intake and adequacy, choosing interventions, and measuring compliance and/or desired change. A critical need still exists, however, for a validated and simplified instrument that will reliably and quickly help us to assess not only the quantitative value of diets with regard to nutrients and change in energy intake, and their dietary adequacy with regard to food groups and dietary balance, but also the qualitative aspects of eating patterns and specific behaviors having long-term importance for managing food intake. Insofar as treatment programs are accountable for their dietary claims, the ability to assess and monitor dietary changes at critical points during a program will be important to its success.

Many weight-management programs have clients keep food records as a self-monitoring strategy. However, if these records are to be useful in evaluating the overall effectiveness of a diet intervention, care must be taken to properly instruct clients in how to keep accurate records and periodically evaluate their skills at this task. Future studies should give further consideration to this potential of combining intervention and monitoring with ongoing assessment efforts. For a recent review of dietary assessment methods, see Buzzard and Willett, 1994.

### Measures of Dietary Assessment

#### Questionnaires

A wide variety of questionnaires are available to assess an individual's past and current dietary patterns, food likes and dislikes, use of dietary supplements, presence of food allergies, and general knowledge and attitudes about food and nutrition issues (Dwyer, 1994; St. Jeor, in press; Willett, 1990). The results of these assessments help an individual to set realistic dietary goals and develop interventions to achieve them.

## Dietary Interviews

In typical 24-hour dietary recalls, a trained interviewer uses a standardized protocol and props (e.g., food models, cups, and spoons) to prompt a respondent to recall all foods and beverages consumed over a 24-hour period, as well as the specific amounts consumed and, as appropriate, the preparation methods. The recall takes about 15–30 minutes to administer but considerably more time to analyze. It is a more objective assessment tool than a dietary questionnaire, providing a quantitative assessment of energy and nutrient intakes on one day as well as qualitative insight into the foods eaten and timing of food intake. Dietary recalls are generally used to assess the dietary intakes of groups rather than individuals. The number of days needed to obtain accurate data on nutrient intakes varies by nutrient. A minimum of three 24-hour recalls on nonconsecutive days is generally recommended to assess the energy and nutrient intake of an individual. Recalls are useful in clinical settings. A major problem with their use is that individuals can under- or overreport their food intake. In addition, a provider cannot be certain that even several days of 24-hour recalls can represent one's typical dietary pattern. Useful references pertaining to 24-hour recalls include Basiotis et al. (1987), Dwyer (1994), and Tarasuk and Beaton (1991).

## Dietary Records and Diaries

With these assessment tools, a client records everything he or she eats and drinks for a specified period of time, such as 3–4 days, 1 week, or periodically over a longer time. The client is usually asked to record information about mood and behavior at the time food is consumed. As with 24-hour recalls, dietary records and diaries provide a quantitative assessment of energy and nutrient intakes (with accuracy increasing the longer they are kept) and a qualitative assessment of food-related behaviors. To assess the diet of an individual, a 7-day record is recommended, to include both weekdays and the weekend. In practice, however, 3–4-day records are kept to minimize the time and costs of analysis. Dietary records and diaries are the most objective methods available for evaluating dietary patterns. For further information, see Dwyer (1994), St. Jeor et al. (1983), and Willett (1990).

## Food Frequencies

Food frequencies are lists of frequently consumed foods (typically 100–130 items). Respondents administered a food frequency list are expected to note the frequency with which they consume each food over a specified period of time (e.g., one consumed broccoli approximately three times per week in the course of the month). With this assessment tool, a typical nutrient intake of an individual can be determined. Food frequencies are quick to administer and not very tedious to analyze. They tend to be used in research studies. Correlation coefficients with food records for varying lengths of time range of 0.4 to 0.7. For further information, see Block (1982), Dwyer (1994), Longnecker et al. (1994), and Willett (1990).

### Food Lists

Food lists are specialized tools in which foods are listed in various groupings by category (e.g., dairy foods) or dietary constituent (e.g., fat- or fiber-containing foods) to learn subjects' intake of particular kinds of foods or nutrients. Information on portion sizes, frequency of consumption, and method of preparation within each group is also obtained. Food lists are useful in the clinical setting as a quick and inexpensive means of assessing diets and identifying areas where the subject might benefit from dietary counseling.

### Computerized Programs

An increasing amount of computer software is available containing information on the nutrient composition of foods. Features and price vary among programs. Some are available to the public for self-assessments, while the more sophisticated and feature-laden programs are marketed to health-care providers. The programs are used to calculate the nutrient content of a person's diet, usually comparing nutrient intake to a reference such as Recommended Dietary Allowances (RDAs); they are of particular benefit because they can perform the calculations in seconds and provide immediate feedback on the results. The size of the nutrient database and data-analysis capabilities of the programs vary tremendously, so the validity and reliability of these programs vary.

## ASSESSING PHYSICAL ACTIVITY

Health behaviors are difficult to measure, and physical activity is no exception. Existing methods, while relatively crude, nonetheless provide valid and reliable estimates of participation in physical activity and total energy expenditure. The most valid methods of physical activity assessment (doubly-labeled water, direct calorimetry, individual observation, and electronic monitoring) are complicated, technically daunting, intrusive, and expensive, and they are not feasible for use in weight-management programs. Questionnaire assessments of physical activity are the most widely used technique in clinical and epidemiological studies.

Of the variety of questionnaires available to assess physical activity (Blair et al., 1985; Paffenbarger et al., 1993; Sallis et al., 1985; Taylor et al., 1978; Wilson et al., 1986), most are self-administered, although some require a trained interviewer. Simple one- or two-item questionnaires provide a quick classification of low, moderate, and high activity levels, and these methods show reduced risk of morbidity and mortality in the more active individuals (Lindsted et al., 1991). These simple questionnaires, while useful in epidemiological studies of activity and health, are not sufficiently precise to estimate energy expenditure and changes in energy expenditure for individuals in weight-management programs. To be useful for weight-management programs, questionnaires need to provide estimates of total energy expenditure. In themselves, the frequency of exercise sessions and the intensity of the activity are relatively unimportant for weight loss. The most important aspect is the total amount of activity.

There are questionnaires that do provide valid estimates of total energy expenditure (TEE), or at least the physical activity component of TEE (Blair et al., 1985; Paffenbarger et al., 1993; Sallis et al., 1985). These methods typically involve obtaining estimates of the amount of time individuals spend performing activities of various intensities and using these data to calculate total energy expenditure. Major sources of error are inaccurate recall or recording of time intervals and underestimating the intensity of the effort.

### The MET Approach

The concept of metabolic-equivalent units (METs) is a useful way to estimate the intensity of physical activity. A MET is the energy expended during quiet seated rest, generally considered to be an oxygen uptake of 3.5 ml per kg of body weight per minute. This is approximately 1 kcal per kg per hour. Energy expenditure of other physical activities can be expressed as multiples of this resting energy expenditure (working metabolic rate divided by resting metabolic rate). Thus, an activity requiring a threefold increase in metabolism (walking at 3 mph, for example) would be classified at 3 METs and, for a 70-kg person, would result in an energy expenditure of 210 kcal per hour.

Rates of energy expenditure have been verified for many activities, usually by indirect calorimetric methods. Estimates of energy expenditure for activities where the body is moved through space at a constant rate (such as walking, running, or stair climbing at different speeds) are reasonably accurate. Although sport, recreational, household, and occupational activities can be typically performed over a broad range of intensities (e.g., competitive singles tennis versus casual weekend doubles play), common activities as performed by most individuals can nonetheless be assigned to a category of MET values with some confidence. For example, most housework is in the range of 2 to 5 METs, and light office work typically requires 1.5 to 3 METs. Jogging, cycling, and sports involving running, such as basketball or soccer, demand an average of 6 to 12 METs, depending on skill and fitness levels of the participant. An extensive list of the MET cost of common physical activities is available (Ainsworth et al., 1993).

It also is necessary to obtain information on time spent in physical activities in order to calculate daily or weekly energy expenditure. The typical method is to multiply the time spent in the activity (in hours) by the MET value of the activity times the body weight (in kg) of the individual, which yields an estimate of kilocalories expended over the period. It is not necessary to ask individuals to account for every waking minute when assessing their physical activity. Rather, it is sufficient to identify and measure the amount of time they spend doing activities that result in energy expenditure above a moderate level, perhaps 3 METs or more. This level has significance inasmuch as laborsaving devices make it possible to spend virtually the entire day in activities requiring 3 METs or less, which leads to the relatively low levels of TEE prevalent in the United States.

All of the several physical activity questionnaires that provide estimates of energy expenditure, either for voluntary physical activity or for TEE (Blair et al., 1985; Paffenbarger et al., 1993; Sallis et al., 1985; Taylor et al., 1978), use some variation of the MET approach described above. These methods are acceptable for use in population-based studies and for clinical applications. Used properly, they can enhance obesity treatment programs by providing an assessment of the energy expenditure side of the energy-balance equation. The concepts involved are simple and can be understood by most participants with a minimum of instruction.

In addition to the importance of assessing energy balance in order to evaluate treatment outcome, the MET approach is useful in the physical activity intervention aspect of the weight-management program. Most individuals entering obesity treatment are already quite familiar with the caloric value of food, and teaching them about the caloric value of physical activity is not difficult. The multiples of resting energy expenditure method (the MET approach) is easily communicated by the example that even strolling (at 2 mph) doubles energy expenditure (to 2 METs), and brisk walking (at 3–4 mph) triples or quadruples it (to 3 or 4 METs).

The remainder of this appendix presents an annotated list of references for studies using most of the principal methods now available for measuring physical activity.

## Measures of Activity[*]

As stated earlier, questionnaire assessments are the most widely used method for measuring physical activity in epidemiological studies. Unfortunately, whereas diets are assessed periodically in many weight-management programs, physical-activity assessments are not nearly as common. Both diet and exercise should be evaluated routinely. References are given here for the best known and most thoroughly validated questionnaires that are applicable to large population studies. Specific papers on activity assessment in children and elderly individuals are included. Several major review papers on physical activity assessment are included on the list of references. These reports can provide an overview of issues related to the topic of activity assessment, and also present a broad array of additional techniques and methods. Physical activity monitors may be suitable for some studies and several papers on these devices are included. The gold standard for physical activity measurement is by the doubly-labeled water method. This technique provides a reliable estimate of total energy expenditure, but cost and complexity limit its usefulness. Three references describing the doubly-labeled water method are included. Physical fitness measurement may be used as a marker for habitual physical activity, and several references are listed for this topic. Finally, several references on blood pressure response to exercise are given. The list of references annotated here is not exhaustive, but includes most of the principal techniques on activity assessment that are currently in use.

### Questionnaires

*Taylor et al., 1978* Subjects review a checklist of household, recreational, and sports activities and indicate the activities in which they have participated over the past year. A trained interviewer reviews the checklist with the subject, and details regarding the frequency and duration of each activity are recorded. The interview takes approximately 20 minutes. Time spent in each activity is multiplied by an activity intensity code to estimate the energy expenditure for each activity. Energy expenditure is

---

[*]The following is by Steven N. Blair and will be published in a slightly altered form in the *Annotated Bibliography of Epidemiological Methods of Cardiovascular Research, 2nd edition*, by the American Heart Association.

summed across all activities to obtain total expenditure over the year. Energy expenditure subgroup scores also are calculated for light, moderate, and heavy intensity activities. Administration and scoring instructions are included in the article. This questionnaire has been used in several large studies including the Multiple Risk Factor Intervention Trial.

*Folsom et al., 1986*  The Minnesota Leisure-Time Physical Activity (MLTPA) questionnaire was developed from a year-long study on leisure time physical activity, ranging from household home repair to sports and conditioning activities. The MLTPA, used extensively in epidemiological studies, yields an estimate of energy expenditure, typically in kilocalories expended per week. Folsom and colleagues administered the MLTPA two times over a five-week interval to 140 adults from the general population and two times over a two-week interval to 150 men who were participating in the Multiple Risk Factor Intervention Trial. Energy expenditure estimates were slightly, but not significantly, lower at the second administration of the questionnaire. Rank order correlations were high (0.79 to 0.88) for total activity.

*Blair et al., 1985; Sallis et al., 1985*  The questionnaire described in these papers is an interviewer-administered recall of physical activity participation over the past seven days. Subjects are asked to estimate the number of hours spent sleeping and in moderate, hard, and very hard intensity activities. Light physical activity hours are obtained by subtraction. All physical activities are surveyed, including occupational, household, recreational, and sports. Total daily energy expenditure in kcal per kg of body weight is calculated. The questionnaire was validated in a randomized exercise training study, by comparison of energy expenditure and energy intake, and by showing an association between energy expenditure and physical fitness. Instructions for administration and scoring are included in the articles.

*Paffenbarger et al., 1993*  This paper presents the latest version of the questionnaire used for activity assessment in the Harvard Alumni Study, which has been in operation for more than 20 years. Evidence for validity of the method derives from the strong and consistent association of physical activity measured by this technique with several important health outcomes, including non-insulin-dependent diabetes mellitus, coronary heart disease, some site-specific cancers, and all-cause mortality.

*Washburn et al., 1991*  Physical activity data from the Harvard Alumni Activity Survey were significantly correlated with high density lipoprotein cholesterol and body mass index in a large general population sample in Boston. Test-retest reliability coefficients for two administrations 7 to 12 weeks apart were 0.58 to 0.69. These associations and reliability coefficients are comparable to data reported for more complicated and labor intensive questionnaire procedures.

Bouchard et al., 1983   Energy expenditure estimates are derived from a three-day activity record. Subjects code their activity intensity (from one of nine intensity categories ranging from sleeping [1.0 MET] to intense manual work [> 7.8 METs]) every 15 minutes on a data form. A reliability study in 61 subjects who completed the record twice within 6 to 10 days yielded an intraclass coefficient of 0.96. Validity of the procedure is supported by associations with physical fitness and body fatness.

Godin and Shephard, 1985; Owen et al., 1988; Schechtman et al., 1991; Washburn et al., 1987, 1990; Weiss et al., 1990   These six papers present evidence that crude assessments of physical activity can be valid. The questions used in these research projects were simple, short, and easily completed. The various studies used from one to four questions. The questions could be completed within several seconds or at most a minute or two.

Blair et al., 1989a   Subjects were 3,943 women and 15,627 men who performed a maximal exercise test on a treadmill and received a clinical examination. Physical fitness, as determined by the treadmill test, was associated with the sedentary traits. When smoking habit, a simple physical activity index, and the sedentary traits were included in a multiple regression model with physical fitness as the dependent variable, $R^2$ values ranged from 0.20 to 0.53 in women and 0.45 to 0.61 in men across age groups. These data suggest that the addition of data on sedentary traits to a simple physical activity index can sharpen the prediction of physical fitness in epidemiologic studies.

Kohl et al., 1988   Self-reported physical activity habits from a mail survey were correlated with data from a maximal exercise test in 375 men. The exercise test was administered within 60 days of the receipt of the mail questionnaire. Validity of the mail questionnaire physical activity assessment was supported by a multiple correlation of 0.65 between physical fitness and age and physical activity questions.

Baecke et al., 1982   This questionnaire includes 16 questions that cover three components of physical activity: physical activity at work, sports during leisure time, and physical activity during leisure time excluding sports. The questionnaire was given to a group of 306 young (ages 20 to

32 years) Dutch men and women. Test-retest reliability for the three activity components ranged from 0.74 to 0.88.

Jacobs et al., 1989 CARDIA is a large biracial study of more than 5,000 young (ages 18 to 30 years) men and women. The CARDIA questionnaire includes items about physical activity participation over the past three months and over the past year. The questionnaire is interviewer administered, and can be administered by a telephone interview. Validity of the method is supported by comparison of body composition, energy intake, physical fitness, and blood lipids across physical activity groups. Test-retest reliability is reported to range from 0.77 to 0.84.

Williams et al., 1989 This study compared the reliability and convergent validity of the seven-day physical activity recall, the Caltrac monitor, and a daily physical activity log for 45 subjects over a three-week interval. Reliability was high for the seven-day recall and the activity log, but not for the Caltrac. Convergent validity was high for the seven-day recall and the daily log, but was low for both of these measures when compared with the Caltrac.

## Physical Activity Monitors

LaPorte et al., 1979 This study evaluated the Large-Scale Integrated Motor Activity Monitor. The unit is slightly larger than a wristwatch, and it uses a mercury switch to detect bodily movement. The instrument was validated by comparing movement counts from the instrument in sedentary and active groups. The subjects also maintained an activity log while wearing the movement sensor. There was a significant correlation ($r = 0.65$) between activity log reports and movement counts from the instrument.

Kalkwarf et al., 1989 Twelve young women wore heart rate monitors and completed 24-hour activity diaries for a four-week period. Resting metabolic rate and the energy cost of various activities were assessed by indirect calorimetry with simultaneous recording of heart rates. These data were used in conjunction with the activity diaries and heart recordings to estimate energy expenditure. The standard of comparison for energy expenditure was energy intake calculated from weighed food intake and changes in body energy stores. Heart rate monitors overestimated group energy expenditure by 2 to 9 percent. Activity diaries underestimated energy expenditure by 2 to 6 percent. The authors conclude that heart rate monitoring and activity diaries may be accurate enough for group estimates of energy expenditure, but not for individual estimates.

Avons et al., 1988 Subjects wore three actometers (modified self-winding watches, one each on an arm, leg, and waist) and had heart rates recorded during a stay in a whole-body calorimeter. Additional data from the actometers were collected during seven days in the free-living condition. The actometers provided a satisfactory estimate of energy expenditure.

Taylor et al., 1982, 1984 These two studies used the Vitalog monitor, which is a microprocessor device that records heart rate and bodily movement. The instrument has been used in several exercise trials, and its reproducibility has been established both within weeks and between weeks. Validity has been shown by monitoring changes in exercise groups in controlled studies. Objective data from both heart rate and bodily movement presumably provide more precise estimates of energy expenditure than for either used alone.

Montoye et al., 1983; Wong et al., 1981 These two papers describe a portable accelerometer that is worn on the waist to measure bodily movement. The instrument has good reproducibility ($r = 0.94$). The standard error of estimate for predicting oxygen uptake is reported to be 6.6 ml min$^{-1}$ kg$^{-1}$.

### Children

Baranoski et al., 1984 This study evaluated six different forms of self-report of aerobic activity in third- to sixth-grade children. Self-report data were compared to behavioral observations. Greatest agreement with the criterion measure was obtained when the self-report method that segmented the day into functional components was used. The average percentage of agreement across all forms of self-report was 73.4.

Klesges and Klesges, 1987 The investigators evaluated physical activity in 30 young children (ages 24 to 48 months) with a portable accelerometer and by direct observation by trained observers. Correlations between hourly accelerometer readings and observation ranged from 0.62 to 0.95. The best predictor of all-day accelerometer readings was with the observed behavior of walking, which accounted for 32 percent of the variance in the accelerometer data.

O'Hara et al., 1989 Heart rates were compared with behavioral observations in 36 children (ages 8–10) during physical education class. Heart rate was obtained from a wristwatch-size monitoring unit that recorded heart rate every 15 seconds from the ECG. Trained observers recorded physical activity in four categories of movement each minute. The average correlation for minute-by-minute heart rates and observations was 0.64. Interobserver agreement was high ($r = 0.96$).

*Sallis et al., 1990* Body movement (by the Caltrac) and heart rates (by a portable monitor) were recorded in elementary-school-age children. Correlations between the instruments were 0.54 for day one and 0.42 for day two. Inter-instrument reliability in the field setting was 0.96. Data from the accelerometers and heart rate monitors were significantly correlated with physical activity recalls of the same day.

### Elderly

Several of the questionnaires described above have been used in populations across the age range. In this section, two papers are listed that were specifically used with older groups.

*Cartmel and Moon, 1992* Two questionnaires (Minnesota Leisure-Time Physical Activity [MLTPA] and seven-day recall) were administered to 24 older men and women (ages 59 to 83 years). Each person also kept a physical activity diary over four consecutive days. Data from the diaries were compared with each questionnaire. The MLTPA was more accurate than the seven-day recall for moderate/heavy activities, and the seven-day recall was more accurate than the MLTPA for time spent sitting.

*Cauley et al., 1987* The investigators used five different methods for measuring physical activity in a population of 255 white, postmenopausal women. Both questionnaires and an activity monitor were used. The activity measures were only weakly correlated. The authors recommend that several different types of activity assessment be used to obtain adequate data on different types of physical activity patterns.

### Review Papers

*Caspersen, 1989; Lamb and Brodie, 1990; Saris, 1986; Tremblay and Bouchard, 1987; Wilson et al., 1986* These five review papers present information on most of the commonly used methods for the assessment of physical activity and physical fitness in population based studies. Methods applicable across the age range are presented.

### Doubly-Labeled Water

*Klein et al., 1984; Livingstone et al., 1992; Stein et al., 1987* These three papers describe the doubly-labeled water method of estimating energy expenditure in humans. Validation of the technique is by comparison with directly measured energy expenditure in a whole body calorimeter. The doubly-labeled water method is considered by many to be the "gold standard" for energy expenditure. Unfortunately, the method is quite complex and very expensive, and it is not suited for epidemiological studies. The doubly-labeled water technique has great promise for validating physical activity questionnaires.

### Physical Fitness

*Montoye et al., 1970; Siconolfi et al., 1982; Sidney et al., 1992* These three reports describe and discuss various methods of assessing aerobic power (physical fitness) in population-based studies. Maximal and submaximal testing protocols are described. Both cycle ergometry and treadmill testing are included.

### Blood Pressure Response to Exercise

*Jones et al., 1985* One hundred healthy subjects representing an even distribution of sex, age, and height underwent a progressively incremental exercise test to obtain standards for the various physiological measures. Systolic blood pressure was measured by cuff methods. Age and sex specific normal values are provided.

*Ekelund et al., 1990* Approximately 4,300 representative healthy black and white men and women aged 20–69 years performed a standardized treadmill exercise test (to 85 percent of age-specific predicted maximal heart rate). Systolic blood pressure was measured at rest and at each stage of exercise using a mercury manometer and stethoscope. Data on age, sex, and race specific values are presented, demonstrating that black men have higher systolic blood pressures during exercise that white men even after adjustments for resting values.

*Morris et al., 1978* The incidence of decreases in peak systolic blood pressure during treadmill exercise was investigated in 460 patients with definite or suspected coronary heart disease. Systolic blood pressure was measured at rest, at each stage of exercise, and at peak exercise. Also, all patients were studied with coronary cineangiography. A sustained exercise-induced decrease in peak systolic blood pressure of 10 mm Hg or more is a highly specific sign of multiple vessel coronary artery disease.

*Franz, 1982* Systolic and diastolic blood pressures were measured using

1st and 4th phase Korotkoff sounds at rest and during each minute of cycle ergometry in healthy normotensive men ($n$ = 173) and women ($n$ = 130) aged 20 to 50 years. A similar protocol was performed by smaller numbers of borderline and frank hypertensive patients. The mean and standard deviation for blood pressure responses during an exercise load ranging from 100 to 600 watts are presented by sex, age, and resting blood pressure status.

Wolthuis et al., 1977 Systolic and diastolic blood pressures were measured using the Korotkoff method in 704 healthy asymptomatic aircrewmen at rest and at each stage of a maximal treadmill exercise test using a Balk-c-Ware protocol. The mean, 10th, and 90th percentiles for systolic and diastolic blood pressures are presented for several submaximal workloads, maximal exercise, and at 2 and 5 minutes of recovery. These data provide good "normal" values for blood pressure responses to treadmill exercise in healthy younger men.

# B

## The Diet Readiness Test and the General Well-Being Schedule

In Chapters 7 and 8, we recommended that all individuals assess their psychological status prior to beginning a weight-management program or have it assessed by the program. We suggested use of the Dieting Readiness Test or a comparable test to help point out potential problems with motivation and attitudes toward dieting and exercise. In addition to the Dieting Readiness Test, we recommended that clinical programs administer the General Well-Being Schedule or a comparable test to their potential clients to identify any psychological pathologies (e.g., depression) and determine whether an individual should be referred for more in-depth psychological assessment before beginning the program. This appendix provides both the Dieting Readiness Test and the General Well-Being Schedule in their entirety.

### THE DIETING READINESS TEST

Answer the questions below to see how well your attitudes equip you for a weight-loss program. For each question, circle the answer that best describes your attitude. As you complete each of the six sections, add the numbers of your answers and compare them with the scoring guide at the end of each section.

### Section 1: Goals and Attitudes

1. Compared to previous attempts, how motivated to lose weight are you this time?
   1. Not at all motivated
   2. Slightly motivated
   3. Somewhat motivated
   4. Quite motivated
   5. Extremely motivated

2. How certain are you that you will stay committed to a weight loss program for the time it will take you to reach your goal?
   1. Not at all certain
   2. Slightly certain
   3. Somewhat certain
   4. Quite certain
   5. Extremely certain

3. Consider all outside factors at this time in your life (the stress you're feeling at work, your family obligations, etc.). To what extent can you tolerate the effort required to stick to a diet?
   1. Cannot tolerate
   2. Can tolerate somewhat
   3. Uncertain
   4. Can tolerate well
   5. Can tolerate easily

4. Think honestly about how much weight you hope to lose and how quickly you hope to lose it. Figuring a weight loss of 1 to 2 pounds per week, how realistic is your expectation?
   1. Very unrealistic
   2. Somewhat unrealistic
   3. Moderately unrealistic
   4. Somewhat realistic
   5. Very realistic

5. While dieting, do you fantasize about eating a lot of your favorite foods?
   1. Always
   2. Frequently
   3. Occasionally
   4. Rarely
   5. Never

6. While dieting, do you feel deprived, angry and/or upset?
   1. Always
   2. Frequently
   3. Occasionally
   4. Rarely
   5. Never

**Section 1—TOTAL Score** _____

If you scored:

**6 to 16:**    This may not be a good time for you to start a weight loss program. Inadequate motivation and commitment together with unrealistic goals could block your progress. Think about those things that contribute to this, and consider changing them before undertaking a diet program.

**17 to 23:**    You may be close to being ready to begin a program but should think about ways to boost your preparedness before you begin.

**24 to 30:**    The path is clear with respect to goals and attitudes.

### *Section 2: Hunger and Eating Cues*

7. When food comes up in conversation or in something you read, do you want to eat even if you are not hungry?
   1. Never
   2. Rarely
   3. Occasionally
   4. Frequently
   5. Always

8. How often do you eat because of physical hunger?
   1. Always
   2. Frequently
   3. Occasionally
   4. Rarely
   5. Never

9. Do you have trouble controlling your eating when your favorite foods are around the house?
   1. Never
   2. Rarely
   3. Occasionally
   4. Frequently
   5. Always

**Section 2—TOTAL Score** _____

If you scored:

**3 to 6:**    You might occasionally eat more than you would like, but it does not appear to be a result of high responsiveness to environmental cues. Controlling the attitudes that make you eat may be especially helpful.

**7 to 9:**    You may have a moderate tendency to eat just because food is available. Dieting may be easier for you if you try to resist external cues and eat only when you are physically hungry.

**10 to 15:**    Some or most of your eating may be in response to thinking about food or exposing yourself to temptations to eat. Think of ways to minimize your exposure to temptations, so that you eat only in response to physical hunger.

### _Section 3: Control Over Eating_
If the following situations occurred while you were on a diet, would you be likely to eat more or less immediately afterward and for the rest of the day?

10. Although you planned on skipping lunch, a friend talks you into going out for a midday meal.
   1. Would eat much less
   2. Would eat somewhat less
   3. Would make no difference
   4. Would eat somewhat more
   5. Would eat much more

11. You "break" your diet by eating a fattening, "forbidden" food.
   1. Would eat much less
   2. Would eat somewhat less
   3. Would make no difference
   4. Would eat somewhat more
   5. Would eat much more

12. You have been following your diet faithfully and decide to test yourself by eating something you consider a treat.
   1. Would eat much less
   2. Would eat somewhat less
   3. Would make no difference
   4. Would eat somewhat more
   5. Would eat much more

**Section 3—TOTAL Score** _____

If you scored:

**3 to 7:**     You recover rapidly from mistakes. However, if you frequently alternate between eating out of control and dieting
very strictly, you may have a serious eating problem and
should get professional help.

**8 to 11:**    You do not seem to let unplanned eating disrupt your program. This is a flexible, balanced approach.

**12 to 15:**   You may be prone to overeat after an event breaks your control or throws you off the track. Your reaction to these prob-
lem-causing eating events can be improved.

### *Section 4: Binge Eating and Purging*

13. Aside from holiday feasts, have you ever eaten a large amount of food
rapidly and felt afterward that this eating incident was excessive and out
of control?
    2.  Yes
    0.  No

14. If you answered yes to #13 above, how often have you engaged in
this behavior during the last year?
    1.  Less than once a month
    2.  About once a month
    3.  A few times a month
    4.  About once a week
    5.  About three times a week
    6.  Daily

15. Have you ever purged (used laxatives, diuretics or induced vomiting) to control your weight?
    5.  Yes
    0.  No

16. If you answered yes to #15 above, how often have you engaged in
this behavior during the last year?
    1.  Less than once a month
    2.  About once a month
    3.  A few times a month
    4.  About once a week
    5.  About three times a week
    6.  Daily

**Section 4—TOTAL Score** _____

If you scored:

**0 to 1:** It appears that binge eating and purging is not a problem for you.

**2 to 11:** Pay attention to these eating patterns. Should they arise more frequently, get professional help.

**12 to 19:** You show signs of having a potentially serious eating problem. See a counselor experienced in evaluating eating disorders right away.

## _Section 5: Emotional Eating_

17. Do you eat more than you would like to when you have negative feelings such as anxiety, depression, anger, or loneliness?
    1. Never
    2. Rarely
    3. Occasionally
    4. Frequently
    5. Always

18. Do you have trouble controlling your eating when you have positive feelings—do you celebrate feeling good by eating?
    1. Never
    2. Rarely
    3. Occasionally
    4. Frequently
    5. Always

19. When you have unpleasant interactions with others in your life, or after a difficult day at work, do you eat more than you'd like?
    1. Never
    2. Rarely
    3. Occasionally
    4. Frequently
    5. Always

**Section 5—TOTAL Score** _____

If you scored:

**3 to 8:** You do not appear to let your emotions affect your eating.

**9 to 11:** You sometimes eat in response to emotional highs and lows. Monitor this behavior to learn when and why it occurs and be prepared to find alternate activities.

**12 to 15:**     Emotional ups and downs can stimulate your eating. Try to deal with the feelings that trigger the eating and find other ways to express them.

### *Section 6: Exercise Patterns and Attitudes*
20. How often do you exercise?
    1. Never
    2. Rarely
    3. Occasionally
    4. Somewhat
    5. Frequently

21. How confident are you that you can exercise regularly?
    1. Not at all confident
    2. Slightly confident
    3. Somewhat confident
    4. Highly confident
    5. Completely confident

22. When you think about exercise, do you develop a positive or negative picture in your mind?
    1. Completely negative
    2. Somewhat negative
    3. Neutral
    4. Somewhat positive
    5. Completely positive

23. How certain are you that you can work regular exercise into your daily schedule?
    1. Not at all certain
    2. Slightly certain
    3. Somewhat certain
    4. Quite certain
    5. Extremely certain

**Section 6—TOTAL Score** _____

If you scored:
**4 to 10:**     You're probably not exercising as regularly as you should. Determine whether your attitudes about exercise are blocking your way, then change what you must and put on those walking shoes.
**11 to 16:**    You need to feel more positive about exercise so you can do

it more often. Think of ways to be more active that are fun and fit your lifestyle.

**17 to 20:**  It looks like the path is clear for you to be active. Now think of ways to get motivated.

After scoring yourself in each section of this questionnaire, you should be able to better judge your dieting strengths and weaknesses. Remember that the first step in changing eating behavior is to understand the conditions that influence your eating habits.

SOURCE: Brownell, 1990. Reprinted with permission.

## GENERAL WELL-BEING SCHEDULE

This section of the examination contains questions about how you feel and how things have been going with you. For each question, fill in the circle next to the answer which best applies to you.

1. How have you been feeling in general? (DURING THE PAST MONTH)
   - ○  In excellent spirits
   - ○  In very good spirits
   - ○  In good spirits mostly
   - ○  I have been up and down in spirits a lot
   - ○  In low spirits mostly
   - ○  In very low spirits

2. Have you been bothered by nervousness or your "nerves"? (DURING THE PAST MONTH)
   - ○  Extremely so—to the point where I could not work or take care of things
   - ○  Very much so
   - ○  Quite a bit
   - ○  Some—enough to bother me
   - ○  A little
   - ○  Not at all

3. Have you been in firm control of your behavior, thoughts, emotions OR feelings? (DURING THE PAST MONTH)
   - ○  Yes, definitely so
   - ○  Yes, for the most part
   - ○  Generally so

○ Not too well
○ No, and I am somewhat disturbed
○ No, and I am very disturbed

4. Have you felt so sad, discouraged, hopeless, or had so many problems that you wondered if everything was worthwhile? (DURING THE PAST MONTH)
○ Extremely so—to the point that I have just about given up
○ Very much so
○ Quite a bit
○ Some—enough to bother me
○ A little bit
○ Not at all

5. Have you been under or felt you were under any strain, stress, or pressure? (DURING THE PAST MONTH)
○ Yes—almost more than I could bear or stand
○ Yes—quite a bit of pressure
○ Yes—some, more than usual
○ Yes—some, but about usual
○ Yes—a little
○ Not at all

6. How happy, satisfied, or pleased have you been with your personal life? (DURING THE PAST MONTH)
○ Extremely happy—could not have been more satisfied or pleased
○ Very happy
○ Fairly happy
○ Satisfied—pleased
○ Somewhat dissatisfied
○ Very dissatisfied

7. Have you had any reason to wonder if you were losing your mind, or losing control over the way you act, talk, think, feel, or of your memory? (DURING THE PAST MONTH)
○ Not at all
○ Only a little
○ Some—but not enough to be concerned or worried about
○ Some and I have been a little concerned
○ Some and I am quite concerned
○ Yes, very much so and I am very concerned

8. Have you been anxious, worried, or upset?
   - ○ Extremely so—to the point of being sick or almost sick
   - ○ Very much so
   - ○ Quite a bit
   - ○ Some—enough to bother me
   - ○ A little bit
   - ○ Not at all

9. Have you been waking up fresh and rested? (DURING THE PAST MONTH)
   - ○ Every day
   - ○ Most every day
   - ○ Fairly often
   - ○ Less than half the time
   - ○ Rarely
   - ○ None of the time

10. Have you been bothered by any illness, bodily disorder, pains, or fears about your health?
    - ○ All the time
    - ○ Most of the time
    - ○ A good bit of the time
    - ○ Some of the time
    - ○ A little of the time
    - ○ None of the time

11. Has your daily life been full of things that were interesting to you? (DURING THE PAST MONTH)
    - ○ All the time
    - ○ Most of the time
    - ○ A good bit of the time
    - ○ Some of the time
    - ○ A little of the time
    - ○ None of the time

12. Have you felt down-hearted and blue? (DURING THE PAST MONTH)
    - ○ All the time
    - ○ Most of the time
    - ○ A good bit of the time
    - ○ Some of the time
    - ○ A little of the time
    - ○ None of the time

13. Have you been feeling emotionally stable and sure of yourself? (DUR-ING THE PAST MONTH)
   - ○  All the time
   - ○  Most of the time
   - ○  A good bit of the time
   - ○  Some of the time
   - ○  A little of the time
   - ○  None of the time

14. Have you felt tired, worn out, used up, or exhausted? (DURING THE PAST MONTH)
   - ○  All the time
   - ○  Most of the time
   - ○  A good bit of the time
   - ○  Some of the time
   - ○  A little of the time
   - ○  None of the time

For each of the four scales below, note that the words at each end of the 0 to 10 scale describe opposite feelings. Fill in the circle along the bar which seems closest to how you have generally felt DURING THE PAST MONTH.

15. How concerned or worried about your HEALTH have you been? (DURING THE PAST MONTH)

| 0 | 1 | 2 | 3 | 4 | 5 | 6 | 7 | 8 | 9 | 10 |
|---|---|---|---|---|---|---|---|---|---|----|
| ○ | ○ | ○ | ○ | ○ | ○ | ○ | ○ | ○ | ○ | ○ |

Not
concerned
at all

Very
concerned

16. How RELAXED or TENSE have you been? (DURING THE PAST MONTH)

| 0 | 1 | 2 | 3 | 4 | 5 | 6 | 7 | 8 | 9 | 10 |
|---|---|---|---|---|---|---|---|---|---|----|
| ○ | ○ | ○ | ○ | ○ | ○ | ○ | ○ | ○ | ○ | ○ |

Very
relaxed

Very
tense

17. How much ENERGY, PEP, and VITALITY have you felt (DURING THE PAST MONTH)

| 0 | 1 | 2 | 3 | 4 | 5 | 6 | 7 | 8 | 9 | 10 |
|---|---|---|---|---|---|---|---|---|---|----|
| O | O | O | O | O | O | O | O | O | O | O |

No energy at all, listless

Very energetic, dynamic

18. How DEPRESSED or CHEERFUL have you been? (DURING THE PAST MONTH)

| 0 | 1 | 2 | 3 | 4 | 5 | 6 | 7 | 8 | 9 | 10 |
|---|---|---|---|---|---|---|---|---|---|----|
| O | O | O | O | O | O | O | O | O | O | O |

Very depressed

Very cheerful

## Scoring

For questions 1, 3, 6, 7, 9, 11, and 13, score 1=5, 2=4, 3=3, 4=2, 5=1, and 6=0.

For questions 2, 4, 5, 8, 10, 12, and 14, score 1=0, 2=1, 3=2, 4=3, 5=4, and 6=5.

For questions 15 and 16, score 0=10, 1=9, 2=8, 3=7, 4=6, 5=5, 6=4, 7=3, 8=2, 9=1, and 10=0.

For questions 17 and 18, score 1=1, 2=2, 3=3, 4=4, 5=5, 6=6, 7=7, 8=8, 9=9, and 10=10.

## Interpretation of Scores

0 to 60 equals "Severe distress."
61 to 72 equals "Moderate distress."
73 to 110 equals "Positive Well-Being."

SOURCE: NCHS, 1977; McDowell and Newell, 1987

# C

# Pediatric Obesity

*Beatrice S. Kanders, Ed.D., M.P.H., R.D.*

$\mathbf{P}$ediatric obesity is a significant public health issue and a prevalent nutritional problem in the United States. The prevalence of obesity among children and adolescents has increased markedly since 1964, possibly affecting 20–27 percent of them (Gortmaker et al., 1987). Recent data from the Third National Health and Nutrition Examination Survey (NHANES III) indicate that these trends have continued for adolescents despite national efforts to reduce overweight (Harlan, 1993). Although it can be explained in part by environmental and economic factors, the cause of the rising incidence of pediatric obesity over the past three decades is not readily apparent. The current literature on childhood and adolescent obesity is reviewed here, focusing on its causes, consequences, treatment, and prevention. As there is still much to be learned about pediatric obesity, research needs are also identified.

## OVERVIEW

Obesity is characterized by an excess of adipose tissue in relation to lean body mass. However, a standard clinical definition of childhood (6–

COMMITTEE'S NOTE: Time constraints prevented us from being able to address the important subject of pediatric obesity. However, given its importance and the fact that obesity among children and adolescents is increasing as it is among adults, we asked obesity specialist Beatrice Kanders to prepare the following background paper on the subject. We hope it helps stimulate further study and research towards preventing and treating obesity during the formative years of childhood and adolescence.

10 years) and adolescent (11–21 years) obesity does not exist. Generally, obesity is defined as weight-for-height above the 90th percentile on the growth charts from the National Center for Health Statistics (NCHS) or weight in excess of 120 percent of the median weight for a given height (Leung and Robson, 1990). The 85th percentile of triceps skinfolds is also used (Garn and Clark, 1976; Gortmaker et al., 1987), and skinfolds correlate well with percentage of body fat in children of both sexes (Forbes and Amirhakimi, 1970; Roche et al., 1981). It may be difficult to measure skinfolds, as evidenced by the mere 8 percent of pediatricians and family practitioners who take these measures (Greecher, 1993).

The Quetelet index or body mass index (BMI) is an indirect measure of body fat, but it is easily and reliably measured, correlating well with more precise estimates of subcutaneous and total body fat (Deurenberg et al., 1991; Roche et al., 1981). In 1985, the National Institutes of Health (NIH) Consensus Conference on Obesity recommended that BMI plus relative weight be used in clinical and public health settings (Burton et al., 1985). Although arbitrary, the 85th and 95th percentiles of BMI have been used to define obesity and superobesity, respectively (Garn and Clark, 1975; Harlan, 1993; Must et al., 1991), and these definitions are used in Table C-1. However, use of the 85th percentile may incorrectly label a large group of children obese, and a BMI in the 90th or 95th percentile may be more appropriate (Dietz and Robinson, 1993; Williams et al., 1993).

The Committee on Clinical Guidelines for Overweight in Adolescent Preventive Services recently proposed specific criteria for defining overweight and obesity in adolescents (Himes and Dietz, 1994), recommending routine use of BMI in screening. The committee also recommended

**TABLE C-1** Body Mass Index (BMI) Cutoff Values for Obesity for Children 6–10 Years of Age by Sex

| Age | Males | | Females | |
|---|---|---|---|---|
| | 85th Percentile | 95th Percentile | 85th Percentile | 95th Percentile |
| 6 | 16.6 | 18.0 | 16.2 | 17.5 |
| 7 | 17.4 | 19.2 | 17.2 | 18.9 |
| 8 | 18.1 | 20.3 | 18.2 | 20.4 |
| 9 | 18.9 | 21.5 | 19.2 | 21.8 |
| 10 | 19.6 | 22.6 | 20.2 | 23.2 |

SOURCE: Adapted from Must et al., 1991. Reprinted with permission of the authors and the American Society for Clinical Nutrition.

**TABLE C-2**   Recommended BMI Cutoff Values for
Adolescents Who Are at Risk of Overweight or Are
Overweight

| Age (years) | At Risk of Overweight | | Overweight | |
|---|---|---|---|---|
|  | Males | Females | Males | Females |
| 10 | 20 | 20 | 23 | 23 |
| 11 | 20 | 21 | 24 | 25 |
| 12 | 21 | 22 | 25 | 26 |
| 13 | 22 | 23 | 26 | 27 |
| 14 | 23 | 24 | 27 | 28 |
| 15 | 24 | 24 | 28 | 29 |
| 16 | 24 | 25 | 29 | 29 |
| 17 | 25 | 25 | 29 | 30 |
| 18 | 26 | 26 | 30 | 30 |
| 19 | 26 | 26 | 30 | 30 |
| 20–24 | 27 | 26 | 30 | 30 |

SOURCE: Adapted from Himes and Dietz, 1994, and Must et al., 1991.
Reprinted with permission of the authors and the American Society for
Clinical Nutrition.

that BMI be used routinely to screen for overweight adolescents. Adolescents with either a BMI in the 95th percentile and higher or a BMI greater than 30 (whichever is smaller) should be considered overweight and referred for in-depth medical follow-up. Adolescents whose BMI is greater than or equal to the 85th percentile but less than the 95th percentile or whose BMI is equal to 30 (whichever is smaller) should be considered at risk for overweight and referred for further screening. The recommended cutoff values are shown in Table C-2. Similar guidelines have yet to be developed for younger children.

### Prevalence

Table C-3 shows estimates of the prevalence of obesity and superobesity among children 6–17 years old using data gathered during 1976–1980. In 1987, the prevalence of obesity and superobesity in children was estimated at 27.1 and 11.7 percent (6–11 years) and 21.9 and 9.0 percent (12–17 years) (Gortmaker et al., 1987). Obesity and superobesity were defined as 85th and 95th percentile of triceps skinfolds, respectively. A comparison of the 1976–1980 levels and the 1987 levels shows that, depending on the age, sex, and race of the group studied, the prevalence of obesity has increased by 54 percent in 6- to 11-year-olds and by 64 per-

**TABLE C-3**  Estimate of Prevalence of Obesity in the United States by Race and Sex in Children 6–17 Years of Age (1976–1980)

|  | 85th Percentile | 95th Percentile |
|---|---|---|
| Males | 17.9 | 5.8 |
| Females | 17.3 | 6.1 |
| Blacks | 8.8 | 2.7 |
| Whites | 19.1 | 6.5 |
| Total | 17.6 | 7.1 |

NOTE: Data are from the Second National Health and Nutrition Examination Survey (1976–1980) (NHANES II).

SOURCE: Adapted from Gortmaker et al., 1987.

cent in 12- to 17-year-olds, and the prevalence of superobesity has increased 98 percent in 6- to 11-year-olds and 64 percent in 12- to 21-year-olds. The 1987 data also indicated that not only was the pediatric population getting fatter, but the fatter members were becoming more obese (Gortmaker et al., 1987).

Sex and racial differences in obesity have also been noted. Girls had an increased prevalence of obesity compared with boys in all age groups and degrees of obesity (Harlan, 1993). More recent data from NHANES III indicate that these trends for adolescents have continued (DHHS, 1991; Harlan, 1993). Similarly, with respect to racial differences, obesity and superobesity are less prevalent among African-American than white children (see Table C-3); however, higher than average rates of obesity have been reported in other minority populations, including Native Americans, Puerto Ricans, and Cuban-Americans (Kumanyika, 1993).

### Ethnicity

The prevalence of obesity varies among children of different ethnic groups. In this country, approximately 20 percent of the population is made up of ethnic minorities. A high prevalence of obesity has been reported among children of certain minority groups, although this finding depends on the age and sex of the group studied as well as the data used to obtain the information (Kumanyika, 1993). A high prevalence of obesity has been reported in preschool and school-aged Native American children. Increases in the prevalence of obesity among preschoolers have also been reported among Puerto Rican males and females and Cuban-American females. Among school-aged children, increases in obesity have been reported among African-American and Puerto Rican girls; Mexican, Puerto Rican, and Cuban boys; and Native Hawaiian boys and girls. Additional information on ethnicity and pediatric obesity is provided by Kumanyika (1993).

## ETIOLOGY

### Energy Intake

Obesity results from an energy imbalance in which energy intake exceeds energy expenditure. This imbalance can result from excessive energy intake, low energy expenditure, or some combination of both. The relative importance of each of these factors in children and adolescents in causing and sustaining the obese state remains a matter of debate (Gutin and Manos, 1993).

Although there has been considerable debate over the issue of whether the obese consume more calories than the nonobese (Griffiths et al., 1987; Rolland-Cachera and Bellisle, 1986; Stefanick et al., 1959; Sunnegardh et al., 1986), there is little evidence to support this theory, and no general consensus exists. For example, several studies have reported a lack of association between energy intake and body weight in adults (Braitman et al., 1985; Romieu, 1988). With regard to children and adolescents, energy intake (as measured by self-report) does not appear to differ significantly among obese, obesity-prone, and normal-weight youths (Corbin and Fletcher, 1968; Eck et al., 1992; Johnson et al., 1956; Stefanick et al., 1959; Wilkinson et al., 1977). Excessive fat intake has been proposed as a determinant of obesity, and data indicate that obese children may consume more calories as fat than do nonobese children (Eck et al., 1992), although these results remain equivocal (Obarzanek et al., 1994; Rose and Mayer, 1986). In addition, self-report data on dietary intake may not be a valid measure of habitual energy intake (Bandini et al., 1990b; Lichtman et al., 1992).

Indeed, using doubly-labeled water techniques, Bandini et al. (1987) found that both obese and nonobese adolescents underreport habitual energy intake. While the self-report estimates of intake of the obese and lean subjects were similar, the doubly-labeled water results showed that obese adolescents underreported caloric intake by 40 percent, while nonobese adolescents underreported caloric intake by only 20 percent. The doubly-labeled water technology allows researchers to assess energy expenditure of free-living individuals accurately over repeated days. Since obesity can result from even a small imbalance in energy intake, a variety of accurate and readily accessible methods for measuring caloric intake must be developed. Additionally, further research is needed to clarify our understanding of the role of energy intake and macronutrient composition in the development of childhood and adolescent obesity.

## Energy Expenditure

There has been much interest in the role of energy expenditure in the development and maintenance of obesity. Total energy expenditure (TEE) is divided into three main components: resting metabolic rate, thermogenesis, and physical activity. If any of these components were reduced, it theoretically could predispose an individual to obesity.

Three prospective investigations have examined the role of low energy expenditure in the development of obesity in children (Griffiths and Payne, 1976; Griffiths et al., 1990; Roberts et al., 1988). In one, 18 infants of lean and obese mothers were studied during their first year of life (Roberts et al., 1988). Total energy expenditure and metabolizable energy intake were measured using doubly-labeled water over a period of 7 days when the infants were 3 months of age; postprandial metabolic rate was measured by indirect calorimetry when the infants were 3 days and 3 months of age. No significant differences with respect to weight, length, skinfold thicknesses, metabolic rate (at 0.1 and 3 months), and metabolizable energy intake (at 3 months) were observed between infants who became overweight by the age of 1 year (50 percent of infants born to overweight mothers) and those who did not. However, total energy expenditure at 3 months was 20.7 percent lower in the infants who became overweight than in infants who remained normal weight. These findings indicate that at 3 months of age, low energy expenditure (rather than high energy intake) was the principal cause of rapid weight gain, which is consistent with prospective studies of weight gain in adult Pima Indians (Ravussin et al., 1988). The authors attributed this energy difference to diminished physical activity and/or arousal rather than resting metabolic rate.

Two additional studies support the hypothesis that low energy expenditure contributes to weight gain in infancy and childhood. In the first study, 3- to 5-year-old children of obese parents were found to have lower resting metabolic rates and energy intake (on average 22 percent lower) per kilogram of body weight than did children of normal-weight parents, even though the children were matched for size and fatness (Griffiths and Payne, 1976). These results suggested that children who have a family history of obesity maintain normal weight by consuming fewer calories per day than do children without a family history. Although these results do not demonstrate any relationship between low energy expenditure and the development of obesity (since the children were normal weight at the time of the study), they might be predictive of obesity at some later time.

A recent follow-up investigation of this same population at ages 15 and 16 years showed that the children of the obese parents gained substantially more weight than did the children of normal-weight parents (Griffiths et al., 1990), suggesting that low energy expenditure earlier in life did contribute to weight gain. Boys with obese parents were taller and heavier (but not fatter) than boys with nonobese parents. However, resting metabolic rate per kilogram of body weight was significantly lower in the boys with obese parents compared with those with nonobese parents; no differences were noted between girls with obese and nonobese parents, though body fat was greater in the girls with the obese parents (not statistically significant, possibly owing to the small sample size) (Griffiths et al., 1990).

Physical activity represents a significant variable in total energy expenditure and the only component that can be directly controlled by the individual. Several studies have reported lower levels of physical activity among obese infants (Roberts et al., 1988; Rose and Mayer, 1986), children (Johnson et al., 1956), and adolescents (Bullen et al., 1964) but have been contradicted by other studies (Bandini et al., 1990a; Berkowitz et al., 1985). The issue of physical activity and obesity is complicated by several factors that make it difficult to draw conclusions. First, free-living physical activity is difficult to measure (Gutin and Manos, 1993). In addition, obese children use more energy for the same amount of movement. Defining physical activity as energy used may lead to the conclusion that the obese child engages in more activity than a lean child, while defining physical activity as movement may lead to the conclusion that the obese child engages in less physical activity (Dietz, 1992). Finally, levels of physical activity may vary over a lifetime. Just as periods of overeating may precede the development of obesity, periods of reduced activity may likewise precede the development of obesity.

Currently, it appears that fatter children move less than leaner children. With the use of more precise measurement techniques, the role of physical activity in the development and/or maintenance of obesity will become clearer. One hypothesis that needs further testing is that a low energy output is in some way corrected by an increase in food intake and subsequent weight gain (Hirsch and Leibel, 1988). The short-term imbalance of energy intake and expenditure required for the development of obesity may be small, making it difficult to identify as the cause. Measures of inactivity (e.g., time spent in a car or watching TV) may also be related to obesity independent of activity (Gortmaker et al., 1990). Further investigations are needed to identify the mechanisms that cause energy expenditure to be reduced early in life and to characterize more accurately the role of energy intake in promoting obesity.

## Genetic Factors

Convincing evidence now shows that body size and fatness have a strong genetic component (Stunkard et al., 1986). If both parents are overweight, approximately 80 percent of the offspring will be overweight. If neither parent is overweight, fewer than 10 percent of the children will be overweight (Bray, 1987). If children remain obese as they age, a greater percentage of them will become obese adults, especially among teenage children (Abraham and Nordsieck, 1960). In addition, the weight status of other family members may affect childhood obesity; obese children are more likely to have obese siblings (Garn et al., 1980, 1981).

The weight status of the parents may also affect the response of the obese child to treatment. Epstein et al. (1987) have reported that obese children of heavy parents do not lose weight as successfully as obese children of thin parents. In addition, in the absence of any treatment effort, a young obese child with two obese parents is much more likely to remain obese than an obese child of lean parents (Garn et al., 1981).

Studies of nuclear families and adoption data report heritability levels for BMI of about 20 to 30 percent (Bouchard and Pérusse, 1993a). However, twin studies have yielded higher heritability estimates of 60 to 90 percent (Feinleib et al., 1977; Stunkard et al., 1986, 1990). Taken together, the research to date suggests an important genetic component in the development of obesity. This genetic component interacts with environmental agents, primarily diet and level of physical activity, to produce obesity in susceptible people.

## Environmental Factors

Several environmental factors have been linked to obesity in children. Childhood obesity has been associated with season, geographic region, and population density. Prevalence is higher in the winter and spring and is lower in the summer and fall. The highest geographic rate of obesity occurs in the Northeast, followed by the Midwest, South, and West. Finally, the prevalence of obesity in urban areas is greater than in rural areas (Dietz, 1983; Dietz and Gortmaker, 1984).

Childhood obesity has also been associated with family characteristics (Dietz and Gortmaker, 1984) such as socioeconomic class (Rolland-Cachera and Bellisle, 1986; Rolland-Cachera, et al. 1988), family size (Ravelli and Belmont, 1979), and education (Sobal and Stunkard, 1989). Sobal and Stunkard (1989) showed that weight was inversely related to socioeconomic status for women but directly related to socioeconomic status for men and children. Jacoby et al. (1975) have shown the prevalence of obesity to be inversely related to family size. Children from high-income families have likewise been found to be fatter than those from lower-income families until late adolescence, when low-income girls become fatter while the girls from high-income families become leaner (Garn and Clark, 1976).

As role models and food providers, parents and other family members offer the first and most powerful influence on a child's eating and activity behavior (Garn et al., 1984). This area has been extensively reviewed by Ray and Klesges (1993). However, nonshared familial influences (defined as certain influences on eating and activity that are not shared among all family members) on body weight and obesity have also been noted (Grilo and Pogue-Geile, 1991). Waxman and Stunkard (1980) have reported that parents will feed obese children more than their thin siblings, claiming that obese children need more food because they are bigger. In another study, encouragement to eat from parents was more frequently directed at obese children compared with their lean siblings (Klesges et al., 1983). Thus, shared and nonshared family influences can affect the development of obesity in children.

Television represents another environmental factor with significant influence on the development of obesity. Dietz and Gortmaker (1985) reported a direct, positive relationship between television viewing and childhood obesity in a national sample of children and adolescents from diverse socioeconomic backgrounds. The average child 6–11 years old watches more than 20 hours of television a week (A. C. Nielsen Company, 1990), more time than attending school (Dorr, 1986). Children will be exposed to hundreds of commercials during this time, the majority of which are for food products (Ray and Klesges, 1993). Television may contribute to obesity by displacing more vigorous activities (Ross et al., 1987; Tucker, 1986), thereby reducing physical activity (or promoting inactivity) and increasing food and snack consumption, particularly of the nonnutritious foods frequently advertised (Clancy-Hepburn et al., 1974; Taras et al., 1989). Television viewing has been shown to be associated with significant reductions in resting metabolic rate among obese and nonobese girls (Klesges et al., 1993), although these results were not replicated in a more recent study (Dietz et al., 1994). Restriction of television viewing has been suggested to reduce body fat and prevent the development of obesity (Gortmaker et al., 1990). Clearly more research is needed to improve our understanding of how television influences both eating and activity behavior as well as body weight.

## Dieting Behaviors and Weight Preoccupation

Children as young as elementary school age appear to be responding to the societal and health pressures against obesity and are dieting to lose weight. Thus, dieting in childhood has become a very common behavior (Lifshitz et al., 1993). In one survey, almost 40 percent of high school children in an upper-class suburban area were dieting on the day of the survey, and almost two-thirds reported dieting during the preceding 4 to 8 weeks (Moses et al., 1989).

Children not only diet but also worry about their appearance. Children who are concerned about their weight and who undertake dieting can adversely affect their physical as well as psychological well-being. Inappropriate nutrient intake may lead to nutritional dwarfing and to a variety of other nutrition problems, as has been described elsewhere (Lifshitz, 1993). Children and adolescents can develop eating disorders such as anorexia and bulimia as a consequence of their weight and dieting preoccupation, which can lead to a variety of medical complications (Palla and Litt, 1988).

## HEALTH CONSEQUENCES OF OBESITY

### Medical

Obesity is an independent risk factor for the development of a number of chronic diseases that are the leading causes of morbidity and mortality in the United States, including atherosclerotic cardiovascular disease, hypertension, diabetes mellitus, gallbladder disease, and some cancers (NRC, 1989a). Childhood obesity is accompanied by significant morbidity and is acknowledged as a precursor to several risk factors for adult chronic disease. In addition, compared with adult-onset obesity, the persistence of child-onset obesity has been associated with higher rates of morbidity and mortality (Mellin, 1993). Thus, childhood obesity is a public health concern owing both to its immediate impact on health status and to its potential impact on adult body weight.

Childhood obesity is a major determinant of elevated blood pressure levels (Clarke et al., 1986; Lauer et al., 1991) and serum lipids and lipoproteins (Aristimuno et al., 1984; Wattigney et al., 1991). Childhood obesity is also associated with lower levels of high-density lipoprotein cholesterol, high levels of insulin, and increased heart rate and cardiac output (Freedman et al., 1987; Soto et al., 1989; Srinivasan et al., 1993). In addition, obese children are at greater risk for psychosocial dysfunction (Kimm et al., 1991; Wallace et al., 1993), respiratory disease (Simpser et al., 1977; Tracey et al., 1971), certain orthopedic problems (Figueroa-

Colon et al., 1992), and possibly diabetes (Deschamps et al., 1978). Data from longitudinal studies suggest that persistent childhood obesity can predict later health risks and adult mortality (Javier Nieto et al., 1992; Mossberg, 1989; Must et al., 1992). For example, school-age children, initially 13 to 18 years of age, were followed for up to 55 years. Follow-up mortality was greater among those who were overweight in adolescence; except for diabetes, the risks appear to be independent of overweight in adulthood (Must et al., 1992).

### Psychosocial

The most prevalent consequences of childhood obesity are psychosocial. Obese children have been shown to suffer depression (Sheslow et al., 1993) and problems with self-esteem (Sallade, 1973). Children as young as 5 years old learn to associate obesity with a variety of negative characteristics, using adjectives like "ugly," "lazy," "stupid," and "dirty" to describe the obese body type. By the time children reach the first grade, they prefer other disabilities over obesity (Richardson et al., 1967). In addition, parents themselves may have negative perceptions of their obese child (Waxman and Stunkard, 1980). Although the literature in this area is sparse and inconsistent, at least some children classified as obese perceive themselves negatively (Sheslow et al., 1993; Wadden et al., 1990a). Additional research is necessary to clarify our understanding of the psychosocial aspects of this disease in children and adolescents. At the present time, however, obesity should be viewed as a heterogeneous disease that may require a psychological evaluation to rule out associated social and emotional problems.

### Longitudinal

Several longitudinal studies tracking obesity in children indicate that overweight children are more likely than nonobese children to become obese as adults (Mossberg, 1989; Stark et al., 1981; Zack et al., 1979). The relative risk of an obese child becoming an overweight adult increases with the child's age. Approximately one-fourth of obese infants will become obese adults, whereas 80 percent of obese adolescents will become obese adults (Charney et al., 1976; Garn et al., 1989; Mossberg, 1989). Severity of childhood obesity also predicts adult obesity. In one study, one-third of children who were 120 percent of ideal body weight were normal weight by follow-up (approximately 9 years later); but none of those children who were greater than 160 percent of ideal body weight were normal weight at follow-up (Börjeson, 1962).

## HEALTH CONSEQUENCES OF DIETING

### Growth

One of the most debated side effects of the treatment for obesity in children is the effect of weight control on linear growth. Fueling this debate are several reports that suggest that dieting in obese children can influence short-term growth (Dietz and Hartung, 1985; Wolff, 1955). Two important facts must be considered when interpreting the data on this issue. First, obese children tend to be taller and reach their growth spurt sooner than their nonobese counterparts (Garn et al., 1974), underscoring the importance of looking at the long-term effects of dieting on linear growth. Obese and nonobese adults, however, have similar heights (Abraham and Johnson, 1980). Thus, longitudinal studies may actually show slower growth and a decrease in height percentiles in obese compared with nonobese children as they approach adulthood (Epstein et al., 1990a). Second, in evaluating the effect of diet on linear growth, parental height must also be considered since parental height is an important determinant of child height (Tanner et al., 1970).

Two long-term studies have assessed the growth patterns of children who received treatment for their obesity. Epstein et al. (1990b) treated children (6–12 years) in a behaviorally oriented family-based treatment program. Weight change did not correlate with growth when adjusted for parental height, and the children resembled their parents with respect to stature at 5 years of follow-up (Epstein et al., 1990a). After 10 years of follow-up, child height continued to be strongly related to the height of the parents of the same sex with no apparent effect of dieting on linear growth. This study is the first to provide long-term evidence on the effects of weight regulation during development on final height achieved.

These results are in agreement with a more recent study by Epstein and colleagues (1993). In this 10-year follow-up study of 158 obese children (6–12 years old), moderate energy restriction in conjunction with dietary guidance did not negatively influence long-term growth. Comparison of obese children who had dieted with normal-weight children (who had not dieted) at 10 years showed no differences in growth. It is prudent, however, when modifying diets of growing children to ensure adequate nutrition, and, as always, the child's height should be regularly monitored.

### Psychosocial Consequences

It is commonly believed that dieting is related to the development of eating disorders (Brownell, 1991b; Garner and Wooley, 1991) and that overweight and obese children and young adults may be at increased risk for subsequent development of eating disorders (Hsu, 1990), including body weight dissatisfaction, anorexia and bulimia, and binge eating disorder.

Body weight dissatisfaction, which is common among adolescent girls, is more severe in obese girls (Wadden and Stunkard, 1993). Many report that their bodies are "ugly and despicable and that others view them with hostility and contempt" (Stunkard and Mendelson, 1967). Further, histories obtained from persons with bulimia nervosa indicate that their first binge usually occurred when they were dieting, while anorexia is often defined as a diet that never ends (Wadden and Stunkard, 1993). Binge eating disorder, defined by the occurrence of eating binges with the absence of vomiting or other purging behavior, is common among obese persons entering weight-reduction programs (30 percent) but less common among obese persons in the community at large (5 percent). Although little is known about the specific incidence in children and adolescents, one study reported that 30 percent of obese adolescent girls seeking treatment for obesity engaged in binge eating (Berkowitz et al., 1993).

The effect of dieting on the development of eating disorders among obese children and adolescents is largely unknown. One study reported six children (3.8 percent) developing eating disorders (all with bulimia) following participation in a weight-control program (Epstein, 1993a). Thus, while eating disorders are a recognizable risk of obesity treatment, more research is clearly needed to improve our understanding of the relationship between dieting and the psychosocial consequences of obesity treatment, particularly in the pediatric population.

## TREATMENT

Despite the rising prevalence of obesity in the United States and the fact that childhood obesity is an important public health problem, few obesity treatment programs are available for children and adolescents (Dietz, 1994b). Research on the treatment of childhood obesity has been quite limited, particularly when compared with treatment for adults. As yet, no consensus exists on what constitutes the most effective treatment strategy for children and adolescents. Current programs for children are similar to adult treatment programs and are generally multidisciplinary in nature. This section reviews the literature on the basic components for treatment of childhood and adolescent obesity in both clinics and school settings.

Simply stated, the goals of the treatment of childhood obesity are weight loss without adverse health effects, followed by weight maintenance at the reduced body weight. In moderately overweight young children, the goal may simply be to maintain body weight since future growth will normalize the body weight. While treatment combines dietary change, an increase in exercise and physical activity, and behavior modification, what is unique to childhood treatment programs is the inclusion of parent training.

## Effect of Age

Because of the wide variation in developmental capabilities between the ages of 1 and 18, the age of the obese child must be considered when planning the treatment (Epstein, 1985). The child's capacity for understanding the disease is limited by his or her cognitive and motor abilities, which vary with age (Epstein, 1993a, b). In the very young child (1–5 years of age), parents have major control over the child's eating and activity and therefore represent an important focus of treatment in terms of food selection, preparation, and availability. In later years, the responsibility shifts from parents to the child, particularly as the adolescent strives to achieve autonomy. In fact, research among adolescents has shown that the outcome improves when parents and children are treated separately (Brownell et al., 1983). To date, little research has been devoted to age-appropriate intervention programs, though Epstein (1985) has developed a multistage model for the treatment of childhood obesity in which the responsibility for habit change is shifted from the parent to the child on the basis of the child's age and stage of development.

Most intervention studies have focused on treatment of preadolescent children (6–12 years of age) as compared to younger children (1–5 years) or adolescents (13–19 years) (Epstein, 1993b; Epstein and Wing, 1987). Future studies must focus on younger children and adolescents to fill in these gaps in our understanding of treatment and its outcome, to identify an optimal or preferred age to initiate treatment, and to develop treatment strategies that would be age appropriate.

## Parent Training

Since obesity is a familial disorder (Garn and Clark, 1976), the family, particularly the parents, is important in the treatment of the disease. As previously discussed, family influence is both environmental (e.g., modeling, food availability, and food and activity habits) as well as genetic. Epstein and Wing (1987) have demonstrated in numerous investigations the importance of family involvement in the treatment of obesity. The most impressive of these studies showed that targeting both obese children and their parents during treatment results in lower body weights and significantly less obesity at 5 and 10 years of follow-up than in a comparison group (Epstein et al., 1990c). In addition, more participants in the parent-plus-child group approached or achieved normal weight after 10 years than in the comparison group. Although participants were treated for a relatively short period of time (eight weekly visits and six monthly visits), these data provide the first evidence that a behavioral, family-based treatment program initiated when the child is 6 to 12 years of age can produce long-term effects that persist into young adulthood.

### Exercise

Physical activity has an important role in the treatment and prevention of obesity in children (Epstein et al., 1984a). Despite the controversy on the effect of inactivity in the development of obesity, physical activity in combination with dietary change has been shown to be effective in reducing obesity in children (Epstein, 1992; Epstein et al., 1985b). The inclusion of exercise has been shown to help preserve fat-free mass and to retard the reduction in metabolic rate that occurs among adults who are dieting (Whatley and Poehlman, 1994). To date, however, the results are inconclusive in children and require further study.

Some researchers have reported greater weight loss when exercise is combined with a low-calorie diet versus diet treatment alone (Epstein et al., 1985b; Reybrouck et al., 1990). Exercise may exert its greatest influence by promoting a more active lifestyle throughout adolescence and into adulthood (DHHS, 1991). Epstein et al. (1984b, 1985a) have evaluated two types of exercise programs (aerobic versus lifestyle) in conjunction with a hypocaloric diet in obese children. Both programs were isocaloric and included equivalent amounts of energy expenditure through exercise. The goal of the lifestyle program was to increase energy expenditure by increasing the amount of the participant's less structured, less intense daily activities (e.g., walking and climbing stairs). The aerobic exercise program included activities (e.g., running, cycling, swimming, or walking) of a specific duration and intensity. The results demonstrated that the lifestyle exercise program was associated with better weight change over the long term (17 to 24 months) but not over the short term (in which both programs were equal). The lifestyle program may have been more effective because of increased long-term adherence. Research in adults indicates that many people who begin exercise programs drop out (Oldridge, 1982). Epstein (1992) and colleagues (1984a) have shown that exercise intensity is an important determinant in predicting exercise nonadherence (i.e., the greater the intensity, the greater the dropout rate). Thus, exercise programs must always be evaluated with respect to adherence as well as changes in weight, fitness, and body composition.

Finally, data also demonstrate the importance of family involvement with regard to exercise adherence. Family-based programs in which parents are trained to reinforce their children's physical activity have reported increases in both activity and fitness levels in obese children (Epstein et al., 1987, 1990c).

## Diet

As with obesity treatment in adults, diet remains the cornerstone of therapy for the obese child since caloric restriction produces far greater energy deficits than exercise alone. Debate continues, however, about the degree of calorie restriction that should be used in children. Most diet programs for children fall into one of two fundamental types: a balanced hypocaloric diet or the more restrictive protein-sparing modified fast. Clearly, the diet should be matched to the severity of the problem.

A balanced hypocaloric diet, which is low in fat, high in complex carbohydrates, and contains adequate protein, is appropriate for most children and adolescents. This diet should be sufficient to promote growth while concurrently decreasing excess body fat. A reasonable goal on such a program is to lose 1 to 4 pounds per month, with maximal loss of fat and preservation of lean tissue. The diet must provide adequate protein, calories, and micronutrients to ensure normal growth and development (Dietz, 1983; Dietz and Robinson, 1993; Epstein, 1986; Williams et al., 1993). Because pediatric patients who undergo weight loss are in a period of growth and development, it is important to evaluate weight change as a function of stature.

When administered properly, these diets pose no recognized hazard for continued growth during weight reduction (Epstein et al., 1990c, 1993) and have been used by children as young as 5 years of age with good success (Epstein, 1986). Caloric intake may range from 1,200 to 2,000 calories per day or a deficit of 30 to 40 percent of usual intake (Figueroa-Colon et al., 1992), but should be adjusted to promote gradual weight loss (Williams et al., 1993). Children and parents must be taught portion size and food exchanges to provide balance and variety within the restricted intake.

The balanced hypocaloric diet programs can produce a 5-kilogram weight loss over 10 weeks (Figueroa-Colon et al., 1992). In a review of the literature, Epstein and Wing (1987) reported reductions in percentage of overweight that ranged from 3.2 to 28 percent over 2 to 12 months among published controlled studies. Variations in treatment outcome could be explained by the different components of the programs (i.e., family-based, treatment contingencies, or exercise).

The more restrictive protein-sparing modified fast (PSMF) should be limited for use in more serious cases of childhood and adolescent obesity, for which rapid weight reduction is essential. Use of a PSMF must always be carried out under the careful supervision of a physician (Merritt et al., 1980, 1981, 1983; NTF, 1993; Wadden et al., 1990b). In adults, very-low-calorie diets are generally recommended for individuals who are at least 30 percent or more over ideal body weight (Wadden et al., 1990b). In children, although the data are limited, the PSMF has been used on children as young as 6 years of age and by children whose body weight ranges from 120 percent to greater than 200 percent of ideal body weight (Suskind et al., 1993). In England, the PSMF is not recommended for use by children under the age of 13 (Department of Health and Social Security, 1987), though in the United States no consensus exists on what represents appropriate indications for its use in children. Recently, the National Task Force on the Prevention and Treatment of Obesity (1993) suggested that use of the PSMF in children and adolescents should be considered experimental and treatment should be administered by experienced medical staff. The PSMF is contraindicated in children who have renal, hepatic, or cardiac disease, and all patients should be monitored closely for sustained nitrogen losses, cardiac arrhythmias, and cholelithiasis (Dietz and Robinson, 1993).

The PSMF for children and adolescents typically ranges from 600 to 800 calories per day. The diet provides 1.5 to 2.0 grams of high-quality protein per kilogram of ideal body weight per day, which is higher than the level recommended for adults because of the potential for complications from increased nitrogen losses in children (Dietz and Robinson, 1993; Dietz and Wolfe, 1985; Merritt et al., 1980). In addition, at least 2 liters of water or calorie-free fluids are consumed daily, along with 2–4 cups of low-starch vegetables, one multivitamin tablet containing iron, 800 milligrams of calcium, and 25 milliequivalents of potassium. Details of the dietary protocol for the PSMF are given by Dietz (1983), Figueroa-Colon et al. (1992), and Suskind et al. (1993).

An average weight loss of about 10 kilograms in 10 weeks has been reported for use of the PSMF (Figueroa-Colon et al., 1992; Suskind et al., 1993). Long-term data are lacking, though recently Figueroa-Colon et al. (1993) reported that children maintained a 10-kilogram weight loss produced on a PSMF for 14.5 months. In another study, 12 of 17 obese adolescents treated with a PSMF diet were available for follow-up at 1 year (Stallings et al., 1988); of these, 48 percent had maintained their weight loss. Although not frequently used in children or adolescents, a liquid very-low-calorie diet (VLCD) has been shown in one study to have poor compliance and a high dropout rate in eight adolescents (Brownell et al., 1983). Clearly, more short- and long-term studies (with at least 2 years or more of follow-up) are needed to characterize treatment outcome in this population, particularly with regard to the effect of severe caloric restriction on linear growth and development.

## Behavior Modification

Behavior modification facilitates weight-loss efforts by helping patients develop appropriate eating and exercise behaviors and cope with disturbing weight-related thoughts and emotions (Stunkard, 1987). The effectiveness and importance of this treatment component has been documented in more than 100 controlled clinical trials (Brownell and Kramer, 1994). Standard behavioral programs include self-monitoring, positive reinforcement, stimulus control, cognitive restructuring, and nutrition education. The details of the standard behavior modification program have been reviewed extensively by Epstein (1986) and Kramer et al. (1989).

## Long-Term Outcome

The true effectiveness of treatment can be measured only by examining data on long-term outcome. While few studies have attempted to follow patients beyond the initial treatment, results reported to date have been promising, especially compared with 5- and 10-year outcomes in adults (Kramer et al., 1989). Epstein et al. (1990b) evaluated the 5-year outcome results of four prospective, randomized, controlled, multidisciplinary treatment programs that differed with respect to how family-based treatment or exercise was implemented. Subjects were 6–12 years of age at the start of the studies and were randomized to alternative treatments that lasted 8–12 weeks, with monthly meetings continuing for another 6–12 months. One subgroup within each of two of the studies achieved a 10 percent reduction in relative weight at the end of 5 years. The best results were achieved by reciprocal reinforcement of the children and their parents compared with a program that reinforced only the child for success.

Ten-year follow-up data have been reported for a three-arm study of multidisciplinary treatment (Epstein et al., 1990c). The groups differed only in the method of reinforcement for weight and behavior change. Children in the group that reinforced both parents and children showed significantly greater reductions in percentage of overweight after 5 and 10 years (11.2 and 7.5 percent, respectively). In addition, a greater percentage of children in the parent-plus-child treatment group achieved or approached normal weight for height (33 percent) than of the children treated without their parents (5 percent).

Nuutinen and Knip (1992) conducted a 5-year follow-up study of 48 obese children who participated in a multidisciplinary weight-reduction program. They defined a successful weight loser as a child with at least a 10 percent reduction in relative weight after 2 years of active treatment. At 5 years' follow-up, 49 percent (n = 22) of subjects who had been treated and defined as successful weight losers after 2 years were still able to maintain at least a 10 percent decrease in relative weight, and 31 percent (n = 14) of children were not obese after 5 years. Favorable changes in cardiovascular risk factors (e.g., reduced total cholesterol, triglycerides, and plasma insulin levels and increased HDL cholesterol levels) were also reported.

### School-Based Studies

Few obesity intervention studies have been conducted in the schools. However, schools provide an excellent opportunity for preventing and treating this disease, as children spend a significant amount of their first two decades of life in school and more than 95 percent of American youth aged 5–17 are enrolled in school (NCES, 1990). In contrast to clinic programs, school programs require no financial commitment from parents and may reach children who might otherwise not seek treatment. In addition, children eat one or two meals at school, which offers the opportunity to expose them to nutritious foods and to teach healthful eating habits.

Over the past 12 years, only four large controlled studies have been conducted in schools (Brownell and Kaye, 1982; Foster et al., 1985; Lansky and Brownell, 1982; Lansky and Vance, 1983). Each program included nutrition education, exercise, and behavior modification strategies, and interventions lasted from 10 to 18 weeks. The programs were administered only to overweight or obese children. Three of the studies compared the intervention group with a no-treatment control (Brownell and Kaye, 1982; Foster et al., 1985; Lansky and Brownell, 1982); one study compared the intervention with a standard health-education program as the comparison group (Lansky and Brownell, 1982). In all four studies, the intervention group had a significantly greater reduction in percentage of overweight compared with the control group (see Table C-4). A more in-depth summary of these studies is provided by Epstein and Wing (1987) and Resnicow (1993).

Unfortunately, few follow-up data are available from these studies, and the long-term effects remain unknown. School-wide programs that would include both nonobese and obese children may also have an impact on children not currently obese but at risk (e.g., thin children of two obese parents). Thus the school represents a potentially useful setting for

**TABLE C-4**  Summary of Multidisciplinary School-Based Intervention Studies

| Study | Age (years) | Treatment Group | Randomized | Number | Treatment Duration (months) | Change in % Overweight |
|---|---|---|---|---|---|---|
| Brownell and Kaye, 1982 | 5–12 | beh mod | yes | 63 | 10 | -15.4 |
|  |  | control |  | 14 | — | -2.8 |
| Foster et al., 1985 | 5–12 | beh mod | no | 43 | 3 (6)[a] | -5.4 (-3.6)[a] |
|  |  | control |  | 41 | — | +0.3 (-0.2)[a] |
| Lansky and Brownell, 1982 | 12–15 | beh mod | yes | 36 | 3.5 | -3.0 |
|  |  | health ed |  | 35 | — | -2.1 |
| Lansky and Vance, 1983 | 11–14 | beh mod | no | 30 | 12 | -5.7 |
|  |  | control |  | 25 | — | +2.4 |
|  |  | ss control |  | 59 | — | -1.5 |

NOTE:  Beh mod = behavior modification; control = no treatment control; health ed = health education program which includes nutrition and exercise education; ss control = self-selected control.

[a]6-month follow-up data are available and denoted in parentheses.

SOURCE:  Epstein, L.H., and R.R. Wing. 1987. Behavioral treatment of childhood obesity. Psychology Bulletin 101:331–342. Copyright 1987 by the American Psychological Association. Adapted by permission.

the primary and secondary prevention of obesity, and more research needs to be initiated in this setting.

## PREVENTION

Because of the refractory nature of obesity, prevention remains the treatment of choice (Council on Scientific Affairs, 1988). Preventing childhood obesity may, in fact, be an effective way to prevent adult obesity. However, to date little research has addressed the prevention of pediatric obesity. In the only controlled study specifically investigating the prevention of obesity in children, Pisacano et al. (1978) gave parents of infants health education emphasizing a low-fat, prudent diet. Compared with a usual-care control group, the prevalence of obesity was significantly reduced for intervention group children from 3 months to 3 years.

Available epidemiologic data make it possible to identify individuals at increased risk for obesity in whom preventive measures could be implemented. Parental obesity is an important risk factor for childhood obesity (Garn and Clark, 1976). In children of obese parents, careful monitoring of weight change could help to identify children for whom alterations in diet and physical activity are needed to prevent the disease. Recently, specific periods for the development of obesity and its health sequels have been identified (Dietz, 1994a). These include the period of adiposity rebound that occurs between the ages of 5 and 7, adolescence, and possibly the period of gestation and early infancy. However, it is unclear whether these periods represent critical periods of the onset of persistent obesity. Further research is needed to identify the most effective time to initiate treatment of childhood obesity and possibly prevent adult obesity; the most effective time to initiate preventive efforts for childhood obesity could also be the focus of research. Prevention interventions could be adapted from existing treatment programs (Epstein and Wing, 1987; Epstein et al., 1990c).

With respect to prevention, two important interventions are altering diet and increasing physical activity. Decreasing the amount of inactivity, possibly by limiting television exposure, may also be effective (Gortmaker et al., 1990). A recent study has suggested that early and frequent (more than four visits) intervention among preschool children (ages 1–5 years) was effective at reducing the degree of obesity over a 1-year period (Davis et al., 1993a). These results, while provocative, suggest that future research must address the effect of frequency and timing of the intervention on the long-term outcome of preventive treatment. School-based prevention programs would likewise offer an excellent setting for intervention and education (Resnicow, 1993). Although many gaps exist in our current knowledge of the etiology and treatment of obesity, the foundation is in place to develop and evaluate the primary prevention of obesity in the pediatric population.

## SUMMARY AND DIRECTIONS FOR FUTURE RESEARCH

In its Healthy People 2000 report, the federal government proposed the goal of reducing obesity to a prevalence of no more than 15 percent among adolescents aged 12 to 19 years (DHHS, 1991). From a health perspective, obesity treatment in children and adolescents seeks a reduction in body fat that is safe; involves minimal hunger; preserves lean body mass; and allows for normal growth, development, and activity. As with adult programs, comprehensive treatment for childhood and adolescent obesity includes a hypocaloric diet, an exercise program, and a behavior management program. The program must be appropriate for the child's age and stage of development and include the parents and family in treatment.

Few data address the etiology, treatment, and prevention of childhood and adolescent obesity. More studies must be conducted to develop a consensus in a number of areas. Six general areas have been identified for future studies: definition, etiology, treatment, eating behavior, weight maintenance, and prevention. Although not exhaustive, the following observations summarize the most salient research agendas in each of these areas.

### Definition

Although new guidelines have been issued by the Expert Committee on Clinical Guidelines for Overweight in Adolescent Preventive Services, the expected sensitivity, specificity, and predictive value of the two-level screening remains unknown. In addition, no consensus exists for equivalent values in preschool (ages 1–5 years) and preadolescent (ages 6–9 years) children. Further research is clearly needed to provide standard guidelines for the screening of at-risk and overweight children of all ages.

### Etiology

Despite several theories, the causes of obesity in children remain unclear, particularly those related to energy imbalance and age of onset. Fundamental to answering these questions is the development of improved techniques for measuring subtle changes in energy expenditure (including total energy expenditure, physical activity, resting metabolic rate, thermogenesis, and energy intake). Some evidence suggests that obese children consume a greater percentage of calories as fat than do normal weight children, thus making the effect of macronutrient composition on the development of obesity another area of potential interest.

## Treatment

What is the optimal approach to treating childhood obesity? Standard programs tend to be modeled after adult treatment programs and include dietary change, increasing physical activity, and behavior modification along with parent training. However, future work must continue to examine the efficacy of each component and to test variations in intervention in different populations. For example, continued investigation of the short- and long-term (into adulthood) effects of use of a PSMF or liquid VLCD is needed, as is research into the role of duration of treatment. A large body of work has come from Leonard Epstein and his colleagues at the University of Pittsburgh, who have explored different behavioral strategies and their effect on treatment outcome. This work needs to be continued and effective treatment models refined. Other important research questions include the identification of appropriate treatment goals for children and adolescents as well as identifying the optimal age for treatment.

Interventions must also be tailored to the child's age and level of cognitive, social, and emotional development. Because of the psychological consequences of adolescent-onset obesity and the disproportionate share of adult obesity that originates in adolescence, treatment for this group deserves special emphasis. Research must be undertaken to determine the most effective methods for intervention during adolescence, bearing in mind the vulnerability of adolescents to eating disorders. Treatment programs also need to be culturally and ethnically appropriate. Much research is needed in the area of minority food preference, preparation habits, and parental influence to develop effective treatment programs for different ethnic groups.

## Eating Behavior

More research must explore the effect of family, social/cultural, and environmental factors on eating behavior. Epstein et al. (1990c) have shown that children can lose and maintain weight over an extended period of time and that parental participation is essential to a positive outcome. It is likely, however, that the motivation structures within the family that affect behavior change may be as important as the behaviors being modified (Epstein, 1993a). Future research must identify methods that mobilize family support for behavior change. In addition, descriptive research is needed to clarify our understanding of how the family contributes to or can help mitigate the development of obesity. Research into how environmental factors (e.g., television, video games, cars, and readily available snack foods) affect behavior and body weight must also continue.

## Weight Maintenance

Strategies for promoting maintenance of weight loss and preventing relapse have been largely ignored in the pediatric population. Future studies must address both maintenance and relapse prevention in children and adolescents.

## Prevention

Almost no research has been done in the area of prevention, although prevention of pediatric obesity may be the only effective treatment of adult obesity. By adapting existing treatment protocols, programs directed at primary prevention of obesity can be developed. Issues to be resolved include who should be targeted (all children or just those at risk) and where these programs would be administered (e.g., in schools, in communities, through physicians' offices). Schools clearly represent a cost-effective setting, but intervention programs must be developed and tested in other locations as well.

At least two or three critical periods have been identified during childhood for the development of obesity and its putative health consequences (diabetes, hypertension, hypercholesterolemia, and cardiovascular disease). These periods represent potential treatment targets for the prevention of adult obesity, and additional research is needed to identify the most effective time to target efforts to prevent and treat childhood obesity.

# D

# Accrediting Providers of Weight-Management Services

*Arthur Frank, M.D.*

The weight-loss industry is largely unregulated. Health-care providers are required to maintain their own licensure, but commercial and nonprofessional programs have essentially no license or regulatory requirements. Anyone can provide weight-loss services in almost any context. Skills, training, and the maintenance of standards are not required, monitored, or assessed in any way.

Accreditation systems have been successful in hospitals, colleges, and universities, and in many other aspects of health care. Typically, these are voluntary accreditation systems, but since government agencies, insurance companies, and many physicians and consumers would not tolerate an unaccredited hospital (or college or university), no hospital could survive without accreditation. I believe such a system could be made to work in the control of weight-loss programs. Without much involvement of government agencies, a voluntary accreditation system could be established as follows:

---

COMMITTEE'S NOTE: In Chapter 1, we describe several efforts and initiatives to influence and regulate the practices and advertising claims of the weight-loss industry. Committee member Arthur Frank believes strongly in a voluntary accreditation system for weight-management programs to accomplish these goals. While the committee does not endorse Dr. Frank's proposal as described above, we feel it represents a point of view that merits wider attention and debate.

1. A national commission could be established by an appropriate authority to formulate reasonable standards of care, to characterize the types of services provided, to establish a nongovernmental accrediting agency, and then to go out of business.

2. The commission would identify different levels of weight-loss care and develop reasonable standards within each of these levels.

3. Programs and providers may elect to be accredited according to these standards or choose not to be accredited and then answer to their clients. The programs would specify the types of services they provide and the qualifications of the providers. The accrediting agency would not tolerate the mislabeling of professional skills, the promotion of exaggerated claims, or the misrepresentation of services provided.

4. Much like the system of hospital accreditation, the programs would pay for the privilege of accreditation and would need continuing recertification at appropriate intervals. The system should be financially self-sufficient and not require government funds.

5. The accreditation system should be able to provide guidelines for consumers about the kinds of services and how to select from among them. Overweight people should be able to identify who is providing the care, the intensity and cost of the program, and the skills and training of those involved.

Regulators, particularly those involved with hospital regulation, have questioned whether there would be enough incentive in such a system to pressure weight-loss companies into participating, particularly when the sanctions of withholding financial benefits are not available as a weapon. It is worth considering whether the marketplace would provide the needed incentive. There is sustained and intense competition among weight-loss companies. Each is looking for an edge in its direct promotions to consumers. Perhaps many would consider this certification to provide significantly better leverage in reaching consumers than traditional flashy advertising promotions alone. Perhaps, also, a newly reformed health-care system, with a more enlightened approach to the disease of obesity, could require that benefits be available only to programs that are certified—the kind of leverage that made hospital accreditation mandatory and universal.

# E

## Biographies of Committee Members

**JUDITH S. STERN** (*Chair*) is a Professor in the Department of Nutrition at the College of Agricultural and Environmental Sciences, University of California, Davis. Concurrently, she is a Professor in the Department of Internal Medicine, Division of Clinical Nutrition and Metabolism, at the University of California, Davis, School of Medicine. She also serves as Director for the university's Food Intake Laboratory Group. Dr. Stern is a registered dietitian and is a member of the American Institute of Nutrition, the Vice-President Elect of the American Society for Clinical Nutrition (and past chair of the Public Information Committee), the American Dietetic Association, the Gerontological Society of America, the Institute of Food Technologists, the North American Association for the Study of Obesity (where she is a Past President), and the Society for Ingestive Behavior, among others. She has served on several advisory boards and committees, including the Institute of Medicine's Committee on Nutrition Components of Food Labeling. In addition to her many journal publications, Dr. Stern frequently writes for popular magazines as well. She is currently an executive editor for *Appetite* and is on the editorial board of *Obesity Research* and *Weight Control Digest*. She earned a B.S. in Food and Nutrition at Cornell University and an M.S. and Sc.D. in Nutrition at the Harvard University School of Public Health.

**JULES HIRSCH** (*Vice Chair*) is the Sherman Fairchild Professor at Rockefeller University, Physician-in-Chief at Rockefeller University Hospital, and Senior Attending Physician at St. Luke's-Roosevelt Hospital.

As a senior member of the National Academy of Sciences Institute of Medicine, he has served on the Committee on the Health Consequences of Bereavement, the Board on Biobehavioral Sciences and Mental Disorders, the Panel on Clinical Sciences, and the Panel on Metabolism, Endocrinology, and Hematology. Dr. Hirsch is a Past President of the American Psychosomatic Society and the American Society of Clinical Nutrition. He is a fellow of the American Institute of Nutrition, the Royal College of Physicians in Edinburgh, the New York Academy of Medicine, the American Association for the Advancement of Science, and the American College of Physicians. He has received the McCollum Award and the Herman Award of the American Society for Clinical Nutrition and an Honorary Doctor of Science degree from the State University of New York. In addition to being a section editor for *Obesity Research*, Dr. Hirsch is a member of several editorial boards, including those of the *American Journal of Clinical Nutrition, Journal of Nutritional Biochemistry, Weight Control Digest*, and the *International Journal of Obesity*. He attended Rutgers, the State University of New Jersey, and holds his M.D. from the Southwestern Medical School at the University of Texas, Dallas.

**STEVEN N. BLAIR** is Director of Research and Director of Epidemiology and Clinical Applications at the Cooper Institute for Aerobics Research. For seven years, Dr. Blair served as the exercise epidemiology section editor for *Research Quarterly for Exercise and Sport* and continues work on the editorial boards for several epidemiology, exercise, and sports medicine journals, including the *Macmillan Health Encyclopedia*. He was a contributor and co-principal investigator for the Multiple Risk Factor Intervention Trial. In the past, he was on the Board of Trustees and was a Vice President for the American College of Sports Medicine. Dr. Blair has received several awards from the American Alliance for Health, Physical Education, Recreation, and Dance (AAHPERD), and he received a Citation Award from the American College of Sports Medicine and a Doctor Honoris Causa degree from the Free University of Brussels. He holds a B.A. in Physical Education from Kansas Wesleyan University and an M.S. and P.E.D. in Physical Education from Indiana University, Bloomington. Dr. Blair was a postdoctoral scholar in preventive cardiology at Stanford University and is a certified exercise program director with the American College of Sports Medicine.

**JOHN P. FOREYT** is a Professor in the Department of Medicine at Baylor College of Medicine in Houston, Texas and Director of the DeBakey Heart Center's Nutrition Research Clinic. Concurrently, he is a clinical professor in the Department of Psychology at the University of Houston and is a member of the Medical Scientist Staff for Internal Medicine Service at

The Methodist Hospital. He is licensed by the Texas State Board of Examiners of Psychologists. In addition to serving as a manuscript reviewer for several publications, Dr. Foreyt is currently an editorial board member for the *Journal of the American Dietetic Association; Eating Disorders; Medicine, Exercise, Nutrition and Health; Obesity Research; Journal of Cardiopulmonary Rehabilitation; American Journal of Health Promotion; Journal of Behavioral Medicine;* and *Health Values.* Among his professional affiliations, he is a fellow of the Behavior Therapy and Research Society, the Society of Behavioral Medicine, and the Academy of Behavioral Medicine Research. Dr. Foreyt received his B.S. in Psychology at the University of Wisconsin, Madison, and holds his M.S. in Psychology and Ph.D. in Clinical Psychology from Florida State University, Tallahassee.

**ARTHUR FRANK** is the Medical Director of the Obesity Management Program at the George Washington University School of Medicine in Washington, D.C., where he is also on the faculty in the Department of Medicine. He is an internist and completed his specialty training, including a U.S. Public Health Service Fellowship in Endocrinology and Metabolism, at Stanford University. He studied lipid kinetics as a research fellow at the National Heart Institute. He also served as the Director of the Food and Nutrition Programs for the Office of Economic Opportunity and as a consultant to the Assistant Secretary for Health of the Department of Health and Human Services. He has been on the faculty at Georgetown University School of Medicine and was the first Medical Director of the university's community health plan. In addition to publications in obesity and lipid kinetics, Dr. Frank has written for the public on issues of medical care as a health columnist for *Mademoiselle* and is coauthor of *The People's Handbook of Medical Care.* Dr. Frank holds his B.S. in Chemistry from the Massachusetts Institute of Technology, M.S. in Biochemistry from the University of Pennsylvania, and M.D. from New York University.

**SHIRIKI K. KUMANYIKA** is Professor and Associate Director for Epidemiology, Center for Biostatistics and Epidemiology at the Pennsylvania State University College of Medicine in Hershey, Pennsylvania. Previously, she taught at Cornell University and The Johns Hopkins University. Dr. Kumanyika has a long working relationship with the National Institutes of Health; she served as an investigator for the National Cancer Institute, the National Institute of Allergy and Infectious Diseases, the National Institute on Aging, and the National Heart, Lung, and Blood Institute. Some of her most recent consulting activities have been for the Women's Health Trial at the University of Alabama, Birmingham; the Women's Health and Aging Study at The Johns Hopkins University; the

University of Wisconsin School of Nursing, Milwaukee; and the Clinical Epidemiology Unit at the University Canton Hospital in Geneva, Switzerland. Dr. Kumanyika served on the Institute of Medicine's Committee to Study the Legal and Ethical Issues Relating to the Inclusion of Women in Clinical Studies and is a member of the 1995 Dietary Guidelines Advisory Committee of the U.S. Public Health Service. Among her many professional affiliations, Dr. Kumanyika includes the American Institute of Nutrition, the American Society for Clinical Nutrition, the Gerontological Society of America, the North American Association for the Study of Obesity, and the Society for the Analysis of African American Public Health Issues. She is a registered dietitian and holds her B.A. in Psychology from Syracuse University, M.S. in Social Work from Columbia University, Ph.D. in Human Nutrition from Cornell University, and M.P.H. from The Johns Hopkins University School of Hygiene and Public Health.

**JENNIFER H. MADANS** is Director of the Division of Epidemiology at the National Center for Health Statistics (NCHS), Centers for Disease Control and Prevention (CDC), in Hyattsville, Maryland, where she is also the Acting Chief of the division's Demographic Analysis Staff. She is an Adjunct Associate Professor at the Georgetown University School of Medicine and has been a Lecturer at The Catholic University of America. Dr. Madans was a member of several CDC committees and chairs the Interagency Coordinating Committee of NCHS and the National Heart, Lung, and Blood Institute, and the Health Interview Survey Scientific Advisory Committee. In addition to several student prizes, she received the Public Health Service Superior Service Award, NCHS Directors Award in Methodological Statistics, and NCHS Elijah White Memorial Award. She is a member of the American Sociological Association, the American Statistical Association, the Population Association of America, the American Public Health Association, the Society for Epidemiological Research, and the Gerontological Society of America. Dr. Madans received a B.A. in Sociology from Bard College in Annandale-on-Hudson, New York, and an M.A. and Ph.D. in Sociology from the University of Michigan, Ann Arbor.

**G. ALAN MARLATT** is Professor of Psychology and Director, Addictive Behaviors Research Center, Department of Psychology, at the University of Washington. He has conducted research at the Harvard University Center for Addiction Studies; La Trobe University in Melbourne, Australia; the Addiction Research Unit of the Institute of Psychiatry at Maudsley Hospital, London; and the University of Auckland, New Zealand. Dr. Marlatt served as president of the Association for the Advancement of Behavior Therapy and the Society of Psychologists in Addictive Behaviors. He has also served on the Institute of Medicine's Committee on the Treatment of Alcohol Problems. He is also on the editorial board of several journals, including *Weight Control Digest, Addictive Behaviors,* and *Cognitive Therapy and Research,* and is a consulting editor for *Psychology of Addictive Behaviors.* Dr. Marlatt received an Annual Research Award from the Society of Psychologists in Addictive Behaviors, the Distinguished Psychologist for Professional Contributions to Knowledge award from the Washington State Psychological Association, and Jellinek Memorial Award for Alcohol Studies from the International Council on Alcohol and Addiction. He holds a B.A. in Psychology from the University of British Columbia in Vancouver and a Ph.D. in Clinical Psychology from Indiana University, Bloomington.

**SACHIKO TOKUNAGA ST. JEOR** is Professor of Clinical Medicine and Director of the Nutrition Education and Research Program in the School of Medicine and Professor of Nutrition in the College of Human and Community Sciences at the University of Nevada. Her research interests are weight management, obesity, nutrition assessment, cancer prevention, and nutrition education in medical schools. Dr. St. Jeor has been honored as an outstanding alumna from both the College of Health and Human Development at Pennsylvania State University and the College of Health at the University of Utah. She also received the Award for Excellence in the Practice of Dietetic Research and chaired the Council of Research of the American Dietetic Association and is a founding member of the Council on Renal Nutrition of the National Kidney Foundation. Dr. St. Jeor was a member of the Institute of Medicine's Committee on Opportunities in the Nutrition and Food Sciences and has served in the Behavioral Medicine Study Section and on the Clinical Applications and Prevention Advisory Committee for the National Heart, Lung, and Blood Institute, National Institutes of Health. She is currently a member of the 1995 Dietary Guidelines Advisory Committee of the U.S. Public Health Service. She has served on the editorial boards of *Behavioral Medicine Abstracts, Clinics in Applied Nutrition, Weight Control Digest,* and the *Journal of the American Dietetic Association.* Dr. St. Jeor holds a B.A. in Nutrition from the University of Utah, Salt Lake City; an M.S. in Nutrition from the University of Iowa, Iowa City; and a Ph.D. in Nutrition from Pennsylvania State University, University Park.

**ALBERT J. STUNKARD** is Professor of Psychiatry and former Chairman of the Department of Psychiatry at the University of Pennsylvania. His research has investigated sociological, psychological, metabolic, and genetic determinants of human obesity and treatment of the disorder by behavioral, dietary, pharmacological, and surgical measures. He has twice been awarded the Annual Prize for Research of the American Psychiatric Association and received the Joseph Goldberger Award in Clinical Nutrition of the American Medical Association. He serves on several editorial boards and is Executive Editor of *Appetite*. He is a member of the Institute of Medicine and most recently served on its Committee on Opportunities in the Nutrition and Food Sciences. Dr. Stunkard is also Past President of the American Psychosomatic Society, the Society of Behavioral Medicine, and the Association for Research in Nervous and Mental Disease. He holds a B.S. from Yale University, an M.D. from Columbia College of Physicians and Surgeons, and an honorary Doctor of Medicine degree from the University of Edinburgh.

**PAUL R. THOMAS** (FNB Staff, Project Director) has served as Project Director of the Committee on Opportunities in the Nutrition and Food Sciences and the Committee on Dietary Guidelines Implementation. He was editor for the report *Improving America's Diet and Health: From Recommendations to Action*, co-editor of *Opportunities in the Nutrition and Food Sciences: Research Challenges and the Next Generation of Investigators*, and assisted the FNB subcommittee that produced the *10th Edition of the Recommended Dietary Allowances*. Dr. Thomas also was the co-editor of the popular book *Eat For Life: The Food and Nutrition Board's Guide to Reducing Your Risk of Chronic Disease*. In addition, he co-authored *The Nutrition Debate: Sorting Out Some Answers* with Joan Dye Gussow, Ed.D. Prior to joining the FNB, he established and directed the Division of Nutrition Services at the Monongalia County Health Department in Morgantown, West Virginia. Dr. Thomas holds a B.A. degree in Biology from the State University of New York at Buffalo; an M.S. degree in Public Health Nutrition from Case Western Reserve University, Cleveland; and Ed.M. and Ed.D. degrees in Nutrition Education from Teachers College, Columbia University, New York.

# Bibliography

A. C. Nielsen Company. 1990. 1990 Nielsen Report on TV. Nielsen Co., Northbrook, IL.

Abraham, S., and C. L. Johnson. 1980. Prevalence of severe obesity in the United States. Am. J. Clin. Nutr. 33:364–369.

Abraham, S., and M. Nordsieck. 1960. Relationship of excess weight in children and adults. Public Health Rep. 75:263–273.

ADA and ADA (American Dietetic Association and the American Diabetes Association, Inc.). 1989. Exchange Lists for Weight Management. American Dietetic Association, Chicago, IL.

Adams, S. O., K. E. Grady, C. H. Wolk, and C. Mukaida. 1986. Weight loss: A comparison of group and individual interventions. J. Am. Diet. Assoc. 86:485–490.

Agras, W. S. 1987. Eating Disorders: Management of Obesity, Bulimia, and Anorexia Nervosa. Pergamon Press, New York.

AIN (American Institute of Nutrition). 1994. Report of the American Institute of Nutrition (AIN) Steering Committee on Healthy Weight. J. Nutr. 124:2240–2243.

Ainsworth, B. E., W. L. Haskell, A. S. Leon, D. R. Jacobs Jr., H. J. Montoye, J. F. Sallis, and R. S. Paffenbarger Jr. 1993. Compendium of physical activities: Classification of energy costs of human physical activities. Med. Sci. Sports Exerc. 25:71–80.

Allan, J. D., K. Mayo, and Y. Michel. 1993. Body size values of white and black women. Res. Nurs. Health 16(5):323–333.

Amatruda, J. M., J. F. Richeson, S. L. Welle, R. G. Brodows, and D. H. Lockwood. 1988. The safety and efficacy of a controlled low-energy ("very low-calorie") diet in the treatment of non-insulin-dependent diabetes and obesity. Arch. Intern. Med. 148:873–877.

Anderson, J. J., and D. T. Felson. 1988. Factors associated with osteoarthritis of the knee in the first national Health and Nutrition Examination Survey (HANES I): Evidence for an association with overweight, race, and physical demands of work. Am. J. Epidemiol. 128:179–189.

Anderson, J. W., C. C. Hamilton, and V. Brinkman-Kaplan. 1992. Benefits and risks of an intensive very low-calorie diet program for severe obesity. Am. J. Gastroenterol. 87:6–15.

Andres, R., D. C. Muller, and J. D. Sorkin. 1993. Long-term effects of change in body weight on all-cause mortality. A review. Ann. Intern. Med. 119:737–743.

Apfelbaum, M., P. Björntorp, J. Garrow, W. P. T. James, E. Jéquier, and A. J. Stunkard. 1987. Standards for reporting the results of obesity treatment programs. Am. J. Clin. Nutr. 45:1035–1036.

Archaumbault, F. X. Jr. 1992. Review of the Tennessee Self-Concept Scale [Revised]. Pp. 931–933 in J. J. Kramer and J. C. Conoley, eds. The Eleventh Mental Measurements Yearbook. The University of Nebraska Press, Lincoln, NE.

Aristimuno, G. G., T. A. Foster, A. W. Voors, S. R. Srinivasan, and G. S. Berenson. 1984. Influence of persistent obesity in children on cardiovascular risk factors: The Bogalusa Heart Study. Circulation 69:895–904.

Atkinson, R. L., and V. S. Hubbard. 1994. Report on the NIH Workshop on Pharmacologic Treatment of Obesity. Am. J. Clin. Nutr. 60:153–156.

Avons, P., P. Garthwaite, H. L. Davies, P. R. Murgatroyd, and W. P. James. 1988. Approaches to estimating physical activity in the community: Calorimetric validation of actometers and heart rate monitoring. Eur. J. Clin. Nutr. 42:185–196.

Baecke, J. A., J. Burema, and J. E. Frijters. 1982. A short questionnaire for the measurement of habitual physical activity in epidemiological studies. Am. J. Clin. Nutr. 36:936–942.

Bandini, L. G., D. A. Schoeller, H. N. Cyr et al. 1987. A validation of energy intake and energy expenditure in obese and nonobese adolescents. Int. J. Obes. 11:937A.

Bandini, L. G., D. A. Schoeller, and W. H. Dietz. 1990a. Energy expenditure in obese and nonobese adolescents. Pediatr. Res. 27:198–203.

Bandini, L. G., D. A. Schoeller, H. N. Cyr, and W. H. Dietz. 1990b. Validity of reported energy intake in obese and nonobese adolescents. Am. J. Clin. Nutr. 52:421–425.

Bandura, A., and K. M. Simon. 1977. The role of proximal intentions in self-regulation of refractory behaviors. Cognit. Ther. Res. 1:177–193.

Baranoski, T., R. J. Dworkin, C. J. Cieslik, P. Hooks, D. R. Clearman, L. Ray, J. K. Dunn, and P. R. Nader. 1984. Reliability and validity of self-report of aerobic activity: Family Health Project. Res. Q. Exerc. Sports 55:309–317.

Basiotis, P. P., S. O. Welsh, F. J. Cronin, J. L. Kelsay, and W. Mertz. 1987. Number of days of food intake records required to estimate individual and group nutrient intakes with defined confidence. J. Nutr. 117:1638–1641.

Beck, A. T., C. H. Ward, M. Mendelson, J. Mock, and J. Erbaugh. 1961. An inventory for measuring depression. Arch. Gen. Psychiatry 4:561–571.

Beck, A. T., R. A. Steer, and M. G. Garbin. 1988. Psychometric properties of the Beck Depression Inventory: Twenty-five years of evaluation. Clin. Psychol. Rev. 8:77–100.

Bennion, L. J., and S. M. Grundy. 1975. Effects of obesity and caloric intake on biliary lipid metabolism in man. J. Clin. Invest. 56:996–1011.

Bennion, L. J., and S. M. Grundy. 1978. Risk factors for the development of cholelithiasis in man. N. Engl. J. Med. 299:1221–1227.

Berkowitz, R., A. J. Stunkard, and V. A. Stallings. 1993. Binge-eating disorder in obese adolescent girls. Pp. 200–206 in C. L. Williams and S. Y. S. Kimm, eds. Prevention and Treatment of Childhood Obesity. Ann. NY Acad. Sci., vol. 699.

Berkowitz, R. I., W. S. Agras, A. F. Korner, H. C. Kraemer, and C. H. Zeanah. 1985. Physical activity and adiposity: A longitudinal study from birth to childhood. J. Pediatr. 106:734–738.

Berscheid, E., E. Walster, and G. Bohrnstedt. 1973. The happy American body: A survey report. Psychol. Today 7:119–131.

Bhagat, R. S., S. J. McQuaid, H. Lindholm, and J. Segovis. 1985. Total life stress: A multimethod validation of the construct and its effects on organizationally valued outcomes and withdrawal behaviors. J. Appl. Psychol. 70:202–214.

Björntorp, P. 1993. Visceral obesity: A "civilization syndrome." Obes. Res. 1:206–222.

Björvell, H., and S. Rössner. 1992. A ten-year follow-up of weight change in severely obese subjects treated in a combined behavioural modification programme. Int. J. Obes. 16:623–625.

Blackburn, G. L. 1993. Comparison of medically supervised and unsupervised approaches to weight loss and control. Ann. Intern. Med. 119:714–718.

Blackburn, G. L., and B. S. Kanders. 1987. Medical evaluation and treatment of the obese patient with cardiovascular disease. Am. J. Cardiol. 60:55–58.

Blair, S. N. 1993a. C. H. McCloy Research Lecture: Physical activity, physical fitness, and health. Res. Q. Exerc. Sport 64:365–376.

Blair, S. N. 1993b. Evidence for success of exercise in weight loss and control. Ann. Intern. Med. 119:702–706.

Blair, S. N., W. L. Haskell, P. Ho, R. S. Paffenbarger Jr., K. M. Vranizan, J. W. Farquhar, and P. D. Wood. 1985. Assessment of habitual physical activity by a seven-day recall in a community survey and controlled experiments. Am. J. Epidemiol. 122:794–804.

Blair, S. N., H. W. Kohl, and N. N. Goodyear. 1987. Rates and risks for running and exercise injuries: Studies in three populations. Res. Q. Exerc. Sport 58:221–228.

Blair, S. N., W. B. Kannel, H. W. Kohl, N. Goodyear, and P. W. F. Wilson. 1989a. Surrogate measures of physical activity and physical fitness. Evidence for sedentary traits of resting tachycardia, obesity, and low vital capacity. Am. J. Epidemiol. 129:1145–1156.

Blair, S. N., H. W. Kohl 3rd, R. S. Paffenbarger Jr., D. G. Clark, K. H. Cooper, and L. W. Gibbons. 1989b. Physical fitness and all-cause mortality. A prospective study of healthy men and women. JAMA 262:2395–2401.

Blair, S. N., J. Shaten, K. Brownell, G. Collins, and L. Lissner. 1993. Body weight change, all-cause mortality, and cause-specific mortality in the Multiple Risk Factor Intervention Trial. Ann. Intern. Med. 119:749–757.

Block, G. 1982. A review of validations of dietary assessment methods. Am. J. Epidemiol. 45:492–505.

Blumberg, P., and L. P. Mellis. 1985. Medical students' attitudes toward the obese and the morbidly obese. Int. J. Eating Disord. 4:169–175.

Börjeson, M. 1962. Frequency of overweight children of different grades in the Stockholm population. Acta Paediatr. 51(suppl. 132):23–34.

Bouchard, C., ed. 1994. The Genetics of Obesity. CRC Press, Inc., Boca Raton, FL.

Bouchard, C., and L. Pérusse. 1993a. Genetic aspects of obesity. Pp. 26–35 in C. L. Williams and S. Y. S. Kimm, eds. Prevention and Treatment of Childhood Obesity. Ann. NY Acad. Sci., vol. 699.

Bouchard, C., and L. Pérusse. 1993b. Genetics of obesity. Annu. Rev. Nutr. 13:337–354.

Bouchard, C., A. Tremblay, C. Leblanc, G. Lortie, R. Savard, and G. Theriault. 1983. A method to assess energy expenditure in children and adults. Am. J. Clin. Nutr. 37:461–467.

Bouchard, C., A. Tremblay, J-P. Deprés, A. Nadeau, P. J. Lupien, G. Thériault, J. Dussault, S. Moorjani, S. Pinault, and G. Fournier. 1990. The response to long-term overfeeding in identical twins. N. Engl. J. Med. 322:1477–1482.

Bouchard, C., J-P. Deprés, and A. Tremblay. 1993. Exercise and obesity. Obes. Res. 1:133–147.

Bouchard, C., A. Tremblay, J-P. Deprés, G. Thériault, A. Nadeau, P. J. Lupien, S. Moorjani, D. Proudhomme, and G. Fournier. 1994. The response to exercise with constant energy intake in identical twins. Obes. Res. 2:400–410.

Bowman, K., and E. M. Jellinek. 1941. Alcohol addiction and its treatment. Q. J. Studies on Alcohol. 2:98–176.

Braitman, L. E., E. V. Adlin, and J. L. Stanton Jr. 1985. Obesity and caloric intake: The

National Health and Nutrition Examination Survey of 1971–1975 (NHANES I). J. Chronic Dis. 38:727–732.

Bray, G. A. 1987. Obesity and the heart. Mod. Concepts Cardiovasc. Dis. 56:67–71.

Bray, G. A. 1993a. Fat distribution and body weight. Obes. Rev. 1:203–205.

Bray, G. A. 1993b. The nutrient approach to obesity. Nutr. Today 28(3):13–18.

Bray, G. A. 1993c. Use and abuse of appetite-suppressant drugs in the treatment of obesity. Ann. Intern. Med. 119:707–713.

Bray, G. A., and D. S. Gray. 1988. Obesity. Part 1. Pathogenesis. West. J. Med. 149:429–441.

Brill, P. A., H. W. Kohl, T. Rogers, T. R. Collingwood, C. L. Sterling, and S. N. Blair. 1991. The relationships between sociodemographic characteristics and recruitment, retention, and health improvements in a worksite health promotion program. Am. J. Health Promo. 5:215–221.

Broomfield, P. H., R. Chopra, R. C. Sheinbaum, G. G. Bonorris, A. Silverman, L. J. Schoenfield, and J. W. Marks. 1988. Effects of ursodeoxycholic acid and aspirin on the formation of lithogenic bile and gallstones during loss of weight. N. Engl. J. Med. 319:1567–1572.

Brownell, K. D. 1990. Dieting readiness. Weight Con. Dig. 1:5–10.

Brownell, K. D. 1991a. Dieting and the search for the perfect body: Where physiology and culture collide. Behav. Ther. 22:1–12.

Brownell, K. D. 1991b. Personal responsibility and control over our bodies: When expectation exceeds reality. Health Psychol. 10:303–310.

Brownell, K. D. 1993. Whether obesity should be treated. Health Psychol. 12:339–341.

Brownell, K. D., and F. S. Kaye. 1982. A school-based behavior modification, nutrition education, and physical activity program for obese children. Am. J. Clin. Nut. 35:277–283.

Brownell, K. D., and F. M. Kramer. 1994. Behavioral management of obesity. Pp. 231–252 in G. L. Blackburn and B. S. Kanders, eds. Obesity: Pathophysiology, Psychology, and Treatment. Chapman & Hall, Inc., New York.

Brownell, K. D., and J. Rodin. 1994. The dieting maelstrom: Is it possible and advisable to lose weight? Am. Psychologist 49:781–791.

Brownell, K. D., and A. J. Stunkard. 1981. Couples training, pharmacotherapy, and behavior therapy in the treatment of obesity. Arch. Gen. Psychiatry 38:1224–1229.

Brownell, K. D., and T. A. Wadden. 1991. The heterogeneity of obesity: Fitting treatments to individuals. Behav. Ther. 22:153–177.

Brownell, K. D., and T. A. Wadden. 1992. Etiology and treatment of obesity: Understanding a serious, prevalent, and refractory disorder. J. Consult. Clin. Psychol. 60:505–517.

Brownell, K. D., J. H. Kelman, and A. J. Stunkard. 1983. Treatment of obese children with and without their mothers: Changes in weight and blood pressure. Pediatrics 71:515–523.

Bullen, B. A., R. B. Reed, and J. Mayer. 1964. Physical activity of obese and nonobese adolescent girls appraised by motion picture sampling. Am. J. Clin. Nutr. 14:211–233.

Burton, B. T., W. R. Foster, J. Hirsch, and T. B. VanItallie. 1985. Health implications of obesity: An NIH consensus development conference. Int. J. Obes. 9:155–170.

Buzzard, I.M., and W.C. Willett. 1994. First international conference on dietary assessment methods: assessing diets to improve world health. Am. J. Clin. Nutr. 59:143S–306S.

CCC (Calorie Control Council). 1993. One out of every two women believe they are overweight. Calorie Control Commentary 15(1):5.

Cartmel, B., and T. E. Moon. 1992. Comparison of two physical activity questionnaires, with a diary, for assessing physical activity in an elderly population. J. Clin. Epidemiol. 45:877–883.

Caspersen, C. J. 1989. Physical activity epidemiology: Concepts, methods, and applications to exercise science. Exer. Sport Sci. Rev. 17:423–473.

Caspersen, C. J., and R. K. Merritt. 1992. Trends in physical activity patterns among older adults. The Behavioral Risk Factor Surveillance System, 1986–1990 [abstract]. Med. Sci. Sports Exerc. 24(May suppl.):S26.

Caspersen, C. J., G. M. Christenson, and R. A. Pollard. 1986. Status of the 1990 physical fitness objectives: Evidence from NHIS 1985. Public Health Rep. 101:587–592.

Caspersen, C. J., R. A. Pollard, and S. O. Pratt. 1987. Scoring physical activity composition, and incidence of orthopedic problems. Res. Q. Exerc. Sport 60:225–233.

Cauley, J. A., R. E. LaPorte, R. B. Sandler, M. M. Schramm, and A. M. Kriska. 1987. Comparison of methods to measure physical activity in postmenopausal women. Am. J. Clin. Nutr. 45:14–22.

Charney, E., H. C. Goodman, M. McBride, B. Lyon, and R. Pratt. 1976. Childhood antecedents of adult obesity: Do chubby infants become obese adults? N. Engl. J. Med. 295: 6–9.

Chase, M. 1994 (January 28). Oregon's new health rationing means more care for some but less for others. Wall Street Journal. B1, B2.

Clancy-Hepburn, K., A. A. Hickey, and G. Nevill. 1974. Children's behavior responses to TV food advertisements. J. Nutr. Educ. 6:93–96.

Clark, D. S. 1993a (December 22). United States of America before Federal Trade Commission in the matter of Diet Center, Inc., a corporation. Decision and order. Docket No. C-3475. Federal Trade Commission, Washington, DC.

Clark, D. S. 1993b (December 22). United States of America before Federal Trade Commission in the matter of Nutri/System, Inc., a corporation. Decision and order. Docket No. C-3474. Federal Trade Commission, Washington, DC.

Clarke, W. R., R. F. Woolson, and R. M. Lauer. 1986. Changes in ponderosity and blood pressure in childhood: The Muscatine Study. Am. J. Epidemiol. 124:195–206.

Cleary, M. P., J. R. Vaselli, and M. R. C. Greenwood. 1980. Development of obesity in the Zucker obese (fafa) rat in the absence of hyperphasia. Am. J. Physiol. 238:E292–E301.

Colditz, G. A. 1992. Economic costs of obesity. Am. J. Clin. Nutr. 55:503S–507S.

Coleman, J. A. August 2, 1993. Discrimination at large. Newsweek. 122:9.

Connors, M. E., and C. L. Johnson. 1987. Epidemiology of bulimia and bulimic behaviors. Addic. Behaviors 12:165–179.

Conoley, C. W. 1992. Review of the Beck Depression Inventory [Revised Edition]. Pp. 78–79 in J. J. Kramer and J. C. Conoley, eds. The Eleventh Mental Measurements Yearbook. The University of Nebraska Press, Lincoln, NE.

Cooper, P. J., M. J. Taylor, Z. Cooper, and C. G. Fairburn. 1987. The development and validation of the Body Shape Questionnaire. Int. J. Eat. Disor. 6:485–494.

Cooper, Z., and C. Fairburn. 1987. The Eating Disorder Examination: A semi-structured interview for the assessment of the specific psychopathology of eating disorders. Int. J. Eat. Disor. 6:1–8.

Corbin, C. B., and P. Fletcher. 1968. Diet and physical activity patterns of obese and nonobese elementary school children. Res. Q. 39:922–928.

Council on Scientific Affairs. 1988. Treatment of obesity in adults. JAMA 260:2547–2551.

Danforth, E. Jr. 1985. Diet and obesity. Am. J. Clin. Nutr. 41:1132–1145.

Darga, L. L., L. Carroll-Michals, S. J. Botsford, and C. P. Lucas. 1991. Fluoxetine's effects on weight loss in obese subjects. Am. J. Clin. Nutr. 54:321–325.

Dattilo, A. M., and P. M. Kris-Etherton. 1992. Effects of weight reduction on blood lipids and lipoproteins: A meta-analysis. Am. J. Clin. Nutr. 56:320–328.

Davis, K., K. K. Christoffel, H. Vespa, M. P. Pierleoni, and R. Papanastassiou. 1993a. Obesity in preschool and school-aged children: Early treatment is best. Pp. 262–264 in C. L. Williams and S. Y. S. Kimm, eds. Prevention and Treatment of Childhood Obesity. Ann. NY Acad. Sci., vol. 699.

Davis, P. B. 1994. Evolution of therapy for cystic fibrosis. New Engl. J. Med. 331:672–673.

Davis, S., Y. Gomez, L. Lambert, and B. Skipper. 1993b. Primary prevention of obesity in American Indian children. Pp. 167–180 in C. L. Williams and S. Y. S. Kimm, eds. Prevention and Treatment of Childhood Obesity. Ann. NY Acad. Sci., vol. 699.

Dawson, D. A., and G. B. Thompson. 1990. Breast cancer risk factors and screening: United States, 1987. Vital Health Stat. 10(172):iii–iv, 1–60.

Debusk, R. F., U. Stenestrand, M. Sheehan, and W. L. Haskell. 1990. Training effects of long versus short bouts of exercise in healthy subjects. Am. J. Cardiol. 65:1010–1013.

de Gennes, C. 1993. Osteoarticular pathology and massive obesity. Rev. Prat. 43:1924–1929.

Department of Health and Social Security. 1987. Report on Health and Social Subjects No. 31, Use of Very Low Calorie Diets in Obesity. Her Majesty's Stationery Office, London.

Deschamps, I., J. F. Desjeux, S. Machineot, F. Rolland, and H. Lestradet. 1978. Effects of diet and weight loss on plasma glucose, insulin, and free fatty acids in obese children. Pediatr. Res. 12:757–760.

Deurenberg, P., J. A. Weststrate, and J. C. Seidell. 1991. Body mass index as a measure of body fatness: Age- and sex-specific prediction formulas. Br. J. Nutr. 65:105–114.

DHHS (U.S. Department of Health and Human Services). 1988. The Surgeon General's Report on Nutrition and Health. DHHS (PHS) Publ. No. 88-50210. Public Health Service, U.S. Department of Health and Human Services. U.S. Government Printing Office, Washington, DC.

DHHS (U.S. Department of Health and Human Services). 1991. Healthy People 2000: National Health Promotion and Disease Prevention Objectives. DHHS (PHS) Publ. No. 91-50212. Public Health Service, U.S. Department of Health and Human Services. U.S. Government Printing Office, Washington, DC.

Dietz, W. H. Jr. 1983. Childhood obesity: Susceptibility, cause, and management. J. Pediatr. 103:676–686.

Dietz, W. H. 1992. Role of physical activity in the prevention of obesity. Pp. 85–86 in Physical Activity and Obesity. National Institute of Diabetes, Digestive, and Kidney Diseases, National Institutes of Health. Bethesda, MD.

Dietz, W. H. 1994a. Critical periods in childhood for the development of obesity. Am. J. Clin. Nutr. 59:955–959.

Dietz, W. H. 1994b. Pharmacotherapy for childhood obesity? Maybe for some. Obesity Res. 2:54–55.

Dietz, W. H. Jr., and S. L. Gortmaker. 1984. Factors within the physical environment associated with childhood obesity. Am. J. Clin. Nutr. 39:619–624.

Dietz, W. H. Jr., and S. L. Gortmaker. 1985. Do we fatten our children at the television set? Obesity and television viewing in children and adolescents. Pediatrics 75:807–812.

Dietz, W. H., and R. Hartung. 1985. Changes in height velocity of obese preadolescents during weight reduction. Am. J. Dis. Child. 139:705–707.

Dietz, W. H., and T. N. Robinson. 1993. Assessment and treatment of childhood obesity. Pediatr. Rev. 14:337–343.

Dietz, W. H. Jr., and R. R. Wolfe. 1985. Interrelationships of glucose and protein metabolism in obese adolescents during short-term hypocaloric dietary therapy. Am. J. Clin. Nutr. 42:380–390.

Dietz, W. H., L. G. Bandini, J. A. Morelli, K. F. Peers, and P. L. Ching. 1994. Effect of sedentary activities on resting metabolic rate. Am. J. Clin. Nutr. 59:556–559.

DiPietro, L., and C. Caspersen. 1991. National estimates of physical activity among white and black Americans [abstract]. Med. Sci. Sports Exerc. 23(April suppl.):S105.

Dishman, R. K., ed. 1988. Exercise Adherence: Its Impact on Public Health. Human Kinetics, Champaign, IL.

Dishman, R. K. 1991. Increasing and maintaining exercise and physical activity. Behav. Ther. 22:345–378.

Doar, J. W. H., C. E. Wilde, M. E. Thompson, and P. F. J. Sewell. 1975. Influence of treatment with diet alone on oral glucose-tolerance test and plasma sugar and insulin levels in patients with maturity-onset diabetes mellitus. Lancet 1:1263–1266.

Dohrenwend, B. S., L. Krasnoff, A. R. Askenasy, and B. P. Dohrenwend. 1978. Exemplification of a method for scaling life events: The PERI Life Events Scale. J. Health Soc. Behav. 19:205–229.

Dorr, A. 1986. Television and Children: A Special Medium for a Special Audience. Sage Publications, Beverly Hills, CA.

Dowd, E. T. 1992. Review of the Tennessee Self-Concept Scale [Revised]. P. 933 in J. J. Kramer and J. C. Conoley, eds. The Eleventh Mental Measurements Yearbook. The University of Nebraska Press, Lincoln, NE.

Drewnowski, A. 1990. Toward Safe Weight Loss: Recommendations for Adult Weight Loss Programs in Michigan. Final report of Task Force to Establish Weight Loss Guidelines. K. A. Petersmarck, ed. Michigan Health Council, East Lansing, MI.

Dubbert, P., and G. T. Wilson. 1983. Failures in behavior therapy for obesity: Causes, correlates, and consequences. Pp. 263–288 in W. B. Foa and P. M. G. Emmelkamp, eds. Failures in Behavior Therapy. Wiley, New York.

Dustan, H. P. 1983. Mechanisms of hypertension associated with obesity. Ann. Intern. Med. 98:860–864.

Dwyer, J. T. 1994. Dietary assessment. Pp. 842–860 in M. E. Shils, J. A. Olson, and M. Shike, eds. Modern Nutrition in Health and Disease, 8th ed. Lea & Febiger, Philadelphia.

Dwyer, J. T., and D. Lu. 1993. Popular diets for weight loss from nutritionally hazardous to healthful. Pp. 231–252 in A. J. Stunkard and T. A. Wadden, eds. Obesity: Theory and Therapy, 2nd ed. Raven Press, New York.

Eck, L. H., R. C. Klesges, C. L. Hanson, and D. Slawson. 1992. Children at familial risk for obesity: An examination of dietary intake, physical activity, and weight status. Int. J. Obes. 16:71–78.

Edelstein, S. L., E. L. Barrett-Connor, D. L. Wingard, and B. A. Cohn. 1992. Increased meal frequency associated with decreased cholesterol concentrations; Rancho Bernardo, CA. Am. J. Clin. Nutr. 55:664–669.

Ekelund, L. G., C. M. Suchindran, J. M. Karon, R. P. McMahon, and H. A. Tyroler. 1990. Black-white differences in exercise blood pressure: The Lipid Research Clinics Program prevalence study. Circulation 81:1568–1574.

Eliahou, H. E., A. Iaina, T. Gaon, J. Schochat, and M. Modan. 1981. Body weight reduction necessary to attain normotension in the overweight hypertensive patient. Int. J. Obes. 5:157–163.

Epstein, L. H. 1985. Family-based treatment for preadolescent obesity. Pp. 1–39 in M. L. Wolraich and D. Routh, eds. Advances in Developmental and Behavioral Pediatrics. JAI Press, Inc., Greenwich, CT.

Epstein, L. H. 1986. Treatment of childhood obesity. Pp. 159–197 in K. D. Brownell and J. P. Foreyt, eds. Handbook of Eating Disorders: Physiology, Psychology, and Treatment. Basic Books, Inc., New York.

Epstein, L. H. 1992. Exercise and obesity in children. J. Appl. Sport Psychol. 4:120–133.

Epstein, L. H. 1993a. Methodological issues and ten-year outcomes for obese children. Pp. 237–249 in C. L. Williams and S. Y. S. Kimm, eds. Prevention and Treatment of Childhood Obesity. Ann. NY Acad. Sci., vol. 699.

Epstein, L. H. 1993b. New developments in childhood obesity. Pp. 301–312 in A. J. Stunkard and T. A. Wadden, eds. Obesity: Theory and Therapy, 2nd ed. Raven Press, New York.

Epstein, L. H., and R. R. Wing. 1987. Behavioral treatment of childhood obesity. Psychol. Bull. 101:331–342.

Epstein, L. H., R. Koeske, and R. R. Wing. 1984a. Adherence to exercise in obese children. J. Cardiac. Rehabil. 4:185–195.

Epstein, L. H., R. R. Wing, R. Koeske, and A. Valoski. 1984b. Effects of diet plus exercise on weight change in parents and children. J. Consult. Clin. Psychol. 52:429–437.

Epstein, L. H., R. R. Wing, R. Koeske, and A. Valoski. 1985a. A comparison of lifestyle exercise, aerobic exercise, and calisthenics on weight loss in obese children. Behav. Ther. 16:345–356.

Epstein, L. H., R. R. Wing, B. C. Penner, and M. J. Kress. 1985b. The effect of diet and controlled exercise on weight loss in obese children. J. Pediatr. 107:358–361.

Epstein, L. H., R. R. Wing, R. Koeske, and A. Valoski. 1987. Long-term effects of a family-based treatment of childhood obesity. J. Consult. Clin. Psychol. 55:91–95.

Epstein, L. H., J. McCurley, A. Valoski, and R. R. Wing. 1990a. Growth in obese children treated for obesity. Am. J. Dis. Child. 144:1360–1364.

Epstein, L. H., J. McCurley, R. R. Wing, and A. Valoski. 1990b. Five-year follow-up of family-based behavioral treatments for childhood obesity. J. Consult. Clin. Psychol. 58:661–664.

Epstein, L. H., A. Valoski, R. R. Wing, and J. McCurley. 1990c. Ten-year follow-up of behavioral, family-based treatment for obese children. JAMA 264:2519–2523.

Epstein, L. H., A. Valoski, and J. McCurley. 1993. Effect of weight loss by obese children on long-term growth. Am. J. Dis. Child. 147:1076–1080.

Epstein, L. H., A. Valoski, R. R. Wing, and J. McCurley. 1994. Ten-year outcomes of behavioral family-based treatment for childhood obesity. Health Psychol. 13:373–383.

Faden, R. R., T. L. Beauchamp, and N. King. 1986. A History and Theory of Informed Consent. Oxford University Press, New York.

Farquhar, J. W., N. Maccoby, P. D. Wood, J. K. Alexander, H. Breitrose, B. W. Brown Jr., W. L. Haskell, A. L. McAlister, A. J. Meyer, J. D. Nash, and M. P. Stern. 1977. Community education for cardiovascular health. Lancet 1:1192–1195.

Farquhar, J. W., S. P. Fortmann, J. A. Flora, C. B. Taylor, W. L. Haskell, P. T. Williams, N. Maccoby, and P. D. Wood. 1990. Effects of community-wide education on cardiovascular disease risk factors: The Stanford Five-City Project. JAMA 264:359–365.

Faust, I. M., P. R. Johnson, J. S. Stern, and J. Hirsch. 1978. Diet-induced adipocyte number increase in adult rats: A new model of obesity. Am. J. Physiol. 235:E279–E286.

Fazio, A. F. 1977. A concurrent validational study of the NCHS General Well-Being Schedule. Vital Health Stat. 2(73):1–53.

Feinleib, M., R. J. Garrison, R. Fabsitz, and J. C. Christian, Z. Hruber, N. O. Borhani, W. B. Kannel, R. Rosenmaw, J. T. Schwartz, and J. O. Wagker. 1977. The NHLBI twin study of cardiovascular disease risk factors: Methodology and summary of results. Am. J. Epidemiol. 106:284–295.

Felson, D. T., Y. Zhang, J. M. Anthony, A. Naimark, and J. J. Anderson. 1992. Weight loss reduces the risk for symptomatic knee osteoarthritis in women: The Framingham Study. Ann. Intern. Med. 116:535–539.

Figueroa-Colon, R., T. K. von Almen, and R. M. Suskind. 1992. Clinical considerations in the treatment of childhood obesity. Pp. 181–196 in P. L. Giorgi, R. M. Suskind, and C. Catassi, eds. The Obese Child. Karger, Basel, New York.

Figueroa-Colon, R., T. K. von Almen, F. A. Franklin, C. Schuftan, and R. M. Suskind. 1993. Comparison of two hypocaloric diets in obese children. Am. J. Dis. Child. 147:160–166.

Fischman-Havstad, L., and A. R. Marston. 1984. Weight loss maintenance as an aspect of family emotion and process. Br. J. Clin. Psychol. 23:265–271.

Fitts, W. F. 1964. Tennessee Self-Concept Scale. Western Psychological Services, Los Angeles, CA.

Fitz, J. D., E. M. Sperling, and H. G. Fein. 1983. A hypocaloric high-protein diet as primary therapy for adults with obesity-related diabetes: Effective long-term use in a community hospital. Diabetes Care 6:328–333.

Fletcher, G. F., S. N. Blair, J. Blumenthal, C. Caspersen, B. Chaitman, S. Epstein, H. Falls, E. S. S. Froelicher, V. F. Froelicher, and I. L. Pina. 1992. Statement on exercise. Benefits and recommendations for physical activity programs for all Americans. A statement for health professionals by the Committee on Exercise and Cardio Rehabilitation of the Council on Clinical Cardiology, American Heart Association. Circulation 86:340–344.

Foley, E. F., P. N. Benotti, B. C. Borlase, J. Hollingshead, and G. L. Blackburn. 1992. Impact of gastric restrictive surgery on hypertension in the morbidly obese. Am. J. Surg. 163:294–297.

Folsom, A. R., D. R. Jacobs Jr., C. J. Caspersen, O. Gomez-Marin, and J. Knudsen. 1986. Test-retest reliability of the Minnesota Leisure Time Physical Activity Questionnaire. J. Chronic Dis. 39:505–511.

Forbes, G. B., and G. H. Amirhakimi. 1970. Skinfold thickness and body fat in children. Hum. Biol. 42:401–418.

Foreyt, J. P. 1987. Issues in the assessment and treatment of obesity. J. Consult. Clin. Psychol. 55:677–684.

Foreyt, J. P., and J. H. Cousins. 1993. Primary prevention of obesity in Mexican-American children. Pp. 137–146 in C. L. Williams and S. Y. S. Kimm, eds. Prevention and Treatment of Childhood Obesity. Ann. NY Acad. Sci., vol. 699.

Foreyt, J. P., and G. K. Goodrick. 1991. Factors common to successful therapy for the obese patient. Med. Sci. Sports Exerc. 23:292–297.

Foreyt, J. P., and G. K. Goodrick. 1994. Attributes of successful approaches to weight loss and control. Applied and Preventive Psychol. 3:209–215.

Foster, G. D., T. A. Wadden, and K. D. Brownell. 1985. Peer-led program for the treatment and prevention of obesity in the schools. J. Consul. Clin. Psychol. 53:538–540.

Franz, I. W. 1982. Assessment of blood pressure response during ergometric work in normotensive and hypertensive patients. Acta Med. Scand. 670(suppl.):35–47.

Freedman, D. S., S. R. Srinivasan, G. L. Burke, C. L. Shear, C. G. Smoak, D. W. Harsha, L. S. Webber, and G. S. Berenson. 1987. Relation of body fat distribution to hyperinsulinemia in children and adolescents: The Bogalusa Heart Study. Am. J. Clin. Nutr. 46:403–410.

FTC (Federal Trade Commission). 1993. Nutri/System, Inc.: Proposed consent agreement with analysis to aid public comment. Federal Register 58:52769–52775.

Fuchs, H. J., D. S. Borowitz, D. H. Christiansen et al. 1994. Effect of aerosolized recombinant human DNAse on exacerbations of respiratory symptoms and on pulmonary function in patients with cystic fibrosis. N. Engl. J. Med. 331:637–642.

Galloway, S. McL., D. L. Farquhar, and J. F. Munro. 1984. The current status of antiobesity drugs. Postgrad Med. J. 60(suppl. 3):19–26.

Garmezy, N. 1983. Stressors of childhood. Pp. 43–84 in N. Garmezy and M. Rutter, eds. Stress, Coping, and Development in Children. McGraw Hill, New York.

Garn, S. M., and D. C. Clark. 1975. Nutrition, growth, development, and maturation: Findings from the Ten-State Nutrition Survey of 1968–1970. Pediatrics 56:306–319.

Garn, S. M., and D. C. Clark. 1976. Trends in fatness and the origins of obesity: Ad Hoc Committee to Review the Ten-State Nutrition Survey. Pediatrics 57:443–456.

Garn, S. M., D. C. Clark, and K. E. Guire. 1974. Level of fatness and size attainment. Am. J. Phys. Anthropol. 40:447–449.

Garn, S. M., S. M. Bailey, and I. T. Higgins. 1980. Effects of socioeconomic status, family line, and living together on fatness and obesity. Pp. 187–204 in R. M. Lauer and R. B. Shokelle, eds. Childhood Prevention of Atherosclerosis and Hypertension. Raven Press, New York.

Garn, S. M., S. M. Bailey, M. A. Solomon, and P. J. Hopkins. 1981. Effects of remaining family members on fatness prediction. Am. J. Clin. Nutr. 34:148–153.

Garn, S. M., M. LaVelle, and J. J. Pilkington. 1984. Obesity and living together. Marriage Family Rev. 7(1–2):33–47.

Garn, S. M., T. V. Sullivan, and V. M. Hawthorne. 1989. Fatness and obesity of the parents of obese individuals. Am. J. Clin. Nutr. 50:1308–1313.

Garner, D. M. 1991. Eating Disorders 2. Psychological Assessment Resources, Inc., Odessa, FL.

Garner, D. M., and P. E. Garfinkel. 1979. The Eating Attitudes Test: An index of the symptoms of anorexia nervosa. Psychol. Med. 9:273–279.

Garner, D. M., and S. C. Wooley. 1991. Confronting the failure of behavioral and dietary treatment for obesity. Clin. Psychol. Rev. 11:729–780.

Garner, D. M., M. P. Olmsted, Y. Bohr, and P. E. Garfinkel. 1982. The Eating Attitudes Test: Psychometric features and clinical correlates. Psychol. Med. 12:871–878.

Garrow, J. S. 1981. Treat Obesity Seriously: A Clinical Manual. Churchill Livingstone, New York.

Genuth, S. M., J. H. Castro, and V. Vertes. 1974. Weight reduction in obesity by outpatient semistarvation. JAMA 230:987–991.

Godin, G., and R. J. Shephard. 1985. A simple method to assess exercise behavior in the community. Can. J. Appl. Sports Sci. 10:141–146.

Goldman, B. A., and D. F. Mitchell. 1990. Directory of Unpublished Experimental Mental Measures, Vol. 5. William C. Brown Publishers, Dubuque, IA.

Goldman, B. A., and W. L. Osborne. 1985. Directory of Unpublished Experimental Mental Measures, Vol. 4. Human Sciences Press, Inc, New York.

Goldstein, D. J. 1991. Beneficial health effects of modest weight loss. Int. J. Obes. 16:397–415.

Goldstein, D. J., and J. H. Potvin. 1994. Long-term weight loss: The effect of pharmacologic agents. Am J. Clin. Nutr. 60:647–657.

Goodrick, G. K., and J. P. Foreyt. 1991. Why treatments for obesity don't last. J. Am. Diet. Assoc. 91:1243–1247.

Gordon, R. 1987. An operational classification of disease prevention. Pp. 20–26 in J. A. Steinberg and M. M. Silverman, eds. Preventing Mental Disorders: A Research Perspective. U.S. Department of Health and Human Services, Public Health Service. Government Printing Office, Washington, DC.

Gormally, J., S. Black, S. Daston, and D. Rardin. 1982. The assessment of binge eating severity among obese persons. Addict. Behav. 7:47–55.

Gortmaker, S. L., W. H. Dietz Jr., A. M. Sobol, and C. A. Wehler. 1987. Increasing pediatric obesity in the United States. Am. J. Dis. Child. 141:535–540.

Gortmaker, S. L., W. H. Dietz Jr., and L. W. Cheung. 1990. Inactivity, diet, and the fattening of America. J. Am. Diet. Assoc. 90:1247–1252, 1255.

Gortmaker, S. L., A. Must, J. M. Perrin, A. M. Sobol, and W. H. Dietz. 1993. Social and economic consequences of overweight in adolescence and young adulthood. N. Engl. J. Med. 329:1008–1012.

Greecher, C. P. 1993. Physicians' perception of childhood and adolescent obesity. Pp. 269–270 in C. L. Williams and S. Y. S. Kimm, eds. Prevention and Treatment of Childhood Obesity. Ann. NY Acad. Sci., vol. 699.

Griffiths, M., and P. R. Payne. 1976. Energy expenditure in small children of obese and nonobese parents. Nature 260:698–700.

Griffiths, M., J. P. Rivers, and P. R. Payne. 1987. Energy intake in children at high and low risk of obesity. Hum. Clin. Nutr. 41:425–430.

Griffiths, M., P. R. Payne, A. J. Stunkard, P. J. Rivers, and M. Cox. 1990. Metabolic rate and physical development in children at risk of obesity. Lancet 336:76–78.

Grilo, C. M.,and M. F. Pogue-Geile. 1991. The nature of environmental influences on weight and obesity: A behavior genetic analysis. Psychol. Bull. 110:520–537.

Grilo, C. M., S. Shiffman, and R. R. Wing. 1989. Relapse crises and coping among dieters. J. Consult. Clin. Psychol. 57:488–495.

Grilo, C. M., K. D. Brownell, and A. J. Stunkard. 1993a. The metabolic and psychological importance of exercise in weight control. Pp. 253–273 in A. J. Stunkard and T. A. Wadden, eds. Obesity: Theory and Therapy, 2nd ed. Raven Press, New York.

Grilo, C. M., S. Shiffman, and R. R. Wing. 1993b. Coping with dietary relapse crises and their aftermath. Addict. Behav. 18:89–102.

Grundy, S. M., H. Y. Mok, L. Zech, D. Steinberg, and M. Berman. 1979. Transport of very low density lipoprotein triglycerides in varying degrees of obesity and hypertriglycer-idemia. J. Clin. Invest. 63:1274–1283.

Gutin, B.,and T. M. Manos. 1993. Physical activity in the prevention of childhood obesity. Pp. 115–126 in C. L. Williams and S. Y. S. Kimm, eds. Prevention and Treatment of Childhood Obesity. Ann. NY Acad. Sci., vol. 699.

Guy-Grand, B., M. Apfelbaum, G. Crepaldi, A. Gries, P. Lefebvre, and P. Turner. 1989. International trial of long-term dexfenfluramine in obesity. Lancet 2:1142–1145.

Hadden, D. R., D. A. Montgomery, R. J. Skelly, E. R. Trimble, J. A. Weaver, E. A. Wilson, and K. D. Buchanan. 1975. Maturity onset diabetes mellitus: Response to intensive dietary management. Br. Med. J. 3:276–278.

Haffner, S. M., M. P. Stern, B. D. Mitchell, and H. P. Hazuda. 1991. Predictors of obesity in Mexican Americans. Am. J. Clin. Nutr. 53:1571S–1576S.

Haines, P. S., D. W. Hungerford, B. M. Popkin, and D. K. Guilkey. 1992. Eating patterns and energy and nutrient intakes of U.S. women. J. Am. Diet. Assoc. 92:698–707.

Hamilton, M. 1960. A rating scale for depression. J. Neurol. Neurosur. Psychiat. 23:56–62.

Hamm, P., R. B. Shekelle, and J. Stamler. 1989. Large fluctuations in body weight during young adulthood and twenty-five year risk of coronary death in men. Am. J. Epidemi-ol. 129:312–318.

Hammond, E. C., and L. Garfinkel. 1969. Coronary heart disease, stroke, and aortic aneu-rysm. Arch. Environ. Health 19:167–182.

Hansen, B. C., and N. L. Bodkin. 1993. Primary prevention of diabetes mellitus by preven-tion of obesity in monkeys. Diabetes 42:1809–1814.

Harlan, W. R. 1993. Epidemiology of childhood obesity: A national perspective. Pp. 1–5 in C. L. Williams and S. Y. S. Kimm, eds. Prevention and Treatment of Childhood Obesi-ty. Ann. NY Acad. Sci., vol. 699.

Hayes, D., and C. E. Ross. 1987. Concern with appearance, health beliefs, and eating habits. J. Health Soc. Behav. 28:120–130.

Healy, B. 1993. Foreword. Ann. Intern. Med. 119:641.

Heilbrun, A. B. 1984. Cognitive defenses and life stress: An information-processing analy-sis. Psychol. Rep. 54:3–17.

Helmrich, S .P., D. R. Ragland, R. W. Leung, and R. S. Paffenbarger Jr. 1991. Physical activ-ity and reduced occurence of non-insulin-dependent diabetes. N. Engl. J. Med. 325:147–152.

Henry, R. R., T. A. Wiest-Kent, L. Scheaffer, O. G. Kolterman, and J. M. Olefsky. 1986. Metabolic consequences of very low-calorie diet therapy in obese non-insulin-depen-dent diabetic and nondiabetic subjects. Diabetes 35:155–164.

Herman, C. P., and D. Mack. 1975. Restrained and unrestrained eating. J. Pers. 43:647–660.

Herman, C. P., and J. Polivy. 1984. A boundary model for the regulation of eating. Pp. 141–156 in A. J. Stunkard and E. Stellar, eds. Eating and its Disorders. Raven Press, New York.

Herman, W. H., S. M. Teutsch, and L. S. Geissm. 1987. Diabetes mellitus. Am. J. Prev. Med. 3:72–82.

Himes, J. H., and W. H. Dietz. 1994. Guidelines for overweight in adolescent preventive services: Recommendations from an expert committee. The Expert Committee on Clinical Guidelines for Overweight in Adolescent Prevention Services. Am. J. Clin. Nutr. 59:307–316.

Hirsch, J., and R. L. Leibel. 1988. New light on obesity [editorial]. N. Engl. J. Med. 318:509–510.

Hirsch, J., and R. L. Leibel. 1991. Clinical review 28: A biological basis for human obesity. J. Clin. Endocrinol. Metab. 73:1153–1157.

Holmes, T. H., and R. H. Rahe. 1967. The Social Readjustment Rating Scale. J. Psychosom. Res. 11:213–218.

Horm, J., and K. Anderson. 1993. Who in America is trying to lose weight? Ann. Intern. Med. 119:672–676.

Hsu, L. K. G. 1990. Eating Disorders. Guilford Press, New York.

Hypertension Prevention Trial Research Group. 1990. The hypertension prevention trial: Three year effects of dietary change on blood pressure. Arch. Intern. Med. 150:153–162.

IBNMRR (Interagency Board for Nutrition Monitoring and Related Research). 1993. Nutrition Monitoring in the United States. Chartbook I: Selected findings from the National Nutrition Monitoring and Related Research Program. U.S. Department of Health and Human Services, Public Health Service, Centers for Disease Control and Prevention, National Center for Health Statistics. DHHS (PHS) Publ. No. 93-1255-2. Government Printing Office, Washington, DC.

IFT (Institute of Food Technologists). 1994. Scientific status summary: Human obesity. Food Tech. 48(2):127–138.

IOM (Institute of Medicine). 1990. Broadening the Base of Treatment for Alcohol Problems. Committee for the Study of Treatment and Rehabilitation Services for Alcoholism and Alcohol Abuse, Division of Mental Health and Behavioral Medicine. National Academy Press, Washington, DC.

IOM (Institute of Medicine). 1992. Eat for Life: The Food and Nutrition Board's Guide to Reducing Your Risk of Chronic Disease. C. E. Woteki and P. R. Thomas, eds. National Academy Press, Washington, DC.

IOM (Institute of Medicine). 1993. Opportunities in the Nutrition and Food Sciences: Research Challenges and the Next Generation of Investigators. Report of the Committee on Opportunities in the Nutrition and Food Sciences, Food and Nutrition Board. National Academy Press, Washington, DC.

IOM (Institute of Medicine). 1994. Reducing Risks for Mental Disorders: Frontiers for Preventive Intervention Research. Report of the Committee on Prevention of Mental Disorders, Division of Biobehavioral Sciences and Mental Disorders. National Academy Press, Washington, DC.

Jacobs, D. R. Jr., L. P. Hahn, W. L. Haskell, P. Pirie, and S. Sidney. 1989. Validity and reliability of short physical activity history: Cardia and the Minnesota Heart Health Program. J. Cardiopulmonary Rehabil. 9:448–459.

Jacoby, A., D. G. Altman, J. Cook, W. W. Holland, and A. Elliott. 1975. Influence of some social and environmental factors on the nutrient intake and nutritional status of school-children. Br. J. Prev. Soc. Med. 29:116–120.

Javier Nieto, F., M. Szklo, and G. W. Comstock. 1992. Childhood weight and growth rate as predictors of adult mortality. Am. J. Epidemiol. 136:201–213.

Jeffery, R. W. 1991. Weight management and hypertension. Ann. Behav. Med. 13:18–22.

Jeffery, R. W., P. D. Thompson, and R. R. Wing. 1978. Effects on weight reduction of strong monetary contracts for calorie restriction or weight loss. Behav. Res. Ther. 16:363–369.

Jeffery, R. W., W. M. Gerber, B. S. Rosenthal, and R. A. Lindquist. 1983. Monetary contracts in weight control: Effectiveness of group and individual contracts of varying size. J. Consult. Clin. Psychol. 51:242–248.

Jeffery, R. W., W. M. Bjornson-Benson, B. S. Rosenthal, C. L. Kurth, and M. M. Dunn. 1984a. Effectiveness of monetary contracts with two repayment schedules upon weight reduction in men and women from self-referred and population samples. Behav. Ther. 15:273–279.

Jeffery, R. W., A. R. Folsom, R. V. Luepker, D. R. Jacobs Jr., R. F. Gillum, H. L. Taylor, and H. Blackburn. 1984b. Prevalence of overweight and weight loss behavior in a metropolitan adult population: The Minnesota Heart Survey experience. Am. J. Public Health 74:349–352.

Jenkins, D. J., T. M. Wolever, V. Vuksan, F. Brighenti, S. C. Cunnane, A. V. Rao, A. L. Jenkins, G. Buckley, R. Patten, W. Singer et al. 1989. Nibbling versus gorging: Metabolic advantages of increased meal frequency. N. Engl. J. Med. 321:929–934.

JNCDETHBP (Joint National Committee on Detection, Evaluation, and Treatment of High Blood Pressure). 1993. The Fifth Report of the Joint National Committee on Detection, Evaluation, and Treatment of High Blood Pressure. NIH Publ. No. 93-1088. National Heart, Lung, and Blood Institute, National Institutes of Health. Bethesda, MD.

Johnson, D., D. Prud'homme, J-P. Després, A. Nadeau, A. Tremblay, and C. Bouchard. 1992. Relation of abdominal obesity to hyperinsulinemia and high blood pressure in men. Int. J. Obes. Relat. Metab. Disord. 16(11):881–890.

Johnson, J. H., and I. G. Sarason. 1979. Recent developments in research on life stress. Pp. 205–233 in V. Hamilton and D. M. Warburton, eds. Human Stress and Cognition: An Information Processing Approach. Wiley, New York.

Johnson, M. L., B. S. Burke, and J. Mayer. 1956. Relative importance of inactivity and overeating the energy balance of obese high school girls. Am. J. Clin. Nutr. 4:37–44.

Jones, N. L., L. Makrides, C. Hitchcock, T. Chypchar, and N. McCartney. 1985. Normal standards for an incremental progressive cycle ergometer test. Am. Rev. Respir. Dis. 131:700–708.

Kahn, H. S., D. F. Williamson, and J. A. Stevens. 1991. Race and weight change in U.S. women: The roles of socioeconomic and marital status. Am. J. Public. Health 81:319–323.

Kalkwarf, H. J., J. D. Haas, A. Z. Belko, R. C. Roach, and D. A. Roe. 1989. Accuracy of heart-rate monitoring and activity diaries for estimating energy expenditure. Am. J. Clin. Nutr. 49:37–43.

Kanders, B. S., and G. L. Blackburn. 1992. Reducing primary risk factors by therapeutic weight loss. Pp. 213–230 in T. A. Wadden and T. B. VanItallie. Treatment of the Seriously Obese Patient. Guilford Press, New York.

Kanders, B. S., and G. L. Blackburn. 1993. Very-low-calorie diets for the treatment of obesity. Pp. 197–216 in G. L. Blackburn and B. S. Kanders, eds. Obesity, Pathophysiology, Psychology, and Treatment. Chapman and Hall, New York.

Kannel, W. B., N. Brand, J. J. Skinner Jr., T. R. Dawber, and P. M. McNamara. 1967. The relation of adiposity to blood pressure and development of hypertension: The Framingham Study. Ann. Intern. Med. 67:48–59.

Kayman, S., W. Bruvold, and J. S. Stern. 1990. Maintenance and relapse after weight loss in women: Behavioral aspects. Am. J. Clin. Nutr. 52:800–807.

Keesey, R. E. 1989. Physiological regulation of body weight and the issue of obesity. Med. Clin. North Am. 73:15–27.

Kern, P. A., J. M. Ong, B. Saffari, and J. Carty. 1990. The effects of weight loss on the activity and expression of adipose-tissue lipoprotein lipase in very obese humans. N. Engl. J. Med. 322:1053–1059.

Kesaniemi, Y. A., and S. M. Grundy. 1983. Increased low density lipoprotein production associated with obesity. Arteriosclerosis 3:170–177.

Kimm, S. Y., C. Sweeney, and J. Jonosky. 1991. Self-concept measures and childhood obesity: A descriptive analysis. J. Dev. Behav. Pediatr. 19:19–24.

King, A. C., and D. L. Tribble. 1991. The role of exercise in weight regulation in nonathletes. Sports Med. 11(5):331–349.

King, A. C., S. N. Blair, D. E. Bild, R. K. Dishman, P. M. Dubbert, B. H. Marcus, N. B. Oldridge, R. S. Paffenbarger Jr., K. E. Powell, and K. K. Yeager. 1992. Determinations of physical activity and interventions in adults. Med. Sci. Sports Exerc. 24(6 suppl.):S221–S236.

King, A. C., C. B. Taylor, and W. L. Haskell. 1993. Effects of differing intensities and formats of 12 months of exercise training on psychological outcomes in older adults. Health Psychol. 12:292–300.

Kirschner, M. A., G. Schneider, N. H. Ertel, and J. Gorman. 1988. An eight-year experience with a very low-calorie formula diet for control of major obesity. Int. J. Obes. 12:69–80.

Klein, P. D., W. P. James, W. W. Wong, C. S. Irving, P. R. Murgatroyd, M. Cabrera, H. M. Dallosso, E. R. Klein, and B. L. Nichols. 1984. Calorimetric validation of the doubly-labelled water method for determination of energy expenditure in man. Hum. Nutr. Clin. Nutr. 38:95–106.

Klesges, L. M., and R. C. Klesges. 1987. The assessment of children's physical activity: A comparison of methods. Med. Sci. Sports Exerc. 19:511–517.

Klesges, R. C. In press. Relationship between psychological factors and body fat in preschool children. J. Consult. Clin. Psychol.

Klesges, R. C., T. J. Coates, and G. Brown. 1983. Parental influences on children's eating behavior and relative weight. J. Appl. Behav. Anal. 16:371–378.

Klesges, R. C., L. M. Klesges, C. K. Haddock, and L. H. Eck. 1992. A longitudinal analysis of the impact of dietary intake and physical activity on weight change in adults. Am. J. Clin. Nutr. 55:818–822.

Klesges, R. C., M. L. Shelton, and L. M. Klesges. 1993. Effects of television on metabolic rate: Potential implications for childhood obesity. Pediatrics 91:281–286.

Kohl, H. W. 3rd, S. N. Blair, R. S. Paffenbarger Jr., C. A. Macera and J. J., Kronenfeld. 1988. A mail survey of physical activity habits as related to measured physical fitness. Am. J. Epidemiol. 127:1228–1239.

Kohl, H. W. 3rd, K. E. Powell, N. F. Gordon, S. N. Blair, and R. S. Paffenbarger Jr. 1992. Physical activity, physical fitness, and sudden cardiac death. Epidemiol. Rev. 14:37–58.

Kral, J. G. 1992. Surgical treatment of obesity. Pp. 496–506 in T. A. Wadden and T. B. VanItallie, eds. Treatment of the Seriously Obese Patient. The Guilford Press, New York.

Kral, J. G. 1994. Side-effects, complications and problems in anti-obesity [abstract] surgery. Int. J. Obes. 18(suppl. 2):86.

Kramer, F. M., R. W. Jeffery, J. L. Forster, and M. K. Snell. 1989. Long-term follow-up of behavioral treatment for obesity: Patterns of weight regain among men and women. Int. J. Obes. 13:123–136.

Kuczmarski, R. S. 1992. Prevalence of overweight and weight gain in the U.S. Am. J. Clin. Nutr. 55:495S–502S.

Kuczmarski, R. S., K. M. Flegal, S. M. Campbell, and C. L. Johnson. 1994. Increasing prevalence of overweight among U.S. adults: The National Health and Nutrition Examination Surveys, 1960 to 1991. JAMA 272:205–211.

Kumanyika, S. 1993. Ethnicity and obesity development in children. Pp. 81–92 in C. L. Williams and S. Y. S. Kimm, eds. Prevention and Treatment of Childhood Obesity. Ann. NY Acad. Sci., vol. 699.

Kumanyika, S. K. 1994. Obesity in minority populations. Obes. Res. 2:166–182.

Kumanyika, S. K., and L. L. Adams-Campbell. 1991. Obesity, diet, and psychosocial factors contributing to cardiovascular disease in Blacks. Pp. 47–73 in E. Saunders and A. N. Brest, eds. Cardiovascular Diseases in Blacks. F. A. Davis, Philadelphia.

Kumanyika, S. K., E. Obarzanek, V. J. Stevens, R. Hebert, and P. K. Whelton. 1991. Weight-loss experience of black and white participants in NHLBI-sponsored clinical trials. Am. J. Clin. Nutr. 53(6 suppl.):1631S–1638S.

Kumanyika, S. K., C. Morssink, and T. Agurs. 1992. Models for dietary and weight change in African-American women: Identifying cultural components. Ethn. Dis. 2:166–175.

Lamb, K. L., and D. A. Brodie. 1990. The assessment of physical activity by leisure-time physical activity questionnaires. Sports Med. 10:159–180.

Lane, P. W., and M. M. Dickie. 1958. The effect of restricted food intake on the lifespan of genetically obese mice. J. Nutr. 64:549–553.

Lansky, D., and K. D. Brownell. 1982. Comparison of school-based treatments for adolescent obesity. J. Sch. Health 8:384–387.

Lansky, D., and M. A. Vance. 1983. School-based intervention for adolescent obesity: Analysis of treatment, randomly selected control, and self-selected subjects. J. Consult. Clin. Psychol. 51:147–148.

LaPorte, R. E., L. H. Kuller, D. J. Kupfer, R. J. McPartland, G. Matthews, and C. Caspersen. 1979. An objective measure of physical activity for epidemiologic research. 109:158–168.

Lauer, R. M., T. L. Burns, W. R. Clarke, and L. T. Mahoney. 1991. Childhood predictors of future blood pressure. Hypertension 18(suppl.):174–181.

Launer, L. J., T. Harris, C. Rumpel, and J. Madans. 1994. Body mass index, weight change, and risk of mobility disability in middle-aged and older women. The epidemiologic follow-up study of NHANES I. JAMA 271:1093–1098.

Lavery, M. A., and J. W. Loewy. 1993. Identifying predictive variables for long-term weight change after participation in a weight loss program. J. Am. Diet. Assoc. 93:1017–1024.

Lee, I. M., and R. S. Paffenbarger. 1992. Change in body weight and longevity. JAMA 268:2045–2049.

Leibel, R. L., J. Hirsch, B. E. Appel, and G. C. Checani. 1992. Energy intake required to maintain body weight is not affected by wide variation in diet composition. Am. J. Clin. Nutr. 55:350–355.

Leigh, J. P., J. F. Fries, and H. B. Hubert. 1992. Gender and race differences in the correlation between body mass and education in the 1971–1975 NHANES I. J. Epidemiol. Community Health 46:191–196.

Lenfant, C., and N. Ernst. 1994. Daily dietary fat and total food-energy intakes—third National Health and Nutrition Examination Survey, Phase 1, 1988–91. MMWR. 43:116–125.

Leon, G. R., and L. Roth. 1977. Obesity: Psychological causes, correlations, and speculations. Psychol. Bull. 84:117–139.

Leung, A. K., and W. L. Robson. 1990. Childhood obesity. Postgrad. Med. 87:123–130, 133.

Levy, A. S., and A. W. Heaton. 1993. Weight control practices of U.S. adults trying to lose weight. Ann. Intern. Med. 119:661–666.

Lew, E. A., and L. Garfinkel. 1979. Variations in mortality by weight among 750,000 men and women. J. Chronic Dis. 32:563–576.

Lichtman, S. W., K. Pisarska, E. R. Berman, M. Pestone, H. Dowling, E. Offenbacher, H. Weisel, S. Heshka, D. E. Matthews, and S. B. Heymsfield. 1992. Discrepancy between self-reported and actual caloric intake and exercise in obese subjects. N. Engl. J. Med. 327:1893–1898.

Liddle, R. A., R. B. Goldstein, and J. Saxton. 1989. Gallstone formation during weight-reduction dieting. Arch. Intern. Med. 149:1750–1753.

Lifshitz, F. 1993. Fear of obesity in childhood. Pp. 230–236 in C. L. Williams and S. Y. S. Kimm, eds. Prevention and Treatment of Childhood Obesity. Ann. NY Acad. Sci., vol. 699.

Lifshitz, F., O. Tarim, and M. M. Smith. 1993. Nutrition in adolescence. Endocrinol. Metab. Clin. North Am. 22:673–683.

Lindsted, K., S. Tonstad, and J. W. Kuzma. 1991. Body mass index and patterns of mortality among Seventh-day Adventist men. Int. J. Obes. 15:397–406.

Lissner, L., R. Andres, D. C. Muller, and H. Shimokata. 1990. Body weight variability in men: Metabolic rate, health and longevity. Int. J. Obesity 14:373–383.

Lissner, L., P. M. Odell, R. B. D. Agostino, J. Stokes 3d, B. E. Keeger, A. J. Belanger, and K. D. Brownell. 1991. Variability of body weight and health outcomes in the Framingham population. N. Engl. J. Med. 324:1839–1844.

Lissner, L., D. Sjöström, H. Wedel, and L. Sjöström. 1994. Risk factors for mortality in obese adults: The first 32 deaths among S.O.S. controls [abstract]. Int. J. Obes. 18(suppl. 2):15.

Livingstone, M. B. E., W. A. Coward, A. M. Prentice, P. S. W. Davies, J. J. Strain, P. G. McKenna, C. A. Mahoney, J. A. White, C. M. Stewart and M. J. Kerr. 1992. Daily energy expenditure in free-living children: Comparision of heart-rate monitoring with the doubly labeled water ($^2H_2^{18}O$) method. Am. J. Clin. Nutr. 56:343–352.

Longnecker, M. P., M. J. Chen, and B. Cann. 1994. Block vs. Willett: A debate on the validity of food frequency questionnaires [letter]. J. Am. Diet. Assoc. 94:16–19.

Loro, A. D. Jr., and C. S. Orleans. 1981. Binge eating in obesity: Preliminary findings and guidelines for behavioral analysis and treatment. Addict. Behav. 6:155–166.

Lowe, M. R., and G. C. Caputo. 1991. Binge eating in obesity: Toward the specification of predictors. Int. J. Eat. Disor. 10:49–55.

Luepker, R. V., D. M. Murray, D. R. Jacobs, Jr., M. B. Mittelmark, N. Bracht, R. Crow, P. Elmer, J. Finnegan, A. R. Folsom, R. Grimm, P. J. Hannan, R. Jeffery, H. Lando, P. McGovern, R. Mullis, C. L. Perry, T. Pechacek, P. Pirie, J. M. Sprafka, R. Weisbrod, and H. Blackburn. 1994. Community education for cardiovascular disease prevention: Risk factor changes in the Minnesota Heart Health Program. Am. J. Pub. Health 84:1383–1393.

Macera, C. A., K. L. Jackson, G. W. Hagenmaier, J. J. Kronenfeld, H. W. Kohl, and S. N. Blair. 1989. Age, physical activity, physical fitness, body composition, and incidence of orthopedic problems. Res. Q. Exerc. Sport 60:225–233.

MacMahon, S. W., G. J. Macdonald, L. Bernstein, G. Andrews, and R. B. Blacket. 1985. A randomized controlled trial of weight reduction and metoprolol in the treatment of hypertension in young overweight patients. Clin. Exp. Pharmacol. Physiol. 12:267–271.

Manson, J. E., E. B. Rimm, M. J. Stampfer, C. A. Colditz, W. C. Willett, A. S. Krolewski, B. Rosner, C. H. Hennekens, and F. E. Speizer. 1991. Physical activity and incidence of non-insulin-dependent diabetes mellitus in women. Lancet 338:774–778.

Marcus, M. D., R. R. Wing, L. Ewing, E. Kern, M. McDermott, and W. Gooding. 1990. A double-blind placebo-controlled trial of fluoxetine plus behavior modification in the treatment of obese binge-eaters and non-binge-eaters. Am. J. Psychiatry 147:876–881.

Marlatt, G. A., and S. F. Tapert. 1993. Harm reduction: Reducing the risks of addictive behaviors. Pp. 243–273 in J. S. Baer, G. A. Marlatt, and R. McMahon, eds. Addictive Behaviors Across the Lifespan. Sage Publications, Newbury Park, CA.

Marlatt, G. A., M. E. Larimer, J. S. Baer, and L. A. Quigley. 1993. Harm reduction for alcohol problems: Moving beyond the controlled drinking controversy. Behav. Ther. 24:461–503.

Masoro, E. J., B. P. Yu, and H. A. Bertrand. 1982. Action of food restriction in delaying the aging process. Proc. Natl. Acad. Sci. USA 79:4239–4241.

McAuley, E. 1992. The role of efficacy cognitions in the prediction of exercise behavior in middle-aged adults. J. Behav. Med. 15:65–88.

McAuley, E., and L. Jacobson. 1991. Self-efficacy and exercise participation in sedentary adult females. Am. J. Health Promo. 5:185–191, 207.

McDowell, I., and C. Newell. 1987. Measuring Health: A Guide to Rating Scales and Questionnaires. Pp. 125–133. Oxford University Press, New York.

McGinnis, J. M., and W. H. Foege. 1993. Actual causes of death in the United States. JAMA 270:2207–2212.

Mellin, L. 1993. To: President Clinton. Re: Combating childhood obesity. J. Am. Diet. Assoc. 93:265–266.

Merritt, R. J., B. R. Bistrian, G. L. Balckburn, and R. M. Suskind. 1980. Consequences of modified fasting in obese pediatric and adolescent patients: I. protein-sparing modified fast. J. Pediatr. 96:13–19.

Merritt, R. J., G. L. Blackburn, B. R. Bistrian, J. Palombo, and R. M. Suskind. 1981. Consequences of modified fasting in obese pediatric and adolescent patients: Effect of a carbohydrate-free diet on serum proteins. Am. J. Clin. Nutr. 34:2752–2755.

Merritt, R. J., B. R. Bistrian, R. M. Suskind, C. Shalaam, and G. L. Blackburn. 1983. Consequences of modified fasting in obese pediatric and adolescent patients: II. the comparative protein-sparing effect of glucose compared to fat during a three week protein-supplemented fast. Nutr. Res. 3:33–41.

Meyer, J. M., and A. J. Stunkard. 1993. Genetics and human obesity. Pp. 137–149 in A. J. Stunkard and T. A. Wadden, eds. Obesity: Theory and Therapy, 2nd ed. Raven Press, New York.

Miller, W. C., A. K. Lindeman, J. Wallace, and M. Niederpruem. 1990. Diet composition, energy intake, and exercise in relation to body fat in men and women. Am. J. Clin. Nutr. 52:426–430.

Miura J., K. Arai, S. Tsukahara, N. Ohno, and Y. Ikeda. 1989. The long-term effectiveness of combined therapy by behavior modificaton and very low calorie diet: 2 years follow up. Int. J. Obes. 13(suppl. 2):73–77.

MKSAP IX (Medical Knowledge Self-Assessment Program). 1991. American College of Physicians, Philadelphia.

MKSAP X (Medical Knowlege Self-Assessment Program). 1994. American College of Physicians, Philadelphia.

Montoye, H. J., D. A. Cunningham, H. G. Welch, and F. H. Epstein. 1970. Laboratory methods of assessing metabolic capacity in a large epidemiologic study. Am. J. Epidemiol. 91:38–47.

Montoye, H. J., R. Washburn, S. Servais, A. Ertl, J. G. Webster and F. J. Nagle. 1983. Estimation of energy expenditure by a portable accelerometer. Med. Sci. Sports Exerc. 15:403–407.

Morris, J. N., D. G. Clayton, M. G. Everitt, A. M. Semmence, and E. H. Burgess. 1990. Exercise in leisure time: Coronary attack and death rates. Br. Heart J. 63:325–334.

Morris, S. N., J. F. Phillips, J. W. Jordan, and P. L. McHenry. 1978. Incidence and significance of decreases in systolic blood pressure during graded treadmill exercise testing. Am. J. Cardiol. 41:221–226.

Moses, N., M. M. Banilivy, and F. Lifshitz. 1989. Fear of obesity among adolescent girls. Pediatrics 83:393–398.

Mossberg, H. O. 1989. 40-year follow-up of overweight children. Lancet 2:491–493.

Must, A., G. E. Dallal, and W. H. Dietz. 1991. Reference data for obesity: 85th and 95th percentiles of body mass index (wt/ht$^2$) and triceps skinfold thickness. Am. J. Clin. Nutr. 53:839–846.

Must, A., P. F. Jacques, G. E. Dallal, C. J. Bajema, and W. H. Dietz. 1992. Long-term morbidity and mortality of overweight adolescents: A follow-up of the Harvard Growth Study of 1922–1935. N. Engl. J. Med. 327:1350–1355.

Nabro, K., E. Jonsson, H. Waaler, H. Wedel, and L. Sjöström. 1994. Economic consequences of sick-leave and disability pension in obese Swedes [abstract]. Int. J. Obes. 18(suppl. 2):14.

Nader, P. R. 1993. The role of the family in obesity prevention and treatment. Pp. 147–153 in C. L. Williams and S. Y. S. Kimm, eds. Prevention and Treatment of Childhood Obesity. Ann. NY Acad. Sci., vol. 699.

NAS, IOM (National Academy of Sciences, Institute of Medicine) Ad Hoc Advisory Group on Preventive Services. 1978. Preventive Services for a Well Population. National Academy of Sciences, Washington, DC.

Näslund, I. 1994. Effects of weight reduction on the somatic, psychological and social complications of morbid obesity [abstract]. Int. J. Obes. 18(suppl. 2):86.

NCEP (National Cholesterol Education Program). 1993. Second Report of the Expert Panel on Detection, Evaluation, and Treatment of High Blood Cholesterol in Adults. NIH Publ. No. 93-3095. National Heart, Lung, and Blood Institute, National Institutes of Health, U.S. Department of Health and Human Services, Bethesda, MD.

NCES (National Center for Educational Statistics). 1990. Digest of Educational Statistics. NCES publ. 91-660. U.S. Department of Education, Washington, DC.

NCHS (National Center for Health Statistics). 1977. A Concurrent Validation Study of the NCHS General Well-Being Schedule. Data Evaluation and Methods Research, Series 2, Number 73. DHEW Publ. No. (HRA) 78-1347. National Center for Health Statistics, Hyattsville, MD.

NCHS (National Center for Health Statistics). 1994. Health, United States, 1993. Public Health Service, Hyattsville, MD.

NHBPEP (National High Blood Pressure Education Program). 1993. The Fifth Report of the Joint National Committee on Detection, Evaluation, and Treatment of High Blood Pressure. NIH Publ. No. 93-1088. U.S. Department of Health and Human Services, Public Health Service, National Institutes of Health, National Heart, Lung, and Blood Institute, Bethesda, MD.

NHBPEPWG (National High Blood Pressure Education Program Working Group). 1993. National High Blood Pressure Education Program Working Group report on primary prevention of hypertension. Arch. Intern. Med. 153:186–208.

NIDDK (National Institute of Diabetes and Digestive and Kidney Diseases). 1993a. Choosing a Safe and Successful Weight-Loss Program. NIH Publ. No. 94-3700. National Institutes of Health, Rockville, MD.

NIDDK (National Institute of Diabetes and Digestive and Kidney Diseases). 1993b. Understanding Adult Obesity. NIH Publ. No. 94-3680. National Institutes of Health, Rockville, MD.

NIH (National Institutes of Health). 1987. Consensus Development Conference on Diet and Exercise in Non-Insulin-Dependent Diabetes Mellitus. Diabetes Care 10:639–644.

NIH (National Institutes of Health). 1992. Gastrointestinal surgery for severe obesity: National Institutes of Health Consensus Development Conference Statement 1991 March 25–27. Am. J. Clin. Nutr. 55:615S–619S.

NIH (National Institutes of Health). 1993. National Institutes of Health Program in Biomedical and Behavioral Nutrition Research and Training, Fiscal Year 1992, 16th Annual Report. NIH Nutrition Coordinating Committee, Division of Nutrition Research Coordination. NIH Publ. No. 93-2092. National Institutes of Health, Bethesda, MD.

NIH (National Institutes of Health). 1994. Strategy Development Workshop for Public Education on Weight and Obesity. National Heart, Lung, and Blood Institute, NIH. NIH Publication No. 94-3314. National Institutes of Health, Bethesda, MD.

NIH (National Institutes of Health) Technology Assessment Conference Panel. 1993. Methods for voluntary weight loss and control: Technology Assessment Conference Statement. Ann. Intern. Med. 119:764–770.

Noles, S. W., T. F. Cash, and B. A. Winstead. 1985. Body image, physical attractiveness, and depression. J. Consult. Clin. Psychol. 53:88–94.

NRC (National Research Council). 1989a. Diet and Health: Implications for Reducing Chronic Disease Risk. Committee on Diet and Health, Food and Nutrition Board, Commission on Life Sciences. National Academy Press, Washington, DC.

NRC (National Research Council). 1989b. Recommended Dietary Allowances, 10th ed. Report of the Subcommittee on the Tenth Edition of the RDAs, Food and Nutrition Board, Commission of Life Sciences. National Academy Press, Washington, DC.

NTF (National Task Force on the Prevention and Treatment of Obesity, National Institutes of Health). 1993. Very low-calorie diets. JAMA 270:967–974.

NTF (National Task Force on the Prevention and Treatment of Obesity, National Institutes of Health). 1994a. Towards prevention of obesity: Research directions. Obes. Res. 2:571–584.

NTF (National Task Force on the Prevention and Treatment of Obesity, National Institutes of Health). 1994b. Weight cycling. JAMA 272:1196–1202.

Nunez, C., S. Heshka, F. X. Pi-Sunyer, and S. B. Heymsfield. 1992. Weight loss on a low calorie deficiency diet: Safety and effectiveness in healthy overweight adults. FASEB J. 6:4274.

Nuutinen, O., and M. Knip. 1992. Long-term weight control in obese children: Persistence of treatment outcome and metabolic changes. Int. J. Obes. 16:279–287.

O'Hara, N. M., T. Baranoski, B. G. Simons-Morton, B. S. Wilson and G. Parcel. 1989. Validity of the observation of children's physical activity. Res. Q. Exerc. Sport 60:42–47.

O'Neil, P. M., and M. P. Jarrell. 1992. Psychological aspects of obesity and dieting. Pp. 252–270 in T. A. Wadden and T. B. VanItallie, eds. Treatment of the Seriously Obese Patient. Guilford Press, New York.

O'Neil, P. M., H. S. Currey, A. A. Hirsch, F. E. Riddle, C. I. Taylor, R. J. Malcom, and J. D. Sexauer. 1979. Effects of sex of subject and spouse involvement on weight loss in a behavioral treatment program: a retrospective investigation. Addict. Beh. 4:167–177.

O'Reilly, P., and H. E. Thomas. 1989. Role of support networks in maintenance of improved cardiovascular health status. Soc. Sci. Med. 28:249–260.

Obarzanek, E., G. B. Schreiber, P. B. Crawford, S. R. Goldman, P. M. Barrir, N. M. Frederick, and E. Lakatos. 1994. Energy intake and physical activity in relation to indexes of body fat: The National Heart, Lung, and Blood Institute Growth and Health Study. Am. J. Clin. Nutr. 60:15–22.

Oettingen, G., and T. A. Wadden. 1991. Expectation, fantasy, and weight loss: Is the impact of positive thinking always positive? Cognit. Ther. Res. 15:167–175.

Oldridge, N. B. 1982. Compliance and exercise in primary and secondary prevention of coronary heart disease: A review. Prev. Med. 11:56–70.

Ornish, D. 1993. Eat More, Weigh Less. HarperCollins, New York.

Osterman, J., T. Lin, H. R. Nankin, K. A. Brown, and C. A. Hornung. 1992. Serum cholesterol profiles during treatment of obese outpatients with a very low calorie diet: effect of initial cholesterol levels. Int. J. Obes. 16:49–58.

Owen, N, A. W. Sedgwick and M. Davies. 1988. Validity of a simplified measure of participation in vigorous physical activity [letter]. Med. J. Aust. 148:600.

Paffenbarger, R. S. Jr., S. N. Blair, I. M. Lee, and R. T. Hyde. 1993. Measurement of physical activity to assess health effects in free-living populations. Med. Sci. Sports Exerc. 25:60–70.

Palla, B., and I. F. Litt. 1988. Medical complications of eating disorders in adolescents. Pediatrics 81:613–623.

Pamuk, E. R., D. F. Williamson, J. Madans, M. K. Serdula, T. Byers, and J. C. Kleinman. 1992. Weight loss and mortality in a national cohort of adults, 1971–1987. Am. J. Epidemiol. 136:686–697.

Pamuk, E. R., D. F. Williamson, M. K. Serdula, J. Madans, and T. E. Byers. 1993. Weight loss and subsequent death in a cohort of U.S. adults. Ann. Int. Med. 119:744–748.

Pavlou, K. N., S. Krey, and W. P. Steffee. 1989. Exercise as an adjunct to weight loss and maintenance in moderately obese subjects. Am. J. Clin. Nutr. 49:1115–1123.

Pekarik, G., C. Blodgett, R. G. Evans, and M. Wierzbicki. 1984. Variables related to continuance in a behavioral weight loss program. Addict. Behav. 9:413–416.

Perri, M. G. 1992. Improving maintenance of weight loss following treatment by diet and lifestyle modification. Pp. 456–477 in T. A. Wadden and T. B. Vanltallie, eds. Treatment of the Seriously Obese Patient. Guilford Press, New York.

Perri, M. G., D. A. McAllister, J. J. Gange, R. C. Jordan, W. G. McAdoo, and A. M. Nezu. 1988. Effects of four maintenance programs on the long-term management of obesity. J. Consult. Clin. Psychol. 56:529–534.

Perri, M. G., A. M. Nezu, E. T. Patti, and K. L. McCann. 1989. Effect of length of treatment on weight loss. J. Consult. Clin. Psychol. 57:450–452.

Perri, M. G., A. M. Nezu, and B. J. Viegener. 1992. Improving the Long-term Management of Obesity: Theory, Research, and Clinical Guidelines. Wiley, New York.

Petersmarck, K. A. 1992. The Michigan approach: Building consensus for safe weight loss. J. Am. Diet. Assoc. 92:679–680.

Piani, A. L., and C. A. Schoenborn. 1993. Health promotion and disease prevention: United States, 1990. Vital Health Stat. 10(185):1–88.

Pi-Sunyer, F. X. 1993a. Medical hazards of obesity. Ann. Int. Med. 119:655–660.

Pi-Sunyer, F. X. 1993b. Short-term medical benefits and adverse effects of weight loss. Ann. Intern. Med. 119:722–726.

Pisacano, J. C., H. Lichter, J. Ritter, and A. P. Siegal. 1978. An attempt at prevention of obesity in infancy. Pediatrics 61:360–364.

Pories, W. J., K. G. MacDonald Jr., E. J. Morgan, M. K. Sinha, G. L. Dohm, M. S. Swanson, H. A. Barakat, P. G. Khazanie, N. Leggett-Frazier, S. D. Long et al. 1992. Surgical treatment of obesity and its effect on diabetes: 10-year follow-up. Am J. Clin. Nutr. 55(2 suppl.):582S–585S.

Prewitt, T. E., D. Schmeisser, P. E. Bowen, P. Aye, T. A. Dolecek, P. Langenberg, T. Cole, and L. Brace. 1991. Changes in body weight, body composition, and energy intake in women fed high- and low-fat diets. Am. J. Clin. Nutr. 54:304–310.

Price, J. H., S. M. Desmond, R. A. Krol, F. F. Snyder, and J. K. O'Connell. 1987. Family practice physicians' beliefs, attitudes, and practices regarding obesity. Am. J. Prev. Med. 3:339–345.

Puska, P., J. T. Salonen, A. Nissinen, J. Tuomilehto, E. Vartiainen, H. Korhonen, A. Tanskanen, P. Rönnqvist, K. Koskela, and J. Huttunen. 1983. Change in risk factors for coronary heart disease during 10 years of a community intervention programme (North Karelia project). Br. Med. J. 287:1840–1844.

Rahe, R. H. 1975. Epidemiological studies of life change and illness. Int. J. Psychiatry Med. 6:133–146.

Rand, C. S., and J. M. Kuldau. 1992. Epidemiology of bulimia and symptoms in a general population: Sex, age, race, and socioeconomic status. Int. J. Eat. Disord. 11:37–44.

Ravelli, G. P., and L. Belmont. 1979. Obesity in nineteen-year-old men: Family size and birth order associations. Am. J. Epidemiol. 109:66–70.

Ravussin, E., and B. A. Swinburn. 1992. Pathophysiology of obesity. 340:404–408.

Ravussin, E., S. Lillioja, W. Knowler, L. Christin, D. Freymond, W. G. Abbott, V. Boyee, B. V. Howard, and C. Bogardus. 1988. Reduced rate of energy expenditure as a risk factor for body-weight gain. N. Engl. J. Med. 318:467–472.

Ray, J. W., and R. C. Klesges. 1993. Influences on the eating behavior of children. Pp. 57–69 in C. L. Williams and S. Y. S. Kimm, eds. Prevention and Treatment of Childhood Obesity. Ann. NY Acad. Sci., vol. 699.

Reed, G. W., and J. O. Hill. 1993. Weight cycling: A review of the animal literatures. Obes. Res. 1:392–402.

Reisin, E., R. Abel, M. Modan, D. S. Silverberg, H. E. Eliahou, and B. Modan. 1978. Effect of weight loss without salt restriction on the reduction of blood pressure in overweight hypertensive patients. N. Engl. J. Med. 298:1–6.

Resnicow, K. 1993. School-based obesity prevention: Population versus high-risk interventions. Pp. 154–166 in C. L. Williams and S. Y. S. Kimm, eds. Prevention and Treatment of Childhood Obesity. Ann. NY Acad. Sci., vol. 699.

Reybrouck, T., J. Vinckx, G. Van den Berghe, and M. Vanderschueren-Lodeweyckx. 1990. Exercise therapy and hypocaloric diet in the treatment of obese children and adolescents. Acta Paediatr. Scand. 79:84–89.

Richardson, S. A., N. Goodman, and A. H. Hastorf. 1967. Cultural uniformity in reaction to physical disabilities. Am. Sociol. Rev. 26:241–247.

Roberts, S. B., J. Savage, W. A. Coward, B. Chew, and A. Lucas. 1988. Energy expenditure and intake in infants born to lean and overweight mothers. N. Engl. J. Med. 318:461–466.

Roche, A. F., R. M. Sievogel, W. C. Chumlea, and P. Webb. 1981. Grading body fatness from limited anthropometric data. Am. J. Clin. Nutr. 34:2831–2838.

Rodin, J. 1993. Cultural and psychosocial determinants of weight concerns. Ann. Intern. Med. 119:643–645.

Rolland-Cachera, M. F., and F. Bellisle. 1986. No correlation between adiposity and food intake: Why are working class children fatter? Am. J. Clin. Nutr. 44:779–787.

Rolland-Cachera, M. F., M. Deheeger, F. Pequignot, M. Guilloud-Bataille, and F. Vinit. 1988. Adiposity and food intake in young children: The environmental challenge to individual susceptibilty. Br. Med. J. 290:1037–1038.

Romieu, I., W. C. Willett, M. J. Stampfer, G. A. Colditz, R. Sampson, B. Rosner, C. H. Hennekens, and F. E. Speizer. 1988. Energy intake and other determinants of relative weight. Am. J. Clin. Nutr. 47:406–412.

Rose, H. E., and J. Mayer. 1986. Activity, calorie intake, fat storage, and the energy balance of infants. Pediatrics 41:18–29.

Rosenberg, M. 1965. Society and the Adolescent Self-Image. Princeton University Press, Princeton, NJ.

Rosenberg, M. 1979. Conceiving the Self. Basic Books, New York.

Ross, J. G., R. R. Pate, C. J. Casperson, C. L. Camberg, and M. Svilar. 1987. Home and community in children's exercise habits. J. Phys. Educ. Rec. Dance 92:58–85.

Rössner, S. 1992. Factors determining the long-term outcome of obesity treatment. Pp. 712–719 in P. Björntorp and B. N. Brodoff, eds. Obesity. J. B. Lippincott Company, Philadelphia.

Ryckman, R. M., M. A. Robbins, B. Thornton, and P. Cantrell. 1982. Development and validation of a physical self-efficacy scale. J. Pers. Soc. Psychol. 42:891–900.

Sallade, J. 1973. A comparison of the psychological adjustment of obese vs. non-obese children. J. Psychosom. Res. 17:89–96.

Sallis, J. F., W. L. Haskell, P. D. Wood, S. P. Fortmann, T. Rogers, S. N. Blair, and R. S. Paffenbarger Jr. 1985. Physical activity assessment methodology in the Five-City Project. Am. J. Epidemiol. 121:91–106.

Sallis, J. F., R. B. Pinski, R. M. Grossman, T. L. Patterson, and P. R. Nader. 1987. The development of scales to measure social support for diet and exercise behaviors. Prev. Med. 16:825–836.

Sallis, J. F., M. J. Buono, J. J. Roby, D. Carlson and J. A. Nelson. 1990. The Caltrac accelerometer as a physical activity monitor for school-age children. Med. Sci. Sports Exerc. 22:698–703.

Sallis, J. F., T. L. McKenzie, J. E. Alcaraz, B. Kolody, M. F. Hovell, and P. R. Nader. 1993. Project SPARK: Effects of physical education on adiposity in children. Pp. 127–136 in C. L. Williams and S. Y. S. Kimm, eds. Prevention and Treatment of Childhood Obesity. Ann. NY Acad. Sci., vol. 699.

Saris, W. H. M. 1986. Habitual physical activity in children: Methodology and findings in health and disease. Med. Sci. Sports Exerc. 18:253–263.

Schechtman, K. B., B. Barzilai, K. Rost and E. B. Fisher Jr. 1991. Measuring physical activity with a single question. Am. J. Pub. Health. 81:771–773.

Schlundt, D. G., and R. T. Zimering. 1988. The Dieter's Inventory of Eating Temptations: A measure of weight control competence. Addict. Behav. 13:151–164.

Schoenborn, C. A. 1986. Health habits of U.S. adults, 1985: The "Alameda 7" revisited. Public Health Rep. 101:571–580.

Schoenborn, C. A. 1988. Health promotion and disease prevention. Vital Health Stat. 10(163):1–91.

Schotte, D. E., and A. J. Stunkard. 1990. The effects of weight reduction on blood pressure in 301 obese patients. Arch. Intern. Med. 150:1701–1704.

Schwartz, R. S. 1987. The independent effects of dietary weight loss and aerobic training on high density lipoproteins and apolipoprotein A-I concentrations in obese men. Metabolism 36:165–171.

Scoville, B. A. 1973. Review of amphetamine-like drugs by the Food and Drug Administration: Clinical data and value judgments. Pp. 441–443 in G. A. Bray, ed. Obesity in Perspective. National Institutes of Health, Bethesda, MD.

Secord, P. F., and S. M. Jourard. 1953. The appraisal of body-cathexis: Body-cathexis and the self. J. Consult. Psychol. 17:343–347.

Seim, H. C. and K. B. Holtmeier. 1992. Effects of a six-week, low-fat diet on serum cholesterol, body weight, and body measurements. Fam. Pract. Res. J. 12:411–419.

Serdula, M. K., M. E. Collins, D. F. Williamson, R. F. Anda, E. Pamuk, and T. E. Byers. 1993. Weight control practices of U.S. adolescents and adults. Ann. Intern. Med. 119:667–671.

Sheppard, L., A. R. Kristal, and L. H. Kushi. 1991. Weight loss in women participating in a randomized trial of low-fat diets. Am. J. Clin. Nutr. 54:821–828.

Sheslow, D., S. Hassink, W. Wallace, and E. DeLancey. 1993. The relationship between self-esteem and depression in obese children. Pp. 289–291 in C. L. Williams and S. Y. S. Kimm, eds. Prevention and Treatment of Childhood Obesity. Ann. NY Acad. Sci., vol. 699.

Siconolfi, S. F., E. M. Cullinane, R. A. Carleton, and P. D. Thompson. 1982. VO2max in epidemiologic studies: Modification of the Astrand-Ryhming test. Med. Sci. Sports Exerc. 14:335–338.

Sidney, S., W. L. Haskell, R. Crow, B. Sternfeld, A. Oberman, M. A. Armstrong, G. R. Cutter, and L. Van Horn. 1992. Sympton-limited graded treadmill exercise testing in young adults in the CARDIA study. Med. Sci. Sports Exerc. 24:177–183.

Sikand G., A. Kondo, J. P. Foreyt, P. H. Jones, and A. M. Gotto Jr. 1988. Two year follow-up of patients treated with very low calorie diet and exercise training. J. Am. Diet. Assoc. 88:487–488.

Silverstone, T. 1993. The place of appetite-suppressant drugs in the treatment of obesity. Pp. 275–285 in A. J. Stunkard and T. A. Wadden, eds. Obesity: Theory and Therapy, 2nd ed. Raven Press, New York.

Simpser, M. D., D. J. Strieder, M. E. Wohl, A. Rosenthal, and S. Rockenmacher. 1977. Sleep apnea in a child with the pickwickian syndrome. Pediatrics 60:290–293.

Sims, E. A. H. 1988. Exercise and energy balance in the control of obesity and hypertension. Pp. 242–257 in E. S. Horton and R. L. Terjung, eds. Exercise, Nutrition, and Energy Metabolism. Macmillan, New York.

Sjöström, C. D., A. C. Hakangard, L. Lissner, and L. Sjöström. 1994a. Relationships between cardiovascular risk factors and visceral and subcutaneous adipose tissue (AT) distribution [abstract]. Int. J. Obes. 18(suppl. 2):15.

Sjöström, L., L. Lissner, B. Larsson, L. Backman, C. Bengtsson, C. Bouchard, S. Dahlgren, E. Jonsson, R. Lindstedt, K. Narbro, I. Näslund, L. Olbe, D. Sjöström, K. Stenlöf, M. Sullivan, and H. Wedel. 1994b. SOS-Swedish obese subjects: An intervention study of obesity [abstract]. Int. J. Obes. 18(suppl. 2):14.

Slade, P. D., M. E. Dewey, T. Newton, D. A. Brodie, and G. Kiemle. 1990. Development and preliminary validation of the Body Satisfaction Scale (BSS). Psychol. Health 4:213–220.

Smoller, J. W., T. A. Wadden, and A. J. Stunkard. 1987. Dieting and depression: A critical review. J. Psychosom. Res. 31:429–440.

Sobal, J., and A. J. Stunkard. 1989. Socioeconomic status and obesity: A review of the literature. Psychol. Bull. 105:260–275.

Society of Actuaries. 1980. Build Study, 1979. Society of Actuaries and Association of Life Insurance Medical Directors of America, Chicago.

Sorkin, J. D., D. Miller, and R. Andres. In press. Body mass index and mortality in Seventh-day Adventist men. A critique and reanalysis. Int. J. Obes.

Soto, L. F., D. A. Kikuchi, R. A. Arcilla, D. D. Savage, and G. S. Berenson. 1989. Echocardiographic functions and blood pressure levels in children and young adults from a biracial population: The Bogalusa Heart Study. Am. J. Med. Sci. 297:271–279.

Spiegel, T. A., T. A. Wadden, and G. D. Foster. 1991. Objective measurement of eating rate during behavioral treatment of obesity. Behav. Ther. 22:61–67.

Spitzer, R. L., M. Devlin, B. T. Walsh, D. Hasin, R. Wing, M. Marcus, A. J. Stunkard, T. A. Wadden, S. Yanovski, S. Agras, J. Mitchell, and C. Nonas. 1992. Binge eating disorder: A multi-site field trial of the diagnostic criteria. Int. J. Eat. Disord. 11:191–203.

Spitzer, R. L., S. Yanovski, T. Wadden, R. Wing, M. D. Marcus, A. Stunkard, M. Devlin, J. Mitchell, D. Hasin, and R. L. Horne. 1993. Binge eating disorder: Its further validation in a multisite study. Int. J. Eat. Disord. 13:137–153.

Srinivasan, S. R., W. Bao, and G. S. Berenson. 1993. Coexistence of increased levels of adiposity, insulin, and blood pressure in a young adult cohort with elevated very low-density lipoprotein cholesterol: The Bogalusa Heart Study. Metabolism 42:170–176.

St. Jeor, S. T. In press. Measurement of food intake. In K. D. Brownell and C. G. Fairburn, eds. Eating Disorders and Obesity: A Comprehensive Handbook. Guilford Press, New York.

St. Jeor, S. T., H. A. Guthrie, and M. B. Jones. 1983. Variability in nutrient intake in a 28-day period. J. Am. Diet. Assoc. 83:155–162.

Stallings, V. A., E. H. Archibald, P. B. Pencharz, J. E. Harrison, and L. E. Bell. 1988. One year follow-up of weight, total body potassium, and total body nitrogen in obese adolescents treated with the protein-sparing modified fast. Am. J. Clin. Nutr. 48:91–94.

Stallone, D. D., and A. J. Stunkard. 1992. Long-term use of appetite suppressant medication: Rationale and recommendations. Drug Development Res. 26:1–20.

Stampfer, M. J., K. M. Maclure, G. A. Colditz, J. E. Manson, and W. C. Willett. 1992. Risk of symptomatic gallstones in women with severe obesity. Am. J. Clin. Nutr. 55:652–658.

Stark, O., E. Atkins, O. H. Wolff, and J. W. Douglas. 1981. Longitudinal study of obesity in the National Survey of Health and Development. Br. Med. J. 283:13–17.

Stefanick, P. A., F. P. Heald, and J. Mayer. 1959. Caloric intake in relation to energy output of obese and non-obese adolescent boys. Am. J. Clin. Nutr. 7:55.

Stein, T. P., R. W. Hoyt, R. G. Settle, M. O'Toole, and W. D. Hiller. 1987. Determination of energy expenditure during heavy exercise, normal daily activity, and sleep using the doubly-labelled-water ($^2H_2{}^{18}O$) method. Am. J. Clin. Nutr. 45:534–539.

Stephens, T. 1987. Secular trends in adult physical activity: Exercise boom or bust? Res. Q. Exerc. Sport. 58:94–105.

Stephens, T., D. R. Jacobs Jr., and C. C. White. 1985. A descriptive epidemiology of leisure-time physical activity. Public Health Rep. 100:147–158.

Stern, M. P., J. A Pugh, S. P. Gaskill, and H. P. Hazuda. 1982. Knowledge, attitudes, and behavior related to obesity and dieting in Mexican Americans and Anglos: the San Antonio Heart Study. Am. J. Epidemiol. 115:917–928.

Stevens, J., and L. Lissner. 1990. Body weight and variability and mortality in the Charleston Heart Study. Int. J. Obes. 14:385–386.

Stevens, V. J., S. A. Corrigan, E. Obarzanek, E. Bernauer, N. R. Cook, P. Herbert, M. Mattfeldt-Beman, A. Oberman, C. Sugars, A. T. Dalcin et al. 1993. Weight loss intervention in phase 1 of the Trials of Hypertention Prevention: The TOHP Collaborative Research Group. Arch. Intern. Med. 153:849–858.

Stunkard, A. J. 1957. The "dieting depression." Incidence and clinical characteristics of untoward responses to weight reduction regimes. Am. J. Med. 23:77–86.

Stunkard, A. J. 1959. Eating patterns and obesity. Psychiat. Q. 33:284–295.

Stunkard, A. J. 1984. The current status of treatment for obesity in adults. Pp. 157–173 in A. J. Stunkard and E. Stellar, eds. Eating and its Disorders. Raven Press, New York.

Stunkard, A. J. 1987. Conservative treatment for obesity. Am. J. Clin. Nutr. 45:1142–1154.

Stunkard, A. J. 1990. Genetic contributions to human obesity. Pp. 205–219 in P. R. McHugh and V. A. McKusick, eds. Genes, Brains and Behavior. Raven Press, NY.

Stunkard, A. J. 1992. An overview of current treatments for obesity. Pp. 33–43 in T. A. Wadden and T. B. VanItallie, eds. Treatment of the Seriously Obese Patient. Guilford Press, New York.

Stunkard, A. J. 1993. Talking with patients. Pp. 355–363 in A. J. Stunkard and T. A. Wadden, eds. Obesity: Theory and Therapy, 2nd ed. Raven Press, New York.

Stunkard, A. J. In press. Prevention of obesity. In K. D. Brownell and C. G. Fairburn, eds. Eating Disorders and Obesity: A Comprehensive Handbook. Guilford Press, New York.

Stunkard, A. J., and M. Mendelson. 1967. Obesity and the body image: I. Characteristics of disturbances in the body image of some obese persons. Am. J. Psychiatry 123:1443–1447.

Stunkard, A. J., and S. Messick. 1985. The three-factor eating questionnaire to measure dietary restraint, disinhibition, and hunger. J. Psychosom. Res. 29:71–83.

Stunkard, A. J., and J. Rush. 1974. Dieting and depression reexamined. A critical review of untoward responses during weight reduction for obesity. Ann. Intern. Med. 81:526–533.

Stunkard, A. J., and T. I. Sørensen. 1993. Obesity and socioeconomic status: A complex relation [editorial]. N. Engl. J. Med. 329:1036–1037.

Stunkard, A. J., T. I. Sørensen, C. Hanis, T. W. Teasdale, R. Chakraborty, W. J. Schull, and F. Schulsinger. 1986. An adoption study of human obesity. N. Engl. J. Med. 314:193–198.

Stunkard, A. J., J. R. Harris, N. L. Pedersen, and G. E. McClearn. 1990. The body mass index of twins who have been reared apart. N. Engl. J. Med. 322:1483–1487.

Sugerman, H. J., G. L. Londrey, J. M. Kellum, L. Wolf, T. Liszka, K. M. Engle, R. Birkenhauer, and J. V. Starkey. 1989. Weight loss with vertical banded gastroplasty and roux-y gastric bypass for morbid obesity with selective versus random assignment. Am. J. Surg. 157:93–102.

Sullivan, M. J. Karlsson, and L. Sjöström. 1994. Swedish obese subjects (SOS): An intervention study of obesity. Two-year follow-up of health and psychosocial functioning [abstract]. Int. J. Obes. 18(suppl. 2):14.

Sundberg, N. D. 1992. Review of the Beck Depression Inventory [Revised Edition]. Pp 79–81 in J. J. Kramer and J. C. Conoley, eds. The Eleventh Mental Measurements Yearbook. The University of Nebraska Press, Lincoln, NE.

Sunnegardh, J., L. E. Bratteby, U. Hagman, G. Samuelson, and S. Sjolin. 1986. Physical activity in relation to energy intake and body fat in 8- and 13-year old children in Sweden. Acta Pediatr. Scand. 75:955–963.

Suskind, R. M., M. S. Sothern, R. P. Farris, T. K. von Almen, H. Schumacher, L. Carlisle, A. Vargas, O. Escobar, M. Loftin, G. Fuchs, R. Brown, and J. N. Udall Jr. 1993. Recent advances in the treatment of childhood obesity. Pp. 181–199 in C. L. Williams and S. Y. S. Kimm, eds. Prevention and Treatment of Childhood Obesity. Ann. NY Acad. Sci., vol. 699.

Swinburn, B., and E. Ravussin. 1993. Energy balance or fat balance? Am. J. Clin. Nutr. 57:766S–770S.

Tanner, J. M., H. Goldstein, and R. H. Whitehouse. 1970. Standards for children's height at ages 2–9 years allowing for height of parents. Arch. Dis. Child. 45:755–762.

Taras, H. L., J. F. Sallis, T. L. Patterson, R. R. Nader, and J. A. Nelson. 1989. Television's influence on children's diet and physical activity. J. Dev. Behav. Pediatr. 10:176–180.

Tarasuk, V., and G. H. Beaton. 1991. The nature and individuality of within-subject variation in energy intake. Am. J. Clin. Nutr. 54:464–470.

Taylor, C. B., and A. J. Stunkard. 1993. Public health approaches to weight control. Pp. 335–353 in A. J. Stunkard and T. A. Wadden, eds. Obesity: Theory and Therapy, 2nd ed. Raven Press, New York.

Taylor, C. B., H. C. Kraemer, D. A. Bragg, L. E. Miles, B. Rule, W. M. Savin, and R. F. DeBusk. 1982. A new system for long-term recording and processing of heart rate and physical activity in outpatients. Comput. Biomed. Res. 15:7–17.

Taylor, C. B., T. Coffey, K. Berra, R. Iaffaldano, K. Casey, and W. L. Haskell. 1984. Seven-day activity and self-report compared to a direct measure of physical activity. Am. J. Epidemiol. 120:818–824.

Taylor, H. L., D. R. Jacobs Jr., B. Schucker, J. Knudsen, A. S. Leon, and G. Debacker. 1978. A questionnaire for the assessment of leisure time physical activities. J. Chronic Dis. 31:741–755.

Thompson, J. K., G. J. Jarvie, B. B. Lahey, and K. J. Cureton. 1982. Exercise and obesity: Etiology, physiology, and intervention. Psychol. Bull. 91:55–79.

Tracey, V. V., N. C. De, and J. R. Harper. 1971. Obesity and respiratory infection in infants and young children. Br. Med. J. 1:16–18.

Tremblay, A., and C. Bouchard. 1987. Assessment of energy expenditure and physical activity pattern in population studies. Pp. 101–116 in F. E. Johnston, ed. Nutritional Anthropology. A. R. Liss, New York.

Tremblay, A., J-P. Després, J. Maheux, M. C. Pouliot, A. Nadeau, S. Moorjani, P. J. Lupien, and C. Bouchard. 1991. Normalization of the metabolic profile in obese women by exercise and a low fat diet. Med. Sci. Sports Exerc. 23:1326–1331.

Tucker, L. A. 1981. Internal structure, factor satisfaction, and reliability of the Body-Cathexis Scale. Perceptual and Motor Skills 53:891–896.

Tucker, L. A. 1986. The relationship of television viewing to physical fitness and obesity. Adolescence 21:797–806.

Tufts. 1994. But are you ready to lose weight? Tufts University Diet & Nutr. Lett. 12(3):6.

Tyroler, H. A., S. Heyden, and C. G. Hames. 1975. Weight and hypertension: Evans County studies of blacks and whites. Pp. 177–205 in O. Paul, ed. Epidemiology and Control of Hypertension: Papers and Discussions from the Second International Symposium on the Epidemiology of Hypertension. Stratton Intercontinental Medical Book Corp., New York.

Tzankoff, S. P., and A. H. Norris. 1977. Effect of muscle mass decrease on age-related BMR changes. J. Appl. Physiol. 43:1001–1006.

Uchino, H., T. Usami, M. Honda, S. Matsufuji, Y. Mochida, K. Hiroturu, Y. Tokudome, and Y. Arase. 1991. The effect of long-term group education for obese women in a public health center. Nippon Koshu Eisei Zasshi 38:11–19.

U.S. Congress, House. 1990. Deception and Fraud in the Diet Industry, Part I. Pp. 101–150 in hearing before the Subcommittee on Regulation, Business Opportunities, and Energy. Committee on Small Business. 101st Congress, 2nd Session. Government Printing Office, Washington, DC.

USDA (U.S. Department of Agriculture). 1992. USDA's Food Guide Pyramid. Home and Garden Bulletin, no. 252. USDA Human Nutrition Information Service, Washington, DC.

USDA (U.S. Department of Agriculture) and DHHS (U.S. Department of Health and Human Services). 1990. Dietary Guidelines for Americans, 3rd ed. Government Printing Office, Washington, DC.

Vaughn, L., F. Zurlo, and E. Ravussin. 1991. Aging and energy expenditure. Am. J. Clin. Nutr. 53:821–825.

Vega, W. A., J. F. Sallis, T. Patterson, J. Rupp, C. Atkins, and P. R. Nader. 1987. Assessing knowledge of cardiovascular health-related diet and exercise behaviors in Anglo- and Mexican-Americans. Prev. Med. 16:696–709.

Vogler, G. P., T. I. A. Sørensen, A. J. Stunkard, M. R. Srinivasan, and D. C. Rao. In press. Influences of genes and shared family environment on adult body mass index assessed by a comprehensive path model in an adoption study. Int. J. Obes.

Volkmar, F. R., A. J. Stunkard, J. Woolston, and R. A. Bailey. 1981. High attrition rates in commercial weight reduction programs. Arch. Intern. Med. 141:426–428.

Waaler, H. T. 1984. Height, weight, and mortality. The Norwegian experience. Acta Med. Scand. 679(suppl.):1–56.

Wadden, T. A. 1993. Treatment of obesity by moderate and severe caloric restriction: Results of clinical research trials. Ann. Intern. Med. 119:688–693.

Wadden, T. A., and S. J. Bell. 1990. Obesity. Pp. 449–473 in A. S. Bellack, M. Hersen, and A. E. Kazdin, eds. International Handbook of Behavior Modification and Therapy, 2nd ed. Plenum Press, New York.

Wadden, T. A., and G. D. Foster. 1992. Behavioral assessment and treatment of markedly obese patients. Pp. 290–330 in T. A. Wadden and T. B. VanItallie, eds. Treatment of the Seriosly Obese Patient. Guilford Press, New York.

Wadden, T. A., and K. A. Letizia. 1992. Predictors of attrition and weight loss in patients treated by moderate and severe calorie restriction. Pp. 383–410 in T. A. Wadden and T. B. VanItallie, eds. Treatment of the Seriously Obese Patient. Guilford Press, New York.

Wadden, T. A., and A. J. Stunkard. 1985. Social and psychological consequences of obesity. Ann. Intern. Med. 103:1062–1067.

Wadden, T. A., and A. J. Stunkard. 1986. Controlled trial of a very-low-calorie diet, behavior therapy, and their combination in the treatment of obesity. J. Consult. Clin. Psychol. 54:482–488.

Wadden, T. A., and A. J. Stunkard. 1993. Psychosocial consequences of obesity and dieting: Research and clinical findings. Pp. 163–177 in T. A. Wadden and A. J. Stunkard, eds. Obesity: Theory and Therapy, 2nd ed. Raven Press, New York.

Wadden, T. A., A. J. Stunkard, and J. W. Smoller. 1986. Dieting and depression: A methodological study. J. Consult. Clin. Psychol. 54:869–871.

Wadden, T. A., A. J. Stunkard, F. E. Johnston, J. Wang, R. N. Pierson, T. B. VanItallie, E. Costello, and M. Pena. 1988. Body fat deposition in adult obese women: II. changes in fat distribution accompanying weight reduction. Am. J. Clin. Nutr. 47:229–234.

Wadden, T. A., J. A. Sternberg, K. A. Letizia, A. J. Stunkard, and G. D. Foster. 1989. Treatment of obesity by very low-calorie diet, behavior therapy, and their combination: A five-year perspective. Int. J. Obes. 13(suppl. 2):39–46.

Wadden, T. A., A. J. Stunkard, L. Rich, C. J. Rubin, G. Sweidel, and S. McKinney. 1990a. Obesity in black adolescent girls: A controlled clinical trial of treatment by diet, behavior modification, and parental support. Pediatrics 85:345–352.

Wadden, T. A., T. B. VanItallie, and G. L. Blackburn. 1990b. Responsible and irresponsible use of very low-calorie diets in the treatment of obesity. JAMA 263:83–85.

Wadden, T. A., G. D. Foster, K. A. Letizia, and A. J. Stunkard. 1991. A multi-center evaluation of a proprietary weight reduction program for the treatment of marked obesity. Arch. Intern. Med. 152:961–966.

Wadden, T. A., G. D. Foster, and K. A. Letizia. 1994. One-year behavioral treatment of obesity: Comparison of moderate and severe caloric restriction and the effects of weight maintenance therapy. J. Consult. Clin. Psychol. 62:165–171.

Wallace, W. J., D. Sheslow, and S. Hassink. 1993. Obesity in children: Risk for depression. Pp. 301–303 in C. L. Williams and S. Y. S. Kimm, eds. Prevention and Treatment of Childhood Obesity. Ann. NY Acad. Sci., vol. 699.

Wallerstein, R. S. 1956. Comparative study of treatment methods for chronic alcoholism: The alcoholism research project at Winter VA Hospital. Am. J. Psychiatry 113:228–233.

Ward, E. M. 1994. Winners or losers? EN reviews the top weight-loss programs. Environmental Nutrition 17(2):1, 3–5.

Washburn, R. A., L. L. Adams, and G. T. Haile. 1987. Physical activity assessment for epidemiologic research: The utility of two simplified approaches. Prev. Med. 16:636–646.

Washburn, R. A., S. R. W. Goldfield, K. W. Smith and J. B. McKinlay. 1990. The validity of self-reported exercise-induced sweating as a measure of physical activity. Am. J. Epidemiol. 132:107–113.

Washburn, R. A., K. W. Smith, S. R. W. Goldfield, and J. B. McKinlay. 1991. Reliability and physiologic correlates of the Harvard Alumni Activity Survey in a general population. J. Clin. Epidemiol. 44:1319–1326.

Wattchow, D. A., J. C. Hall, M. J. Whiting, B. Bradley, J. Iannos, and J. M. Watts. 1983. Prevalence and treatment of gall stones after gastric bypass surgery for morbid obesity. Br. Med. J. (Clin. Res. Ed.) 286:763.

Wattigney, W. A., D. W. Harsha, S. R. Srinivasan, L. S. Webber, and G. S. Berenson. 1991. Increasing impact of obesity on serum lipids and lipoproteins in young adults: The Bogalusa Heart Study. Arch. Intern. Med. 151:2017–2022.

Waxman, M., and A. J. Stunkard. 1980. Caloric intake and expenditure of obese boys. J. Pediatr. 96:187–193.

Weintraub, M. 1992a. Long-term weight control study: Conclusions. Clin. Pharmacol. Ther. 51:642–646.

Weintraub, M. 1992b. Long-term weight control: The National Heart, Lung, and Blood Institute funded multimodal intervention study. Clin. Pharmacol. Ther. 51:581–585.

Weintraub, M. 1994. Weight control study designs [abstract]. Int. J. Obes. 18(suppl. 2):2.

Weintraub, M., P. R. Sundaresan, B. Schuster, M. Averbuch, E. C. Stein, and L. Byrne. 1992a. Long-term weight control study. V (weeks 190 to 210). Follow-up of participants after cessation of medication. Clin. Pharmacol. Ther. 51:615–618.

Weintraub, M., P. R. Sundaresan, and C. Cox. 1992b. Long-term weight control study. VI. Individual participant response patterns. Clin. Pharmacol. Ther. 51:619–633.

Weiss, T. W., C. H. Slater, L. W. Green, V. C. Kennedy, D. L. Albright, and C. C. Wun. 1990. The validity of single-item, self-assessment questions as measures of adult physical activity. J. Clin. Epidemiol. 43:1123–1129.

Werner, E. E., and R. S. Smith. 1992. Overcoming the Odds: High Children from Birth to Adulthood. Cornell University Press, Ithaca, NY.

Whatley, J. E., and E. T. Poehlman. 1994. Obesity and exercise. Pp. 123–139 in G. L. Blackburn and B. S. Kanders, eds. Obesity: Pathophysiology, Psychology and Treatment. Chapman & Hall, Inc., New York.

Wilkinson, P. W., J. M. Parkin, G. Pearlson, M. Strong, and P. Sykes. 1977. Energy intake and physical activity in obese children. Br. Med. J. 1(6063):756.

Willett, W. 1990. Nutritional Epidemiology. Oxford University Press, New York.

Willett, W. C., M. Stampfer, J. Manson, and T. VanItallie. 1991. New weight guidelines for Americans: Justified or injudicious? [editorial] Am. J. Clin. Nutr. 53:1102–1103.

Williams, C. L., M. Bollella, and B. J. Carter. 1993. Treatment of childhood obesity in pediatric practice. Pp. 207–219 in C. L. Williams and S. Y. S. Kimm, eds. Prevention and Treatment of Childhood Obesity. Ann. NY Acad. Sci., vol. 699.

Williams, E., R. C. Klesges, C. L. Hanson, and L. H. Eck. 1989. A prospective study of the reliability and convergent validity of three physical activity measures in a field research trial. J. Clin. Epidemiol. 42:1161–1170.

Williamson, D. F. 1993. Descriptive epidemiology of body weight and weight change in U.S. adults. Ann. Intern. Med. 119:646–649.

Williamson, D. F., H. S. Kahn, P. L. Remington, and R. F. Anda. 1990. The 10-year incidence of overweight and major weight gain in U.S. adults. Arch. Intern. Med. 150:665–672.

Williamson, D. F., M. K. Serdula, R. F. Anda, A. Levy, and T. Byers. 1992. Weight loss attempts in adults: Goals, duration, and rate of weight loss. Am. J. Public Health 82:1251–1257.

Williamson, D. F., J. Madans, R. F. Anda, J. C. Kleinman, H. S. Kahn, and T. Byers. 1993. Recreational physical activity and ten-year weight change in a U.S. national cohort. Int. J. Obes. 17:279–286.

Wilson, G. T. 1993. Relation of dieting and voluntary weight loss to psychological functioning and binge eating. Ann. Intern. Med. 119:727–730.

Wilson, G. T. 1994a. Behavioral treatment of childhood obesity: Theoretical and practical implications. Health Psychol. 13:371–372.

Wilson, G. T. 1994b. Behavioral treatment of obesity: Thirty years and counting. Adv. Behav. Res. Ther. 16:31–75.

Wilson, G. T., and K. D. Brownell. 1980. Behavior therapy for obesity: An evaluation of treatment outcome. Adv. Behav. Res. Ther. 3:49–86.

Wilson, G. T., C. A. Nonas, and G. D. Rosenblum. 1993. Assessment of binge eating in obese patients. Int. J. Eat. Disord. 13(1):25–33.

Wilson, P. W. F., R. S. Paffenbarger Jr., J. N. Morris, and R. J. Havlik. 1986. Assessment methods for physical activity and physical fitness in population studies: Report of a NHLBI workshop. Am. Heart J. 111:1177–1192.

Wing, R. R. 1992. Weight cycling in humans: A review of the literature. Ann. Behav. Med. 14:113–119.

Wing, R. R., L. H. Epstein, M. D. Marcus, and D. J. Kupfer. 1984. Mood changes in behavioral weight loss programs. J. Psychosom. Res. 28:189–196.

Wing, R. R., R. Koeske, L. H. Epstein, M. P. Nowalk, W. Gooding, and D. Becker. 1987. Long-term effects of modest weight loss in type II diabetic patients. Arch. Intern. Med. 147:1749–1753.

Wing, R. R., M. D. Marcus, R. Salata, L. H. Epstein, S. Miaskewicz, and E. H. Blair. 1991a. Effects of a very low-calorie diet on long-term glycemic control in obese type II diabetic subjects. Arch. Intern. Med. 151:1334–1340.

Wing, R. R., K. A. Matthews, L. H. Kuller, E. N. Meilahn, and P. L. Plantinga. 1991b. Weight gain at the time of menopause. Arch. Intern. Med. 151:97–102.

Wingard, D. L., L. F. Berkman, and R. J. Brand. 1982. A multivariate analysis of health-related practices: A 9-year mortality follow-up of the Alameda County Study. Am. J. Epidemiol. 116:765–775.

Winner, K. 1991. A Weighty Issue: Dangers and Deceptions of the Weight Loss Industry. Department of Consumer Affairs, New York.

Wolf, A. M., and G. A. Colditz. 1994. The cost of obesity: The US perspective. PharmacoEconomics. 5(Supp. 1):34–37.

Wolff, O. H. 1955. Obesity in childhood: A study of the birth weight, the height, and the onset of puberty. Q. J. Med. 24:109–123.

Wolthuis, R. A., V. F. Froelicher Jr., J. Fischer, and J. H. Triebwasser. 1977. The response of healthy men to treadmill exercise. Circulation 55:153–157.

Wong, T. C., J. G. Webster, H. J. Montoye, and R. Washburn. 1981. Portable accelerometer device for measuring human energy expenditure. IEEE Trans. Biomed. Eng. 28:467–471.

Wood, P. D., M. L. Stefanick, D. M. Dreon, B. Frey-Hewitt, S. C. Garay, P. T. Williams, H. R. Superko, S.P. Fortmann, J. J. Albers, K. M. Vranizan et al. 1988. Changes in plasma lipids and lipoproteins in overweight men during weight loss through dieting as compared with exercise. N. Engl. J. Med. 319:1173–1179.

Wood, P. D., M. L. Stefanick, P. T. Williams, and W. L. Haskell. 1991. The effects on plasma lipoproteins of a prudent weight-reducing diet, with or without exercise, in overweight men and women. N. Engl. J. Med. 325:461–466.

Wylie-Rosett, J., S. Wassertheil-Smoller, M. D. Blaufox, B. R. Davis, H. G. Langford, A. Oberman, S. Jennings, H. Hataway, J. Stern, and N. Zimbaldi. 1993. Trial of antihypertensive intervention and management: Greater efficacy with weight-reduction than with a sodium-potassium intervention. J. Am. Diet. Assoc. 93:408–415.

Yanovski, S. Z., M. Leet, J. A. Yanovski, M. Flood, P. W. Gold, H. R. Kissileff, and B. T. Walsh. 1992. Food selection and intake in obese women with binge-eating disorder. Am. J. Clin. Nutr. 56:975–980.

Yanovski, S. Z., J. E. Nelson, B. K. Dubbert, and R. L. Spitzer. 1993. Association of binge eating disorder and psychiatric comorbidity in obese subjects. Am. J. Psychiatry 150:1472–1479.

Young, T., M. Palta, J. Dempsey, J. Skatrud, S. Weber, and S. Badr. 1993. The occurence of sleep-disordered breathing among middle-aged adults. N. Engl. J. Med. 328:1230–1235.

Zabner, J., L. A. Couture, R. J. Gregory, S. M. Graham, A. E. Smith, and M. J. Welsh. 1993. Adenovirus-mediated gene transfer transiently corrects the chloride transport defect in nasal epithelia of patients with cystic fibrosis. Cell 75:207–216.

Zack, P. M., W. R. Harlan, P. E. Leaverton, and J. Cornoni-Huntley. 1979. A longitudinal study of body fatness in childhood and adolescence. J. Pediatr. 95:126–130.

# Index